YOU ARE BEAUTIFUL

Shirley Lord

You are Beautiful
and how to prove it

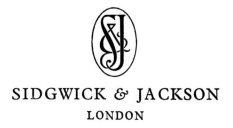

SIDGWICK & JACKSON
LONDON

First published in the U.S.A. as *The Easy Way to Good Looks*
by Thomas Y. Crowell Co. 1976
Revised and enlarged edition first published in Great Britain
by Sidgwick and Jackson Limited, 1978

Line Drawings by Shirley Curzon, Vana Haggerty and Martha Voutas

On pages 17, 45, 95, 106, 109, 295, 323 and 353, photos courtesy of Helena Rubinstein; on pages 24 and 52, photos courtesy of Redken Laboratories; on pages 53 and 229, Dior woman created by Serge Lutens, photo and make-up designed by Serge Lutens for Parfums Christian Dior; on pages 56, 59, 101, 111 and 199, photos by William Silano, courtesy of the Revlon Public Relations Department, for whom they were taken; on pages 63, 119 and 174, photos by Sarah Moon, make-up by Carita; on pages 69, 72 and 91, photos courtesy La Costa Resort Hotel and Spa; on page 125, photo courtesy Lumley's Model Agency; on pages 133, 134, 136, 137, 138 and 139, photos courtesy of Itek Corporation; on pages 168 and 169, photos courtesy of Michaeljohn of London; on page 165, photo courtesy Vidal Sassoon; on page 175, Elura wig by Brentwood, photo courtesy of Monsanto; on page 180, A La Contessa wig, photo courtesy of Monsanto; on page 191, photo by John Cole, colour and hairstyle by Derek Roe of London; on pages 203 and 333, photos by Neal Barr; on page 241, photo courtesy Stewart Model Agency; on page 261, photo courtesy of Clairol Loving Care Colour-Lotion; on page 285, photo courtesy Wilhelmina Model Agency; on page 293, photo courtesy Elite Model Agency; on page 305, photo by Elisabetta Catalno; on page 349, photo by courtesy Carole Gabay.

ISBN 0 283 98418 X

Printed in Great Britain by
The Garden City Press, Letchworth, Herts.
for Sidgwick and Jackson Limited
1 Tavistock Chambers, Bloomsbury Way, London WC1A 2SG

TO DAVID

Contents

YOU ARE BEAUTIFUL

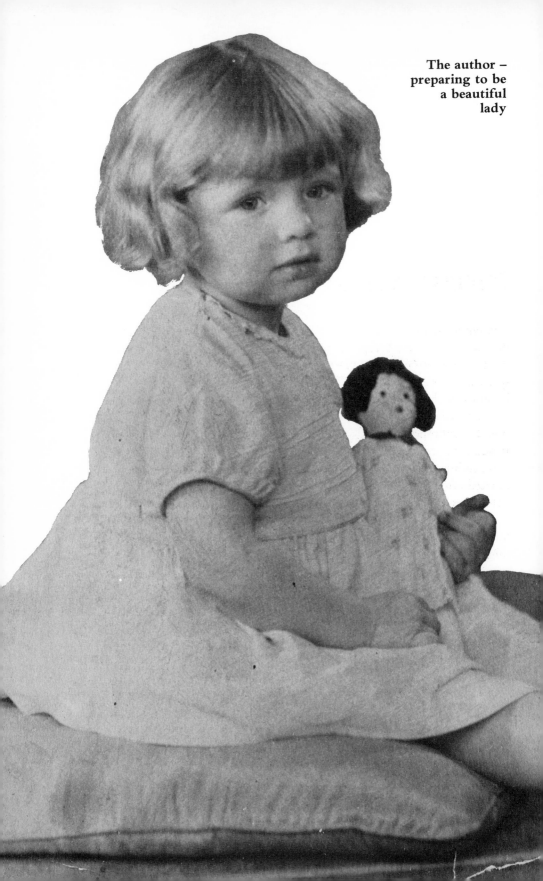

The author –
preparing to be
a beautiful
lady

Introduction

You are beautiful – somebody out there thinks so, although you may not even know it. Accept that statement as fact, knowing that self-doubt is the weevil that can destroy any look – for doubt *shows* and *spoils*, while self-confidence *shows* and *enhances*, when it's built on the knowledge that you've made the best of the raw material that is you.

One of the most famous plastic surgeons in the world once said to me, 'It's not much use lifting a face that belongs to a sagging mentality. It will soon sag again.' It's the same with beauty habits. It's not much use making up a face if you don't really care about the result. Half-hearted attempts with make-up to cope, to keep up, or even to hide behind, end up looking like a permanent apology on the face.

What really matters is what you *do* with what you *have*. Good looks or the lack of them start the day you're conceived, when you inherit the frame on which your skin is going to live, your colouring, your characteristics. Ravishing beauty can be snuffed out by the time your teens are over. Poor nutrition can kill it (too much of the wrong food is as bad as too little of the right); so can poor health, poor habits and (often forgotten as the biggest killer of all) so can an upbringing that neglects to build that invaluable asset *self-confidence*.

When apathy is your attitude it's a warning signal, time to ask yourself 'why'. It's time to reassess yourself, to discover if apathy is the result of constant fatigue, the body's way of telling you to slow down and/or have a complete check-up. It's time to ask yourself whether someone in your life has worn down your self-respect, without which there's no achievement, no enjoyment in life at all.

You are beautiful – but remember it is up to you to give that impression. Every woman at some time or another subconsciously makes the decision either to work at her looks *positively* – developing a style that works with her environment, available time, features and colouring – or to work *negatively* in that every day she lets her looks slide a little, perhaps making the excuse to herself that she was 'never meant to be attractive anyway'. There are other excuses, and 'too busy' leads the field. Too busy is a state of mind rather than of activity. The busiest women are never 'too busy' to put thoughts into action, to take the necessary time, however brief, to help them look as good as they can. It's part of living life to the full, extracting the most potential out of it. It's also the only way to be able to forget about looks, because then you know you've taken care of the job, for the day or night.

HELP YOURSELF

Most of us would like to make changes, but many women don't know how or where to begin. Which is what this book is all about – how to, where to, what to – but not why. Here, every woman has a chance to take stock of herself, and to apply my many solutions to her problems.

We now know that under today's microscopes you can clearly see wrinkles on a two-week-old baby's skin, wrinkles that are pro-grammed genetically, passed on from one generation to another, along with hair colour, bone structure and personality. This isn't reason for a cop-out, however, for the visibility of those programmed wrinkles depends on their depth, and the depth we now know depends on five major points that everyone can tackle:

nutrition,

exercise,

sleep,

sex,

skin care.

Each play a vital part in how we look and how we *can* look. Tension, disease and other assaults on the body speed up ageing. Smoking qualifies as an assault on the body. So does excess drinking, as does, conversely, having a rigidly teetotal personality. So does a job in which frustrations are not absorbed and overshadowed by successes.

Cutting back on the amount of food we eat is generally agreed to be the single most important factor in lengthening Life and im-proving our looks while we live it.

Physical exercise also contributes to good looks and a lengthy lifespan, providing it's a regular part of life. Exercise relaxes and helps us withstand mental frustration, too, for feeling fit has everything to do with feeling young. Keep moving, in other words, and if you can move with a partner so much the better – married people live longer, that's a fact.

When two people live and work together (as in a marriage), what one says and does has an effect upon the other. Generally, there's some 'taking care' of the partner, so that each is likely to gain from health by association. It's interesting to note that married men are expected to outlive single, divorced or widowed men by as much as ten years. For women, the difference is not so dramatic, only three or four years.

It has been suggested that the reason for this difference is that men rarely develop intimate *friendships* (I don't mean love affairs) with other men or women outside marriage, whereas women usually do. This emotional connection has a beneficial effect on health and lifespan, because whereas a typical man-to-man talk is usually about business problems, the stock market or football results, women are more likely to discuss more personal matters, their children, emotional problems.

Our emotions show up on our faces, even if we think we're the inscrutable kind. As you'll read on page 22, the amount of love and/or hate we experience affects our looks more than we'll ever know. If we think of hate as stress and tension, it all becomes more obvious.

The woman who never seems to look any older is the one who is thinking the right way, who through trial and error has worked out the right rhythm for *herself* (the key word, for it is a matter of each to her own). She eats nutritiously, exercises sufficiently, sleeps well, makes love enough (regular sex is important to a woman's looks) and treats skin care as she treats brushing her teeth, as a natural part of daily life.

Over the years, as beauty and health editor of *Harper's Bazaar* on both sides of the Atlantic and as beauty and health editor of American *Vogue*, I've met thousands of women who've proved my point again and again, that to think 'beautiful' contributes enormously to the possibility of being thought of as 'beautiful'.

My present job with Helena Rubinstein, as one of the few female vice-presidents in the cosmetics industry, brings me into still more contact with women the world over and my viewpoint still hasn't changed.

Today we're lucky enough to live in an age when expensive technology works every day towards helping us improve our looks in a way that wasn't possible two decades ago. Scientists with impressive degrees are no longer magisterial about the cosmetics industry. They spend their lives working on products that, for instance, will produce healthy beautiful hair with one quick shampoo.

Did you know that hair growth (at root level) can change from breakfast to lunch and from lunch to dinner, depending on the kind of day you've had? I didn't until I spent a day in a multi-million pound laboratory with the latest whiz-kid of the hair industry. You can read how to improve your own hair with very little effort on pages 153–160.

Other chemists spend their time evaluating the nutritional benefit of our food, so we don't need to be apprehensive when we go to the supermarket. If we keep our eyes open we can easily find the products that will be helpful to our bodies, our strength and our psyches.

Did you know that the body gets bored doing the same exercises every day and can even block shape-up progress if it doesn't get a break or a change, that the same diet day in day out can ruin all chances of getting and staying slim? I didn't until I heard it all from the man responsible for many of the most beautiful bodies in the world. He told me, and I'll tell you (on page 244), how he helps the stars to streamline their bodies with exercises everyone can do. And there are diets here for every mentality (mentality is important: attitude counts) on pages 210–223.

Then there are the research and development scientists who spend their lives improving the gloss and durability of our lipsticks, the moisture in our moisturizers, the benefits of our masks and – above all – making products look as natural on the skin as possible.

Did you know that your skin is your body's personal radar system? It will signal unmistakably 'spot, spot, spot' if your intake of nutritional food is below par. You need to know what you should eat for your skin's sake, too; find out on page 41.

Actress Lois Chiles told me in an interview for *Vogue* that once upon a time she felt a complete failure. 'I was sure I was fat and ugly and decided to bury myself in my studies until I found out what to do with my life.' In fact, she had the decision taken out of her hands. She was spotted by a photographer and after a few months' modelling she was asked to do a screen test in California. As the saying goes, she never looked back. Now she says she feels her looks have improved.

'I never felt attractive and perhaps I wasn't. Now I feel more attractive and people say I am, so perhaps it is just a matter of believing in yourself.'

You are beautiful. Believe and the following pages will make the rest easy.

1

For Woman at Work - 1

CHANNEL YOUR ENERGIES
AND GET TO THE TOP

TIME is the most precious commodity a working woman can have – to spend wisely and well, making five minutes act for ten, carrying out a grooming job like a business commitment, as something to be achieved quickly, efficiently and without fuss in order to be able to move on to the next thing.

The most important thing to realize is what your *priorities* are. If an important part of your job is communicating with the public, how you dress, look and speak is obviously all important. For you to take ten minutes to mend a broken nail isn't necessarily slacking off. For you to get your hair fixed or recoloured can be necessary – and not only because it reflects on your company if the public sees you looking dishevelled or overly casual because of dark roots showing through. It's necessary because *you* know you *need* to have these grooming jobs done, and until they are done you won't perform so efficiently. Your charm can end up needing a touch-up, too.

Rest is as important as exercise for the working woman, particularly if you're one who clocks into another job as soon as you get home to put on your mother hat or housewife apron. It isn't smart to leave sleep out of your priorities because sooner or later lack of sleep can mean you don't operate so well when you're awake (see pages 322-331).

Trying to do too much is a familiar fault of the working woman, for, whatever men say, she still has to prove 'she can do it', often to a boardroom of disbelieving male faces.

One of the simplest facts of life is that if you go to bed early (really early, between 9 and 10 p.m.), not only can you wake up early, but, more important, you will feel ready to tackle the workload that

16

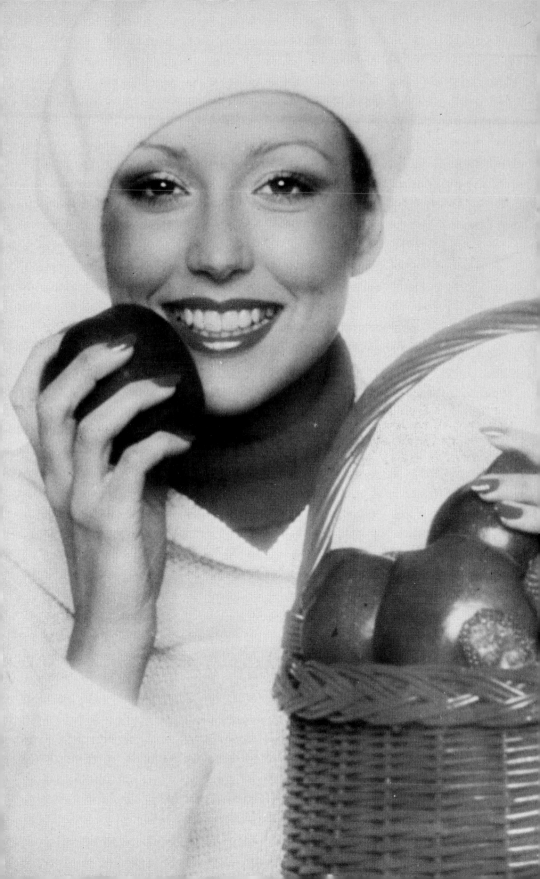

can get you ahead of the crowd. Try it. You'll find it works – but only if it's a regular practice. Don't expect miracles. If your usual schedule runs more like a 1 a.m. shut-eye to a reluctant half-asleep wake-up at 7 a.m. it would take a few dry runs of 9 p.m. to 6 a.m. to work well.

Most working women don't have time to follow a prescribed exercise regime – or let's say it isn't one of their priorities – and yet the experts insist that extra exercise is especially good when you come home after a day wrestling with problems, feeling worn-out and depressed. Instead of a dry martini, exercise is advocated as a guaranteed 'lift' to spirits that have been submerged in rush hour traffic (see page 243).

Learn to plan your priorities in advance. Try to plan a sane schedule with at least two early nights in a working week and one more at weekends if you can.

Planning so that you can take care of your priorities with no fret or fuss is the secret of success.

2

The Basis of Better Looks

A GOOD SKIN: HOW TO ACHIEVE YOUR FIRST GOAL

WE all have good skin as babies because it is skin untramelled by bad habits – and it is largely our habits, good or bad, that determine how fast our skin is going to age.

There's absolutely no set timetable for how and when a face will start to age. Our features – eyes, nose, mouth – don't age and give our birthdays away. Our skin *does*, and heredity, nutrition and environment all have to take part of the responsibility.

To begin with, the way the skin ages is largely the luck of the draw. The baby born into a huge family without sufficient money to feed all the mouths all the time won't have as firm a foundation of good health to build on as the baby born with a 'spoon in its mouth' (whether it's silver or not). The genes may deliver the most beautiful skin in the world to a baby, but it is how it is *maintained* during life that counts.

THE MOST BEAUTIFUL SKIN IN THE WORLD

Who has it? The Baroness de Rothschild for one. Certainly over fifty, Jeanne de Rothschild nevertheless possesses the skin of a girl of twenty-two, truly translucent, pink and white. The redoubtable Barbara Cartland has this kind of skin, too, as do Arlene Dahl, the Begum Aga Khan, Jean Shrimpton and a plethora of 'typical English beauties' from Joanna Naylor-Leyland to Jane Bonham-Carter.

They were all born with stunning skin and they've kept it that way easily. How? First, by avoiding the worst habit of all, sunbathing, knowing what every dermatologist knows, that exposure to the sun damages the skin and ages it faster than bankruptcy – and may produce more serious skin problems such as carcinoma.

Most of the women just mentioned have never deliberately sun-bathed in their lives. Further, to ensure good skin stays in the family, where there are daughters, as in the case of Barbara Cartland, Arlene Dahl and Sally Khan, they have been saying 'don't sunbathe, darling' to their daughters ever since they were old enough to listen. The famous skin of Raine is proof that she listened to every word Mummy – Barbara Cartland – said on the subject.

Skin like Grandmama Used to Have

'My grandmother had the most beautiful skin' is a remark often thrown at me in an accusing tone of voice that suggests the speaker is, in fact, throwing down the glove and challenging me to a verbal duel. The next remark confirms it. 'She never used a cream in her life. She looked fifty when she died and [on a triumphant note of pride] she was actually eighty-eight.'

It doesn't matter how often I point out that grandmama probably spent the first thirty or forty years of her life covered up with high necks, long sleeves, gloves and dresses to the floor, not to mention large shady hats, all protecting her skin, not only from a less polluted atmosphere but also from an enormous amount of light. *All light is ageing, sunlight most of all*. It doesn't matter that I can prove how much damage the change in living conditions has done to the skin or that in grandmama's day it certainly was not the fashion to be tanned – quite the reverse, hence the big cover-up.

There are some women who know full well how much they are improved by the efforts of the cosmetic industry, yet hate admitting it. They will try feverishly to score a Brownie point or two by making that sort of observation, all to no avail as far as I'm concerned.

If grandmama's beautiful, uncreamed skin had to face today's polluted environment, it would soon be in bad shape without any protection. If we had to live with our drying indoor temperatures, carbon dioxide-loaded air, blow-dry dryers and hot rollers without the benefits of all the many ameliorating products available, we would look at least twenty years older than we do now. It's true. You have only to see the neglected skin and dried-out hair of an apathetic woman who has literally let herself go to realize how quickly time can mark its ravages on the few square inches of body we regularly show to the world. The skin on our bodies is generally far superior to that on our faces – again, going back to grandmama, because it is skin that is generally covered up, with no light, or pollution falling directly on it,

Great skin – who has it? Arlene Dahl

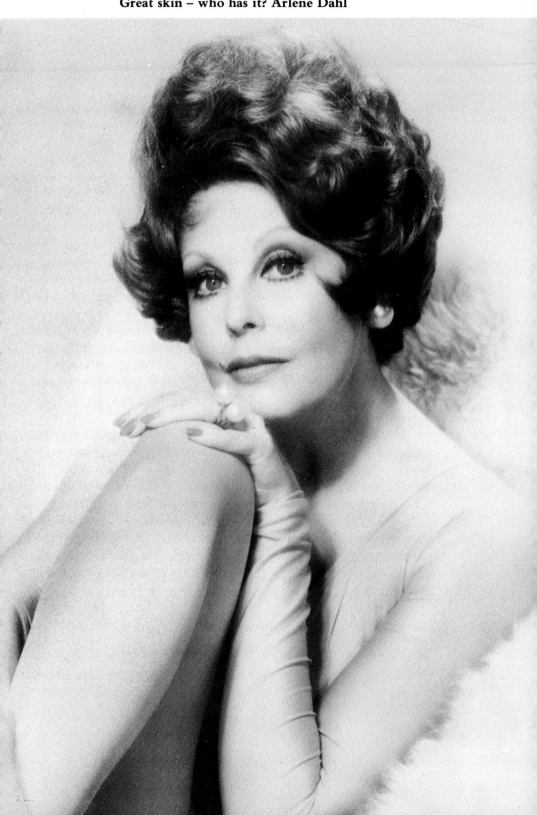

as on our hair, face and hands, and occasionally our exposed limbs. That's why the quality of our body skin is usually lighter, clearer and altogether prettier.

Losing Your Temper Can Age You, Too

There are other factors to ageing, not the least being the way you cope with life – your temperament, and whether you can handle your problems or not. As Dr Joseph Hoffman wrote in his tome *The Life and Death of the Cell*, '. . . if one went to the trouble, it would be feasible to measure the degree of love, hate and anxiety experienced by a human being by the rate of his or her cellular destruction.' You have only to look in the mirror after a row, tears or no tears, to see its effect on your looks, and what you see is your skin disturbed by the signals sent from your brain.

The late cosmetic scientist Marguerite Maury elaborated on Hoffman's theme when she pointed out in *The Secret of Life and Youth*: 'The sexual life of the woman is of the greatest importance to her appearance. Whereas the functions of the man are exogenous and extroverted and he will suffer most from premature old age by abuse of these functions, the woman – being introverted and endogenous – will grow older swifter by *deficiency*.'

How does this relate directly to your skin – dry, greasy, spotty, smooth, whatever it may be? Easily. Skin isn't just a convenient covering for all our component parts. It's as vital to life as the heart, lungs or brain. *It isn't only another organ – it's the largest organ of the body*, wrapping us up in almost 15,000 square inches (97,000 square centimetres). At the embryo stage of life, there is the ectoderm and the endoderm. The ectoderm becomes the skin *and* the brain (the endoderm becomes our 'insides'), creating a link between brain and skin that is far more intimate than that between the brain and any other organ of the body. When we blush, our skin is suffused with blood, because of embarrassed signals from the brain; when we cry our skin gets mottled because of 'unhappy' signals, when we're in love, our skin can look 'radiant' wtih happiness.

YOUR SKIN PICTURE

Your skin consists of three main layers: the *epidermis* at the top that you can see for yourself, the *dermis* beneath, which provides nutrition and oxygen, and the *sub-dermis*, which is the lowest layer. Distributed

Your skin picture

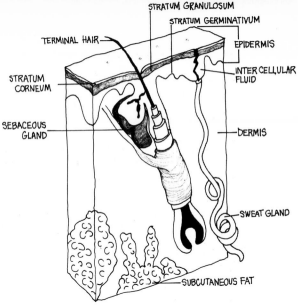

among these three are cells, glands, blood vessels, nerves, hairs and hair follicles.

Your skin does various jobs:

1 It acts as a 'thermostat' for the body, regulating body heat as much as it can to protect the body from destruction, whenever there are *dramatic* swings in temperature.

2 It excretes waste matters the body doesn't need.

3 It keeps in vital fluids the body does need.

4 It keeps out unwanted external fluids – and that means these days that it acts as a first line of defence against pollution.

5 It acts as a control station for sensation, relaying messages to and from the brain faster than the speed of sound – about temperature, touch, pain and pleasure.

This is where Marguerite Maury's and Dr Hoffman's words become appropriate. Think of the skin of the people you love – it's special, whether it's your baby's, your husband's or your lover's. It reflects inner chemistry and you would know that particular skin anywhere, even in the dark when – particularly between lovers – skin can act as super-charged antennae.

How Does Skin Work?

Think of your skin working the way an escalator does. On the 'bottom step' are fresh new cells created deep down in the sub-dermis.

23

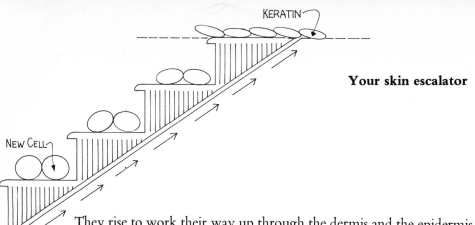

KERATIN

NEW CELL

Your skin escalator

They rise to work their way up through the dermis and the epidermis, and another layer is right behind them – and another and another, just like the escalator steps, never ceasing, always moving upwards on the same route.

When the cells arrive in the epidermis area, they begin to die. They become flat bits of keratin, for living cells can't survive exposure to air or water. Adhering to each other, the keratin bits form the strong shield of dead tissue we see that protects the skin-making machinery and body tissues from the outside world.

Don't blame a cell slow-down for the aging process it's our sebaceous glands (one is seen here in this skin biopsy) that let us down

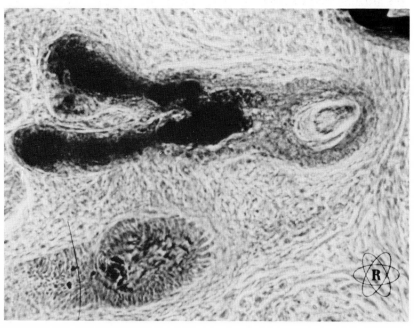

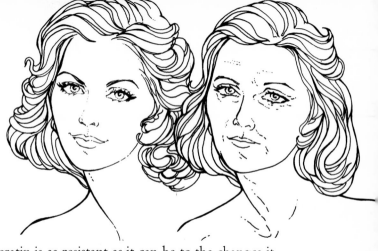

At twenty your skin fits your face like a new suspender belt . . . after a lot of wear and little care, its elasticity is weakened

Tough protein, keratin is as resistant as it can be to the changes it has to face, but it still needs all the help it can get to fight the elements and look its best. Dead cells that stay around too long make skin look dingy, dull. Skin needs a mask or exfoliating cream to whip dead cells away.

Don't Blame a Cell Go-Slow for the Ageing Process

There's never a slowdown in the rate of cell production – often erroneously blamed for signs of old age.

There is a slowdown or weakening of other parts of the skin-making machinery, however. As the years pass, the sebaceous glands, for instance, don't excrete so much sebum, skin's chief lubricant. The amount of sebum in skin's repository makes all the difference between dry and greasy skin – and when skin is dry, its surface 'creases', or shall I say wrinkles, much more easily than if it were moist.

The dermis, the depot in the middle layer, is mostly made up of collagen, the protein fibre responsible for skin's elasticity. It is collagen that allows a smile or an expression to flit on and off a young face leaving no evidence behind. Around forty, when a woman complains she's starting to wrinkle and must do something about it, she isn't just starting to wrinkle. It's been going on for at least twenty years, but the collagen support meant her many expressions left behind no visible trace. Suddenly the collagen starts to sag – and so does her face.

Start as Young as You Can

At twenty your skin fits your face like a new suspender belt. It's firm and gives plenty of control, snapping easily back into place after a yawn, a grimace or a big hello. After a lot of wear (just think how many expressions cross your face in one day) and little care, skin acts like a suspender belt that's been in the washing machine a few times.

25

The 'combination type skin'

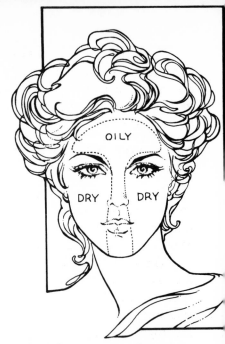

It's looser and thinner, the elasticity is weakened. You can replace your suspender belt. You can't replace skin elasticity, at least not overnight. It takes time, unless you pay a visit to the plastic surgeon to take in a few tucks and darts to restore a taut surface. But that's another story (see pages 318–19).

Recognize Your Type

To help your skin look its best, get to know it. Touch it. Get to understand its *feel* as well as its *look*. Your skin type has to fall into one of the following categories. Choose the one that's most applicable:

I DRY. The most common state of skin in the world (90 per cent of all women have been statistically labelled as having 'too dry skin'). If you're in the majority, your skin is obviously lacking in sebum (oil) and intercellular fluid (moisture). Your skin can *feel* 'fragile'. It can look 'transparent'. It's subject to blotches, little red patches with obvious dry skin in the centre.

2 DEHYDRATED. This is worse than dry. Skin lacks moisture to a painful extent, can wrinkle at the touch of a powder puff, is scaly so that you can see skin flaking – just as if you were peeling after a sunburn.

3 MIXED OR 'NORMAL'. This means you have a 'combination skin'. At its best, it's slightly greasy down the centre panel from forehead to chin with averagely dry sides. At its worst, the centre panel can be excessively greasy with even dehydrated sides.

4 GREASY. Greasy skin has over-active sebaceous glands; the excretion of too much sebum cause the pores to dilate. Skin looks slightly to very coarse, and the general complexion tone is poor and smeary, never quite clear.

5 HYDRATED. If your skin contains too much moisture it's hydrated; it looks and feels swollen, even congested.

Once upon a time the only symbols a woman was expected to know were H_2O and C.O.D. Now many symbols and improbable-sounding names and numbers crop up on cosmetic bottles and jars, all of which are supposed to deliver relevant information to the user.

This is only a beginning; if anything they're going to increase not decrease in the years ahead. Nevertheless, one of the most important symbols to understand is still the pH on the package, two letters that you may have noticed appear time and time again. pH stands for Hydrogen Potential, a form of measurement used by dermatologists to determine skin health. (It also happens to be the measurement used to determine the level of acidity vs alkalinity in practically every substance, not only in skin and hair but in everything from rhubarb to raindrops.)

When skin registers between 5.4 and 6.2 on the pH scale, it's registering a mildly acid condition, which means it's at its peak, beautifully protected from infection by its acid mantle, because bacteria, forever settling on the skin (although we can't see them), cannot live on an acid surface.

Over 6.2 to 7 skin has insufficient acid; it is therefore on the alkaline side, and prone to infection. This state of affairs need treatment (with the right skin care products) to bring it back to its correct slightly acid condition.

At the other end of the skin scale, when pH registers below 5.4, will be a skin that's too acid, extremely sensitive and also in need of special 'balancing' products and/or treatments.

Skin Can Change Its Type, just like Personality

The leopard may not change its spots, but skin can change its identity. It has a lot to do with where you live.

When I moved to New York from London (after a stop-over in Barbados), I was constantly flattered with that old cliché, 'You have that great English complexion, lucky girl.' I took it for granted just as I'd taken my skin for granted all my life – a good skin that never let me down, no spots, no blotches. just smooth and reliable through thick and thin. In Barbados my skin had looked even better, not surprisingly because I was living in the best possible atmosphere, slightly humid, light, clean air, air-conditioned only by soft Atlantic breezes. As I'd learned from early fry-ups to stay out of the sun, the Barbados sun as reliable as clockwork didn't bother my skin. It was really peachy.

After three months of living in New York, I no longer received any 'English skin' compliments, for the simple reason that I didn't have that celebrated type of complexion any more. My skin was dry, hard, even painful on occasions. Nor did it respond to superficial moisturizing with a variety of products.

It needed a lot more than that, but I didn't realize it at the time. My skin was telling me it wasn't used to living in what I now realize is the most punishing environment for skin in the world, a super-controlled atmosphere of constant heat or constant air conditioning, where because the air is de-humidified most natural moisture is extracted.

When I finally followed a new pattern of super-cleansing (with a gentle liquid cleanser and moisturized toner) and extra moisturizing with a regular moisturizer my skin started rewarding me with an occasional trace of bloom. In winter I put two kinds of moisturizer under my make-up, one richer than the other. The skin *can* and *will* change. It isn't only emotional. It's elementary in its approach to weather and the environment. I tell you this to point out that if you've spotted your skin type from the list just given, it doesn't mean you're going to be that type for life. It all depends on where you go to live, or whether you're happy and contented or not, and on what skin care you think corresponds with your geography.

On the Dry Side

You can be born with very dry skin; this is usually a situation needing medical help. More often you inflict dry skin on yourself by washing too much with the wrong soap, thus robbing the skin of its acid mantle and leaving it exposed for the elements to strip it still further of any natural moisture supply. If you're over twenty-five and have a tendency towards dry skin, you should leave soap alone (unless it's a very, *very* mild, non-alkaline one, specially devised for sensitive, dry skin). A moisturized liquid cleanser is a better bet to use for cleansing.

Remember, it's not only prolonged exposure to air conditioning and central heating that hurts skin. Wind velocity and dry air – riding in a fast open car, for instance – can sap skin of its moisture (and hair, too).

Diuretic cures that deliberately set out to dehydrate the body of liquid content in a 'quick diet' (there's really no such thing, see pages 205–210) not surprisingly also dehydrate the skin. Then, as I never get tired of pointing out, the radiation of the sun speeds up oxidation in the cells, drying the skin out just like old leather. You have only to look on a tropical beach to see that I'm speaking the truth. You can polish up old leather to look quite beautiful. Leathery skin is *never* beautiful, however hard you polish.

HOW TO HELP DRY SKIN. As I have said, the predominant skin type everywhere is dry, and a man-made environment doesn't help. When skin has to negotiate rapid changes of temperature and humidity – in offices, planes and cars, not to mention homes – it loses moisture and so gets even drier. The experts say man has been slow to adapt to the changes in his environment, even though he's mainly responsible for creating them. It will take generations to build up the skin's resistance to the deteriorating effects of constant air conditioning and central heating – maybe the hot water bottle wasn't such a bad idea, after all.

The sooner a dry and dehydrated skin starts looking for outside help the better. The help is pretty simple, and can be summed up in one word, now part of the language: MOISTURIZER.

Dr Erno Laszlo, the Hungarian cosmetician, whose beauty principles are still followed slavishly, years after his death, by many of the world's great beauties, used to reiterate, '*If you want skin beauty after forty, you should begin to work at it when you are twenty.*' Luckily for those who didn't know at the time he also said, '*It's never too early or too late to cultivate a better complexion, because the skin has tremendous powers of self-regeneration when properly cared for.*' The late great pioneer for all women, Helena Rubinstein, said the same thing to me herself.

Everything really changed for the better when an unassuming chemist with the even more unassuming name of Dr Irwin Blank, from the University of Massachusetts, discovered in 1931 that to *transmit moisture back into the skin* it was necessary to create an oil-in-water emulsion, even then described as a moisturizer. What else could it have been called?

'Moisturizers have changed everything,' a variety of people have said to me over the last twenty years, from Elizabeth Taylor to H.M. the Queen, and nobody can refute it. The right moisturizer used *regularly*

29

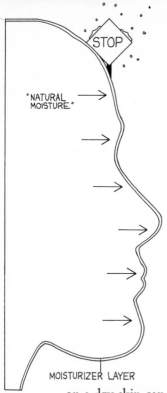

**Moisturizer working as
a barrier to the loss of
'natural moisture'**

MOISTURIZER LAYER

on a dry skin can change even the most arid state of affairs.

How does it work? It increases the water content of the outer layers of the skin. Just as a plant revives with a drink of water, so does skin, the human plant. It blooms, softens, can even have a moist, melting look.

Contemporary moisturizers have advanced to such a point that they don't only *add* extra moisture, they *prevent* any existing moisture escaping. This double dose of treatment is what any dry condition needs, to ward off early wrinkling and to make the skin look prettier. When dermatologists refer to the 'natural moisture', they mean exactly that – it's moisture from the intercellular fluids of the skin's lower layers, which in cold weather easily evaporates in the atmosphere. This means that the 'barrier' part of a moisturizer's work is as essential as anything extra it may add.

There's just no excuse for not combating dry skin, whether you inherited it or brought it on yourself from any of the reasons mentioned.

To maintain skin's natural humidity and prevent further dehydration, a moisturizer is the answer, forming an occlusive film on the skin's surface.

THERE ARE MANY WAYS TO WEAR A MOISTURIZER. If you have very dry skin, you can start the day cleansing with a cleanser that has moisturizer built into its formula.

As your body retains some moisture after a bath or shower (even after you've dried), this is the best time to apply a straight-forward moisturizer or one that's been formulated especially to wear under make-up (usually labelled as an under-make-up moisturizer). This type of product increases the affinity of the skin's surface to make-up, so that it glides on more easily and stays on longer.

Most make-up comes moisturized if you want it that way – a positive answer to the consumer's recent demand for *skin benefit* along with *make-up colour*.

At the end of the day a mask is the newest and most effective way to give the skin that 'drink'. *Make sure it's a moisturizing mask.* Read the labels, that's what they're there for. The reason a mask is such a good – and quick – way to moisturize an overly dry or dehydrated skin is that the skin is a *captive* audience beneath its film.

The skin takes from the mask whatever benefits it has to give, while any moisture present can't escape. Many models, after a gruelling location in a dry, arid place (like Saudi Arabia!), apply a moisturizer liberally beneath a moisturizing mask – this is to 'hydrate' fast the upper layers of the face, and to take any semblance of dryness away. This trick really gives noticeable results.

You can also help dry skin in the bath, when bath oil or an emollient type of bath product should *always* be used. If you're a shower girl, smother yourself in bath oil or gel before you turn on the tap. In winter, for dry skin extra moisturizing this way should be a MUST.

Can the regular use of a moisturizer prevent wrinkles – which appear so easily on dry skin? The superficial kind, yes, especially those tiny sun-lines which look so unattractive out of the sun. If you start at twenty, *regular* – with emphasis on the word – moisturizing can delay the appearance of age's unfortunate insignia.

Remember to study labels. A moisturizer can be different from a product labelled as an emollient. While a *moisturizer* adds moisture, it doesn't necessarily prevent *natural moisture* escaping. An *emollient*, however, both lubricates and traps moisture in the skin. Water is a moisturizer, but can't help your skin keep its own supply. Petroleum jelly and olive oil are emollients with no trace of water, but they both add moisture and prevent its loss. When a product says it's also a humectant, this means it has the ability to attract moisture to the skin from the surrounding atmosphere.

Does Normal Skin Need Care?

Every skin needs care, and in any case 'normal' skin, as I've already described from my own experience, doesn't necessarily stay 'normal'. It all depends on who owns it, and where it lives.

First, it has to be kept clean, wherever it lives, because every day skin collects waste matter on the surface thrown out by the body – gland secretions and cellular debris, in the form of dead skin cells. That rubbish all has to be collected and removed for the skin to stay looking good, whether it's 'normal' or not.

Soap is the most efficient collector. It's also the most drying (except the transparent and/or the especially mild kind), so it shouldn't be a three-times-a-day way of cleaning up. (*Over twenty-five the less soap used on the face the better.*)

What you eat contributes towards maintaining a good skin, and what you drink, too. Nobody has proved yet that alcohol harms the skin, but they're working on it. *Water* is the drink skin likes best, and we don't drink enough say most nutritionists. Eight full glasses a day is the recommended dose for better digestion, better 'flushing' out and so better, unblemished skin.

It isn't only greasy skins that need toners (also called astringents, rinsers, refreshants, scrubs and clean-ups). This type of product does a marvellous tidy-up job after the first cleanse, collecting any left-over debris, and when there's alcohol in the formula (often menthol) this lowers the skin's temperature, thus preparing it for business – which means make-up.

Astringents, by the way, don't reduce pore size. *Pores can't be changed in size with beauty products.* They can be 'tightened', so they look smaller.

Oil Heiress

You need a lot of moisture, but you don't need a lot of oil. The only oil heiress happy to lose her oil deposits is, of course, the girl with oily skin. As she gets older, her skin gets better and easier to cope with, for the simple reason that the excessive sebum flow (that probably made her teens and twenties miserable) generally starts to diminish around twenty-five. By forty her greasy skin may even have been replaced with a really good skin – if she takes care. Then she has to realize that she, too, needs a moisturizer.

Greasy skin can be and often is accompanied by acne, a scourge at any time, but particularly in adolescence. Acne or not, an anti-acne regime can't hurt. This means a low fat, high fruit diet, plenty of sleep and exercise and – difficult to prescribe, but *always* prescribed for acne sufferers – as little tension and anxiety as possible.

You have to wage war on greasy skin; it can't just be ignored or forgotten. The best way to fight it is with vigilant cleansing, using a medicated or soapless cleanser up to six times a day, with *lavish* rinsings. Astringents should follow every cleanse, not only because they remove the 'debris' but also because they give the skin a good send-off for make-up, essential for looks – and morale. The trick is to look for *water-based, no-fat foundations and medicated make-ups*, formulated to cut through oil deposits. Some bases contain powders made to absorb oil all day long.

If your face isn't greasy all over, but only in patches, don't forget to use a moisturizer on the drier spots. They need help, too. A cleansing mask with moisturizing properties is a help for the patchy skin, removing excess oil fast but trapping the moisture skin always needs. There are also blotting lotions available now that 'blot' up oil, but still add moisture.

Never forget oil is *not* moisture.

Never forget that when others are bewailing their early wrinkling, oily skins can be coming into their prime.

Help for the Hydrated

Skin that is too 'hydrated' is congested skin – often needing help from an experienced facialist to reactivate poor circulation, which is responsible for the skin becoming clogged with waste matter that the veins should have carried away. This isn't a time for do-it-yourself techniques. Professional help should be sought and then products chosen with extreme care. This condition rarely occurs in the young. It's more often the result of the skin machinery slowing down and cells not receiving the correct nourishment, so that the skin becomes clogged like a blocked drain with toxins and waste matters. A puffy, bloated look is the result.

Acne and What Can Be Done about It, if Anything

Acne, puberty's scourge, often inherited, is triggered off by a hormonal imbalance that can cause huge hang-ups completely out of proportion to its medical status – all because it generally hits at a time when self-confidence is at its lowest ebb – during the teens.

Doctors agree on what affects acne most – *emotional stress*. This can

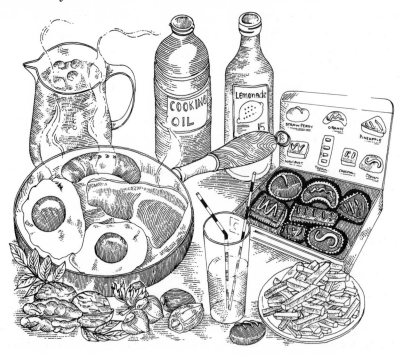

cause the skin to flare up and look disfigured – even overnight.

Diet is controversial. Some doctors think diet has no adverse or advantageous effect, while others ban chocolates (particularly), fried foods, nuts and soft drinks.

Unfortunately, acne is like the common cold, much discussed and highly publicized, but still with no real cure – although certain antibiotic treatments have produced remarkable results in the last few years.

The main stumbling block is the inability to induce acne in any animal for lab tests. We don't need to wonder why there are no human volunteers.

In short, as with greasy skin, acne means too much sebum is produced at too rapid a rate. The pores become clogged, but with acne the sebum production never ceases. Infection sets in, and the result is ugly pimples and spots.

It isn't contagious and, contrary to what many think, dirt is not the cause – although obviously a *lack of proper cleansing* aggravates it. Acne sufferers just can't wash enough – for the more they wash or scrub with medicated soap, the more sebum is removed, reducing bacteria on the skin's surface – producing a drying and peeling effect.

34

THE NEW SOLUTIONS. Although antibiotics are increasingly being tested on acne patients, each case has to be treated independently because patients respond so differently to the same treatment.

The latest *control* methods (but not cures) are medicated soaps, lotions and creams containing sulphur, resorcinol, alcohol, salicylic acid and benzoyl peroxide. Because the male hormone, testosterone, is partly responsible for the trouble, careful doses of female hormones can be used to *decrease* the size of the sebaceous glands, on the theory that the smaller the gland the less sebum gets out. This method is restricted to severe cases, however, and, because of possible feminizing side-effects, only to females.

Ultra-violet light is used to peel and clear up the skin's outer layer, too, while natural sunlight (providing the atmosphere is not humid) can also help.

Vitamin A supplements – the 'good skin' vitamin – are frequently prescribed and vitamin A acid is sometimes used to clear up infected areas.

'No more acne' isn't just a shadowy pipe dream. That day is drawing nearer as research progresses to control excessive sebum, to inhibit the bacteria, and to produce a *topical oestrogen* that works without feminizing or other side-effects.

IS SMOKING BAD FOR THE SKIN?

Are smokers in their forties as wrinkled as non-smokers in their sixties? If they've been smoking for years, yes, yes and yes again. Long-term smoking definitely plays a part in making skin look older than its years. Smokers use a whole lot of mannerisms which non-smokers don't. They purse their lips in different ways, and even if they don't blow smoke rings they certainly blow smoke, which occasionally gets in the way of the eyes. The result? The eyes are continually wrinkling up to avoid it. The heavy smoker is easily recognized, not necessarily by nicotine stains but by tiny lines notching the forehead on either side of the nose.

When you smoke, you also *immediately* take away some of the vitamin C supply of the body, and you need all the vitamin C you can get to keep your bones healthy and to keep teeth and gums in good shape. Vitamin C is also needed to build up your own defence mechanism against illness and infection.

If you aren't a heavy smoker, there are still *immediate* differences in

35

your body's behaviour once you start puffing away. For instance, it's probable the smoker's heart will beat an extra fifteen to twenty-five times a minute, and no one wants to put an extra burden on that miraculous organ. Worse, blood pressure is often raised by as much as ten to twenty points. Many smokers have poor skin tone, a direct result of the noxious gases inhaled, which actually prevent the body from taking in a good supply of oxygen.

Exercise increases oxygen intake, which in turn increases the body's blood supply, so helping extra nutrients to be delivered by the circulation – in particular helping the skin to have a glow and a bloom all its own. When smoking literally 'clouds' the oxygen situation, less blood results, less nutrients are available, and a dingy-looking skin is what you see.

THE PILL – DOES IT AFFECT OUR SKIN?

Yes, it does. Sometimes. I first learned this one summer when a gorgeous model friend and neighbour showed me with alarm little patches of brown pigment that had suddenly turned up on her otherwise, flawless, lightly tanned skin.

There was a patch about the size of an olive above her eyebrow, two more – like odd-size patches on a pair of jeans – on both cheeks. They had appeared faintly the past week, then had deepened after she'd been gardening in the sun one afternoon. I suggested she see a dermatologist, who told her that her patchy problem wasn't unusual, but an increasing phenomenon among women on the pill.

Our melanin (pigment) supply is controlled by the pituitary and adrenal functions, which are also in charge of ovulation. As the pill suppresses ovulation, it can also in an excess of zeal trigger off extra supplies of melanin. The sunlight literally *sets* the patches in place, making them far more visible, as my friend had unwittingly set hers by spending too much time out of doors. In winter, the doctor told her, the patches would fade, and in time, providing she avoided sunlight totally, they could become invisible. Meanwhile, he told her to use a de-pigmenting, bleaching type of cream, with a cover-up base on top.

It was also suggested that she switch pills or stop taking them altogether but, as she told her doctor and me, 'I'd rather be blotchy than pregnant.'

My friend was unfortunate, but statistics show that about 25 per cent of women on the pill do experience the same problem.

On the other hand, another 25 per cent say their skins improved after being on the pill for a few months. Not surprisingly, most of these were acne sufferers, who benefited from the female hormone in the pill, the oestrogen – used, as already described, in acne treatments to combat the harmful effects of too much of the male hormone, testosterone.

Many dermatologists believe that the pill's greatest advantage is a psychological one. When a woman's mind is more relaxed, and she is less fearful of unwanted pregnancies, her skin is more 'relaxed', too, and even blooms. Never forget, skin *is* emotional. It reacts to how you feel and think because of its special affinity to the brain.

ALLERGIES AND WHAT TO DO ABOUT THEM

When the pollen count was high in Donaghadee, County Down, where I used to live, nobody was surprised or even faintly disturbed that my son and I sneezed the day away and often the night as well. It was taken for granted that we were 'allergic' to the pollen and that hay fever was the inevitable result.

When one of the secretaries in my office in London began developing an irritating rash on her hands every two months or so, nobody linked it to an allergic reaction, and yet the peculiar thing was that the rash reappeared like clockwork every time she changed her typewriter ribbon. Eventually, two and two were added together and the secretary changed her typewriter and the ribbon that went with it. End of rash, end of story.

But exactly what causes an allergy? They didn't know yesterday and they don't know today. Heredity is the main factor that gets the dubious credit for causing a person to be 'allergic', a condition that, as we all know, can make itself known suddenly for no apparent reason and with no given warning.

To develop an allergic reaction, the system has to take such a violent dislike to a substance that it sets up immediate defences in the form of antibodies which on next coming into contact with the 'objectionable' object release a form of 'tear-gas' into the bloodstream, composed of one or more chemicals, which in turn produces one or even more of the many miserable reactions we all know and recognize so well.

The most classic is the asthma or hay fever symptom, caused when one of the body's chemical mediators cause the muscles in the air

37

tubes to go into spasm, restricting the amount of air inhaled. When the chemical defence acts on the tiny capillary blood vessels in the brain, violent headaches can occur. If it acts on the nasal passages, sneezing and other strong cold symptoms emerge.

More frustrating is the news that an allergic reaction may or may not necessarily be related to the manner in which the allergen comes into contact with the body. A person can have an asthma attack from eating something, just as something breathed in (smelled) can affect the bloodstream and cause a nasty rash. The most frequent attacks are caused by substances we breathe in – house dust, pollen, cat and dog hairs, perfume. Obviously, the most reliable way of avoiding an allergic reaction is to avoid the things you know might bring one on – even if it means giving Fido or Pussy away to your best friend (who, of course, doesn't have to be troubled at all).

In the beauty industry a huge amount is spent annually to preclude possible allergic reactions to products. As the industry's record shows, the money is well spent because it's a rare occurrence today for an allergic reaction to a product to crop up in any sizeable number of users.

Skin thickness varies over the body's surface, and in general, women have thinner skin than men, but for everyone it becomes thinner and more fragile with age. However, it doesn't always present the same *barrier* to the world.

When people describe their skin as 'sensitive' they really mean they have overly thin skin, allowing greater penetration of unwanted materials. Skin reacts 'irritably' because an irritating element is being forced or injected under it. The thin-skinned know from bitter experience that they have to be especially careful about beauty products. They'll choose, if they know what's good for them, products labelled as 'dermatologically tested' or 'fragrance free'. Fragrance is often the allergy culprit when included in product formulas and it's obvious when you think for a second how intimately related pollen is to fragrance. When fragrance is produced from any natural substance, fruit or animal sources as well as flowers, an allergic reaction may be just round the corner.

Synthetic ingredients are far less likely to produce problems, one reason why more and more perfumes come from test-tube creations and not the flowers blooming in the field. All the same, an allergic reaction can still happen from anything and to anyone, thin- or thick-skinned, and while the thin-skinned should know what and what not to use, the thick-skinned can also be hit with force, although often there are no clues as to what caused the problem.

A leading dermatologist told me that there's a big difference between an irritant and an allergen. An irritant can cause a reaction in at least 80 per cent of the people who use it and it's dose-related – a lot will irritate more than a little. An allergen, however, might cause a reaction in only one person in a million and is not dose-related. The most minute amount is enough to cause a huge allergy.

When you reflect that every time you use your fingers to apply some cream, you leave behind in the jar new bacteria (present on everybody's skin), you begin to appreciate the huge task the cosmetic companies regularly tackle, not only delivering products that do the job they're supposed to do, but also eliminating as far as possible any chance of triggering off something as unpleasant as an allergy.

This is one reason why a cosmetic lab often looks like a hospital clinic or even a moon lab these days. To ensure that products remain fresh, pure and antiseptic, you'll find fragrance-free products being created, manufactured and tested in sealed areas, with double-glazed windows and specially constructed doors so as not to let in any unnecessary outside element – the workers wearing white from top to toe and often masked. If he takes these precautions, the research and development chemist knows he has protected his creation as far as he is able. Once the product is launched and is worn by the consumer he also knows that ninety-nine times out of a hundred there'll be no problems, only hopefully an improved appearance. He can't know, and doesn't profess to, whether there may be one woman who – for one reason or another – has cells that will be sensitive to the product, causing the body to produce antibodies to fight the 'intruder' in the blood-stream, which show themselves in an allergic reaction. Nobody knows just why, but progress marches on as the chemists continue to strive to understand and utilize nature's benefits.

When an Allergy Strikes

What can you do if you suddenly seem to have become allergic to something? First think about your lifestyle and whether or not you have subtly altered it in any way. Think about the products you have bought recently; are there any new ones among them? One could be the culprit. You have to be your own Sherlock Holmes because virtually anything could have caused it, from a new spot remover to the tobacco in your husband's pipe. That's another problem: the strangest (and most frustrating) thing about allergies is that you can suddenly become allergic to something you've lived with for years without trouble. Strange but true – there's documented proof in every dermatologist's consulting room.

If you have the faintest suspicion that any substance of any sort in your life is causing an allergy, get rid of it at once, particularly in the food department. Any food that produces an allergic reaction should be totally avoided – and not only because of the reaction, miserable though it may be. If your body is telling you in unmistakable fashion that seafood shouldn't be on your menu, there's a reason for it. Continued eating of seafood could end you up in hospital or worse.

If you describe your skin as sensitive, it probably means it *is* sensitive and you should stay clear of scented products, because fragrance, as just explained, is composed of so many ingredients and you can't be sure you have the synthetic (and therefore safer) variety.

Learn to read labels. Learn what your skin likes and doesn't like. Don't have a 'hope-for-the-best' approach. When you've found products that work for your sensitive skin, stick to them. Whether your skin is thick or thin, once a product produces a reaction it must be abandoned, but let the manufacturer know. He wants to safeguard *you* as much *as you* want to be safeguarded. For this he needs to know how the cream, lotion or perfume behaves.

On your part, keep products in a cool dark place – even the fridge, though this is not strictly necessary. Don't buy large sizes unless you use them voraciously. Just as the temperature in the manufacturer's formulation room is deliberately kept stable (because a difference up or down can dramatically alter what comes out of the test tubes and eventually what comes out of the jars and bottles you buy), don't move your products about from one atmosphere to another, from extreme heat to extreme cold. That's asking for trouble, and trouble is just what the cosmetic manufacturers want to avoid.

NATURAL PRODUCTS: WHAT DO THEY MEAN AND DO THEY WORK?

During the past few years anything 'natural' as opposed to synthetic has been enjoying a popularity as sweet as mother earth. As far as beauty products are concerned, however, without a synthetic fixative 'shelf life' can be doubtful, and who wants to fill up the deep freeze with moisturizing gels and lotions?

Natural or organic products (the latter refers to anything grown in earth never exposed to fertilizers or chemicals) are formulated from the things you'd expect to find in nature – fruits, vegetables, herbs.

Where a large company is involved, there may be plenty of peaches in the peach night oil, but there's sure to be plenty of *methyl paraben* and *propyl paraben*, too, both preservatives that give a cream long life without having to resort to the deep freeze. If it says avocado on the label and a reputable company's behind it, avocados will have been plucked from the trees by the bushel to serve the needs of mass production. But if it's a moisturizer, some synthetic like *isopropyl myristate* will certainly be part of the formula, helping the avocados to moisturize you more efficiently.

My point is that going the *natural* route can be a fine idea, but it doesn't mean you should turn your back on the companies that know best how to utilize nature's goodies, using them in conjunction with tried and true cosmetic ingredients. The bloom on your cheeks will be better and last longer that way.

Pow - It's a Vitamin!

Tests proved long ago that skin *can absorb pure nutrients and vitamins.* Victims of malnutrition after the second world war, for instance, were often unable to assimilate food through the mouth but received the necessary life-saving nutrients through high calibre food being rubbed on their *skin.*

Many health food lovers I know use face packs of papaya (a natural enzyme), avocado and apricots.

For very dry skin, applications of sunflower seed, sesame, safflower, olive, castor bean, almond or peanut oil are recommended.

From the sea, they believe in treatments from plankton, seaweed and kelp, all naturally packed with minerals, nutritive salts and trace elements.

If you're all for doing-it-yourself, remember your skin type matters just as much when you're dealing with the natural remedies as when you check in at your favourite cosmetics counter.

If your skin is too greasy, you can use a mixture of honey, egg white and ground oatmeal for a homemade cleanser. It will have pulling power (from the honey), attracting blood swiftly to the skin's surface and stimulating circulation; abrasive power (from the oatmeal), clearing up the oil with ease; and finally a bundle of benefits from the egg white to keep the skin better balanced between dry and greasy.

An egg is a beauty armoury – it has protein, iron, vitamin A (the beauty vitamin) and methionine, well documented as a valuable asset to healthy skin.

Mashed papaya acts as a natural enzyme on the skin and has the ability to draw out any oxidized, hardened grit or pollutants from the pores; it is also anti-bacterial, and tightening.

Old black magic prescribes a combination of mashed bananas and peaches worked together in olive oil to deliver plenty of moisture, and keep in what you've got. Use this as a mask, then rinse off with tepid water after fifteen minutes.

No treatment cream need stay on the face longer than fifteen to twenty minutes; in that time it accomplishes the maximum it can do. A longer stay just isn't necessary — though it doesn't do any harm either.

Some models I work with make a kind of mayonnaise for a 'skin snack' whenever their skin looks dreary. They use egg white, unsaturated oil, apple cider vinegar, water and lecithin, normally extracted from the soya bean (lecithin, as many will know, is used as a moisturizing element in many highly regarded cosmetic products). When they're sure the doorbell won't ring, they cover their skin with this mixture (never forgetting the neck), and the skin certainly seems to drink it up. After only a few minutes, texture and elasticity seem improved. They 'tone' or zip up the circulation with cider vinegar, too, using one part vinegar to eight parts water, plus a squeeze of fresh grapefruit juice. The cider vinegar keeps in the natural moisture content while the grapefruit juice (lemon or watermelon would do as well), which contains between 5 per cent and 8 per cent citric acid, is a good pH balancer. This recipe, my model informant tells me, fades blotches, and reduces the chance of blemishes.

Milk, which is an emulsion of 3.8 per cent butterfat in water, stabilized by the additional presence of about 3 per cent casein protein, is helpful, as the big boys in the cosmetic business know. There was even a 'milk war' some time ago, when two of the biggest companies launched milk treatments at the same time – one boosted a 'skimmed milk ingredient', the other a 'whole milk' line. Both were lapped up!

Whatever 'food' we use on our skin, we have to realize that, just like the food we eat, there's a time factor involved in its purity. Let's face it, if the do-it-yourself remedies were as efficacious as the products evolving from the laboratories and top research stations of the world, we would have never deviated from the potions handed down from our grandmothers.

AROMATHERAPY - HOCUS-POCUS OR HELPFUL?

One step back from fruity face packs and milky cleansers is *aromatherapy*, often a normal part of beauty care in Europe, where it's as old as the hills, having arrived there from the East where it began still more hundreds of years ago – though it's a newer, more unexplored form of therapy in Great Britain.

Based on the knowledge of the regenerative powers of certain natural oils, aromatherapy is best explained as the application or massage of these oils on the nerve centres of the face and body. The object? To stimulate the reproductive action of the skin cells and speed up the renewal process, thus recapturing a younger rhythm.

'Rhythm' is the key word. As the late Marguerite Maury often reiterated: '*Ageing is independent of time*. It is our physical and psychological pattern which determines the *real age of our body*.'

She believed that it is possible for women to remain 'ageless' if they take the time to discover and maintain their own perfect rhythm, 'which should stay with them until they die'.

The rhythm she described related to discovering one's sleep requirements, making love enough, eating and drinking the right amount – in fact, leading a perfectly balanced life for *oneself* – for the 'rhythm' differs from person to person.

Once we find the right rhythm for ourselves, she preached, we can then find what she called 'the gift of relaxation' – for without relaxation 'no rejuvenation or regeneration can take place'.

True relaxation is the main object of aromatherapy, practised for many years by Madame Maury in Paris and London, and carried out today by cosmeticians all over the world. Specific massage with a variety of different natural oils induces total relaxation, not inertia but a state in which, energy being freed, one's whole concentration can be directed on to a more perceptive plane.

A truly relaxed person is an extremely alert and conscious one. The natural oil plays its part in treating whatever skin problem exists.

The art of the aromatherapist (Marietta Kavanagh is a well known one in London) is to know which oil is best for which skin. Just as with fingerprints and personality, skin differs from woman to woman and there are hundreds of different oils imported from all parts of the world to choose from. Camomile, mint and lavender are often used to treat sensitive, delicate skin; essence of rose to heal wounds and fade scars; Indian verbena and sandalwood to tighten open pores; geranium

43

oil to stimulate the circulation. Even oil from pulverized tree bark and linseed is used for special problems, while rosewater is an aromatherapist's 'must' for broken capillaries.

The qualified aromatherapist will start the treatment by noting down all details of your medical history, followed by a general examination – blood pressure, heart, lungs and then a blood test. Often highly magnified photographs are taken of the skin for later comparison.

In Europe and the East, where it came from, aromatherapy is still used medically to strengthen skin tissue and muscles before operations and, in the case of severe burns, to reactivate tissue so that scars are minimized.

As far as beauty is concerned, we have only to look at the oriental skin to know that their strict programme of care (which includes aromatherapy) shows results. From childhood the Oriental alternates 'active' days of nourishing and feeding the skin (with many of the oils described) with 'rest' days when the skin is kept scrupulously clean and free of any cosmetic or treatment.

It brings us right back to the main point of this skin section: the earlier you learn about your skin (and how to treat it), the more the question of how to retrieve your looks won't be one you'll ever have to answer.

MASKS – ONE FOR EVERY SKIN

While aromatherapy is a treatment from the past, little changed in its application over the years, the mask – used by the Egyptians more than 2,000 years ago – has been transformed with scientific know-how into one of the most modern skin care products now available.

There are masks for every skin, and today many cosmetic chemists believe that the mask is the one product that will eventually lead to another beauty breakthrough – to produce a wrinkle-free society.

After twenty every third pore is a poor one. Skin can't be nourished from the outside alone. It needs *inside* help to throw off impurities. The best way to make this happen is to *activate* the circulation with masks or massage, the only two ways one can *really* exercise the *skin* on one's face – not to be confused with exercising the facial muscles.

A stimulated circulation brings fresh blood coursing to the surface. This reconditions sluggish cells, sweeps away toxic matters that cause dull skin tone and spots, and brings nourishment to the tissues, cleansing, whitening, softening and refining the pores.

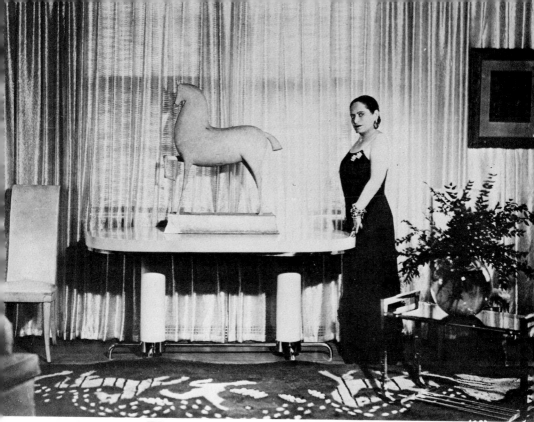

Helena Rubinstein, one of the greatest innovators the cosmetic world has ever known

The first mask we know of – centuries old – was invented by slave women washing clothes at the river's edge. They found their feet, immersed in mud, became soft and white. The smart ones used the mud on their faces and so the mud pack was born, followed later by packs or masks made out of a number of things from narcissus bulbs to butter and grain. Years later Madame de Pompadour used best sirloin to make protein packs for her delicate skin, catching on to the fact that the meat contained an ingredient that helped her skin – protein – plumping it out, and giving it a firmer, younger look.

Helena Rubinstein, after studying every great beauty back to the days of Cleopatra, imported volcanic mud from Ischia into her salons in Paris, London and Rome in the early sixties. There it was used for masks for the body as well as for the face. The mud was a definite circulation zipper-up, for it refreshed tired skin and left it rosy and relaxed.

Now there are almost as many masks available as there are moisturizers and many moisturize beautifully themselves. Their main

45

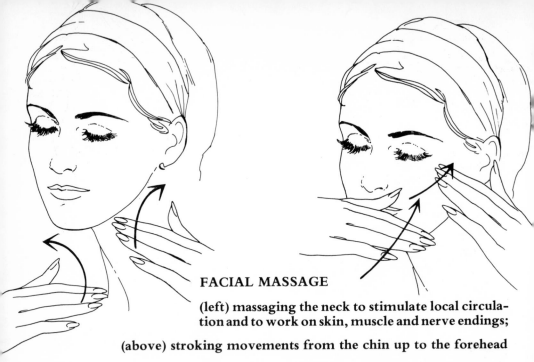

FACIAL MASSAGE

(left) massaging the neck to stimulate local circulation and to work on skin, muscle and nerve endings;

(above) stroking movements from the chin up to the forehead

job, however, is still to *cleanse* more efficiently than any other product, sloughing off dead cells from the surface, firming and tightening temporarily.

A dry or dry-to-normal skin should use a mask *early* in the morning – during the bath or shower is the best idea. That's the time Liza Minnelli puts on a mask, choosing a protein-based one to moisturize and cleanse, to sweep away all the impurities that gather on the skin during the night. It's a good start for make-up – and the day ahead.

If you have a greasy skin you would be better off using a mud or fruit mask *at night*, either before going out or before going to bed, to take away not only the excess sebum produced but also the pollutant build-up that greasy skin invariably attracts (more than a dry one) during the day.

At home, use masks.

At the salon, try a facial, which includes a face massage as well as deep cleansing, steaming (using herbs to get behind deep-rooted grubbiness), lavish moisturizing packs for a dry skin, astringent treatments for a greasy one.

FACIALS

I don't believe in do-it-yourself facial massage unless learned meticulously from a professional.

Elizabeth Arden, who personally inspected the hands of all

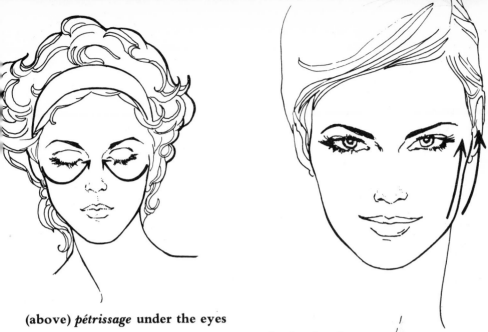

(above) *pétrissage* **under the eyes**

(right) *tapotement* **from the chin up to the forehead**

operators wishing to work in her salons (only employing those with the 'fattest finger pads'), often said, 'Do-it-yourself massage on the face can "sag and bag".' She was right. Traumatizing the skin with the wrong set of movements is ageing.

The best professional facial massage works this way:

1 First, the front and nape of the neck are massaged to relax the client, to stimulate local circulation, to work on skin, muscle and nerve endings.

2 Stroking movements then start from below the chin up to the forehead, never dragging or pushing, only soothing and relaxing the cutaneous nerves and loosening up underlying muscles, using a protein cream for dry skin, vegetable oil for greasy skin.

3 Next comes the more active or '*pétrissage*' part of the massage – kneading. With the hand cupped in the shape of a spoon, the masseur takes up just the *right amount of tissue*, enough to be effective, never enough to give strain. She starts on the lower right cheek under the ear and moves to the left cheek, covering all the peripheral zones of the face, keeping up the same rhythm throughout until the forehead is reached. Here a special technique is employed to relax the frontal muscles, using thumb and middle finger.

4 The massage ends with '*tapotement*', a light and rapid tapping movement designed to tone up the skin completely, leaving it firmer,

47

revived and rosy, the underlying aim is to re-educate the sebaceous glands, whether too active or too lazy.

A facial from an experienced pair of hands and a mask from your own (remember to read the labels) are quick and easy routes to better looks.

LEARN FROM THE MODELS

I've added to and changed my beauty habits over the years, often because of what I've learned from the many models I've worked with – from Lauren Hutton, for instance, one of the highest paid models in the world, who earns over £150,000 a year. Lauren uses herb treatments away from the studio, – herbal steaming to deep cleanse her pores and herbal rinses on her hair, particularly rosemary to give it natural lights.

From superstar Cher I learned to use a bar of transparent soap to

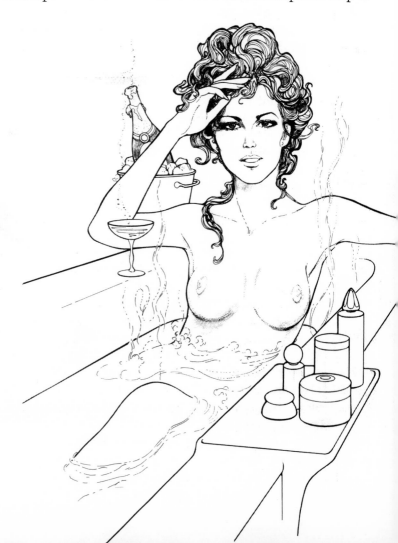

perk up my eyebrows. She brushes a bar up and over the hairs, so they not only glisten but stay put where she wants them.

Cover girl Karen Graham would never dream of putting base all over her face, but only in certain areas where she feels she needs it, to hide a flaw or to produce a special effect.

A good model knows her face as well as a cartographer knows his maps. Increasingly, models arrive at the studio with good skin, not like the 'old days' when a retoucher, the man who takes flaws out of pictures before they're in print, was constantly called in to touch out spots and marks on the faces of the famous – too often signs of too much make-up, not enough cleansing, too much of the wrong food, too much champagne, not enough sleep.

Here are some tips from the top models I worked with at *Vogue* and *Harper's Bazaar*, tips that work and are quick:

'When I take a bath, I make it hot enough to last about an hour and a half, then soak and soak, while I sip a glass of iced water to make me perspire a lot; this cleans out my pores. I use a little baby oil in the water, too, to keep my skin silky. For morale's sake I sometimes substitute cold Dom Perignon for the iced water.'

'I find yogurt makes a great facial mask – so does egg yolk mixed with evaporated milk.'

'I eat lots of avocados for the sake of my skin, because they're full of vitamin A and E. For the sake of my shape, too. If I'm bulging with a few extra pounds I eat nothing but avocados for a couple of days to fine down.'

'If I cry – rough treatment from the photographer or my boyfriend – my eyes get puffy, so I put thin slices of cold potato around them for an hour or so and the puffiness goes completely.' Cold tea bags work too.

'I don't often kick over the traces foodwise, but if I feel queasy the morning after the night before, I drink a mixture of honey, hot water and apple cider vinegar – it helps my digestion and seems to "cleanse" my insides completely, which obviously helps my skin glow. I always have a bottle of mineral water on my dressing table anyway and drink plenty of it all day long to "flush out" bad things from my system – for my skin's sake.'

'I eat lots of fruit and vegetables in the summer, the yellow ones that contain A, the beautiful-skin vitamin. I like rubbing my body with apricot oil or corn oil after bathing. It not only leaves my skin *feeling* like a baby's, but looking like it, too.'

49

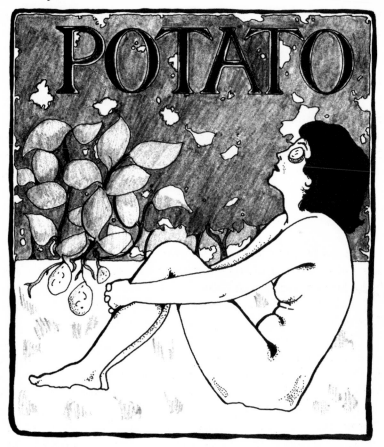

Beauty Secret from Russia

The models learn by trial and error; the beauticians can't afford to. They meet constantly at seminars all over the world to exchange news and views.

Lecturing in Russia at the Institute of Dermatology, beauty authority Aida Grey commented on the good-looking skin of the Russian women – although privately she was appalled at their size. The Russians like their women to weigh in at 10½ stone (67 kg) minimum.

The secret of that skin? Aida finally pinpointed it as the enormous amount of cabbage in the Russian diet. 'There are piles of cabbages at every street corner and at every dinner party I was served cabbage soup. In fact, cabbage is part of every meal, including breakfast on cold days.' When isn't it cold? No wonder the ladies weigh so much. But why is cabbage good for skin? Because of its natural hyaluronic acid content, the same natural acid that *binds* moisture in our skin and, lying in all connective tissues, acts as a shock absorber.

Since her Russian visit Aida has provided cabbage pills in all her salons and urges everyone to eat cabbage, in salad, soup or soufflé form, at least once a week. Interesting note: 2 oz of raw cabbage produces as much vitamin C as 2½ lb of the cooked variety (50 g to 1 kg in metric terms). We often 'cook out' much of the goodness that nature provides.

CHECK YOUR CALENDAR – IT'S TIME TO CHANGE GEAR FOR SUMMER

Summer is potentially the best time for skin – if you know how to take advantage of the great outdoors. Skin acts younger in the summer, like a lot of people we all know.

Take care of your skin properly, and it can help you face the dog days of winter that may lie ahead.

Take the expression 'heating up', when it's applied to making love; it derives from what happens when your *skin 'heats up'* – as it also does in the summer. Adrenalin flows through your veins; you feel more alive. Everything flows faster, including your surface blood level, its speed increasing with each rise in temperature. What is charmingly described as 'cellular rubbish' is collected and carried away faster, while the expression 'in the pink' literally expresses what all this means: your skin *is* pinker, rosier and prettier – though *not* because of a gorge of sunbathing (beware! see below).

With this increased flow of oils and sweat, your skin needs more cleansing, frequent showers, deodorants, fresheners after every cleanse, like a delicious cool frappé after every meal, and light, fresh fragrances.

Sun – Friend or Foe?

The sun *can* be a friend. It all depends on you, because it can also be the most dangerous enemy your skin will ever encounter.

Sun actually makes the skin *stronger* when its rays are at its strongest. Exposed to that amount of ultra-violet, the skin changes colour, but not in the way bread changes to toast under the grill. Tanning results from a process *inside* the skin, when the lower skin cells are provoked into producing extra melanin, that is extra pigment. This is nature's ingenious way of putting up a defence against possible injury from burns, in the same way that the skin protects itself when hurt, thickening into a callus or scab. Without this extra melanin, skin exposed to the full free rays of the sun would shrivel right up and literally 'die'.

When a little extra melanin combines with the skin's own protein to produce a strong healthy shield, *not* burned, not even really tanned, but more slightly flushed (with the extra pigment in force), this makes the skin more resilient and gives it a glorious glow. This amount of sun is fine – about ten minutes back and front, maximum. Then you are also receiving benefits from the sun's infra-red rays, the ones you feel on your body as heat; they nourish certain organs, offer a plus factor in reduced tension and fatigue, and build more vitamin D in your body.

Unfortunately, rarely does enough discipline go along with the sun oil. Too much sun (and too much can be arrived at very speedily) is what most people get, however many times they have read or been told that too much sun eventually spoils the skin *irretrievably*, the extra melanin no longer providing only a healthy strong shield, but rather an ugly piece of skin that looks and feels like leather.

Skin doesn't change colour under the sun in the way bread changes to toast under the grill – here, surface topography of sun-burned skin is seen through a scanning microscope

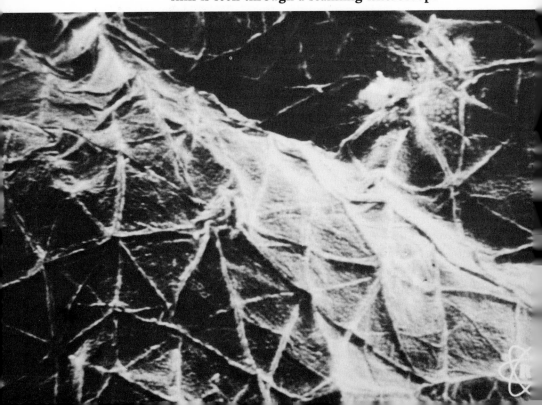

WHY DO WOMEN WANT TO BE BROWN? It's a conundrum that baffles dermatologists, who spend their lives propagating the benefits of shade, for they know – and by now I think *we all know* – that the sun browns, burns and, alas, AGES skin faster than anything else if its rays are allowed free play. The reason is simple: too much sun dries up the corneal layer and melanin produces leathery skin.

More sinister, it has been proved that there's a higher than average incidence of carcinoma (skin cancer) among those who are constantly exposed to sunlight, notably those who because of their work have to spend long periods out of doors.

Once upon a time the paler the skin, the greater the distinction. Up to about the mid-1920s the leisurely affluent lived life indoors rather than out, and lack of a tan meant there was money in the family. Only the working classes changed skin colour with the seasons. They couldn't help it; they worked outside.

Social nuances have changed. There's now something even priggish about the sight of a lily-white girl guarding her complexion beneath a parasol or covering every inch of herself up on the beach. Her very whiteness jars, for today it's a year-round bronze that's wanted.

We don't cultivate tans for health's sake, more for the sake of our looks.

The main problem is that most of us want a tan today, not to-morrow or the day after, yet it can't be rushed. Genetically speaking, some tan faster than others, while there's a whole skin type who can't pigment at all, primarily those of Celtic descent, Irish, Scots and Welsh, who freckle and burn all the way to one big peel no matter what they do. They have 'holes' in their natural sun screen and need the maximum protection from the sun to stay looking pretty.

All suntan preparations are sun screens, but they differ in the amount of ultra-violet they let through. Your genetic make-up sets the speed at which you tan, and if you try to hurry it up you end up *retarding* any increase in colour by developing a burn that blisters off the colour you already have.

Summer isn't the only time to beware. There's an old mountain myth that says you can't get burned in the snow. Each skiing season people learn painfully that it isn't true. As an eminent doctor told me, 'The ultra-violet radiation emitted from the sun that causes sunburn is highly reflected from only two things – sand and snow. Snow is the best reflector, almost 100 per cent reflective. When you are out of doors

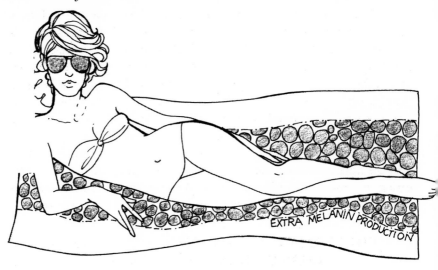

on snow and ice you get double the dose, once from above, once from below. Sand reflects only about 50 per cent, but that's enough to give the skin plenty of trouble.'

The Worst Thing You Can Do to Your Skin

To go after a tan, sitting on a catamaran, holding a reflector, skimming across the water, is like putting your skin in the fire, yet more women than I could pack on to the beach at Bournemouth do just that every year.

Water doesn't reflect ultra-violet (an old fallacy), but it does transmit virtually all of it. When you're out at sea, with no buildings or mountains interfering with the sky, you have the whole globe around you, rays radiating from all directions, so you get far more ultra-violet radiation than if you were on a lake with trees around it or in a pool with your house or somebody else's throwing up some shade.

Because water lets the rays go through, you have to count every minute you're *under* water, swimming or scuba diving, as time spent *in the sun*. You should put on a sun screen when you go in the water, when you come out and when you stay out, for perspiration wears a lot of sun screen away. On a cloudy day you're still not safe. Clouds are made of water vapour, so on a totally cloudy day about 50 per cent radiation is getting through. On a hazy day, you could be getting nearly 100 per cent.

We all have friends who say, 'I don't need any sun screen. I *never* burn. I can take all the sun it wants to give me.' It may not be this year or next that the results of soaking it all up show, but if these people could see their skin in a crystal ball ten to twenty years hence, they might think again. The skin just can't take that kind of third degree year in, year out, without slowly reneging on its identity and turning into a kind of weather-beaten *old* leather – and old is the operative word. Don't let it happen to your skin. It isn't necessary.

If you're taking any medication, check with your doctor that it isn't the kind that can make skin extra sensitive to sunburn. But medication or not, sunbathe only with *proper protection* and always in moderation – however much sun you *think* you can get away with.

CHECK YOUR CALENDAR ... IT'S TIME TO CHANGE GEAR FOR WINTER

The reason why so many house plants do poorly in winter is because of the lack of humidity. Everyone's favourite plant, the human skin, does poorly in winter, too, unless by any chance it's lucky enough to live in a *humidified* atmosphere.

The skin loses less moisture to summer than to winter air, because summer air is obviously more humid. Once you step away from an air conditioner, whatever trouble has been wrought can often be rectified outside. For their skin's sake many models around the world live in unheated houses, using only radiators when the weather gets really arctic. In summer, they turn to air conditioning only to cool the place down when they're going out, switching it firmly off on their return.

Winter skin is different from summer skin; it's thinner, and more vulnerable and sensitive. As winter slowly moves on to spring, the skin's thickness increases according to how much warmth is in the air. It's at its thickest when summer finally comes.

Thin skin needs more help than most women realize. Thin skin is so fragile it can't hold much moisture. It dries *fast* on a cold windy street or in a centrally heated room, and it easily begins to look weather-beaten and old.

The extreme visible result of dehydration is when skin is chapped and cracked anywhere it has a chance to be, at lip corners, around nostrils, even at the corners of the eyes.

Left unchecked, cracks or chapped skin can develop into serious

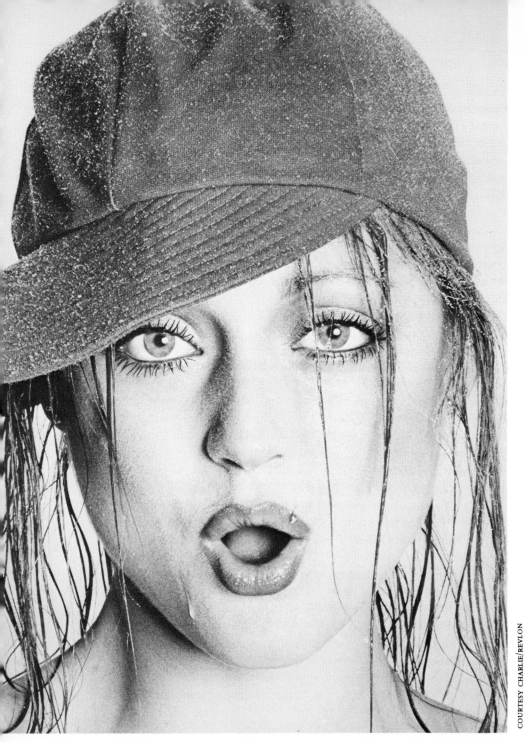

Baby, it's cold outside

problems, but any woman worth her powder puff *knows* they have to be cured fast, with double doses of moisturizer and applications of special creams fortified to increase the skin's capacity to hold more moisture than its thickness usually permits.

As products are refined more and more, the oils used for lotions and potions are light on the skin, yet they have such an affinity for it, they can 'hug' it, ensuring a new 'water supply' is available.

It is basic common sense in winter to take fewer baths, avoiding hot water and soap whenever possible, for that combination removes whatever moisture is lurking about at the surface along with the dirt. Bath at night and, if you must, shower in the morning, a short shower without soap. Bath oil is a must at this time of year, soap or no soap, and you can – and should – be as narcissistic as you like about it, *slathering* rich emollients all over your arms, legs, breast and face while you're soaking.

Don't overclean your face, stripping the skin of any natural oils it would rather hold on to. It's better to cleanse with cream or lotion for safety, leaving it on a few minutes to catch as much debris as it can. Where the skin is thin and vulnerable all the year round, on throat and hands and around the eyes, use even more moisturizer, more creamy, luscious stuff.

If you wash your own hair and like to blow-dry it, wrap your skin up in moisturizer before you start work. Hot, moving air is an extra attack skin doesn't need.

However much cream you put on your skin at night only just so much can be absorbed, so after a generous slathering tissue off what's left on the surface. *Nobody needs to go to bed with a creamy mess on their face.*

Eat high energy food for the sake of your skin, winter and summer, and concentrate on everything containing vitamins A and B2: cheese, liver, eggs, leafy vegetables, fruit.

Doctors say that today people rarely stay out in the cold – skiing, tobogganing, skating – to the frostbite stage, but a pre-frostbite condition can occur without you realizing it. Patches of skin turn white and are then surrounded by a bright red area, and the patches feel like first or second degree burns. When your skin starts to hurt, it's time to get out of the cold – *fast.*

If you wrap your skin up and swaddle it in emollients, just as you wrap your body up in a fur coat, you stand a better chance of defeating old man frost. For those who think to defeat him by migrating with the birds to Barbados and the sun or to the ski slopes and St Moritz, again there's that old man hazard to watch out for – the sun and more sun. *Protect* is the word – in the cold and in the sun.

BLACK SKIN – SLOW TO AGE ... THE BLACK GIRL IS KIND TO HER SKIN

Too much sun ages white skin fast, while the extra melanin content of black skin acts like a filter whenever sun rays are strong, letting less of the damaging ultra-violet through. A black girl rarely sunbathes much anyway, because she generally knows how to look after her skin only too well.

When it comes to skin care, from an early age black women traditionally use many natural substances on their skins. It starts in the cradle, when a mother tenderly applies baby oil, petroleum jelly and cocoa butter to her baby's skin to make it as supple as possible. All these things the dermatologists would love us *all* to use *every day* as shields against the elements that rob our skin so outrageously of its most precious possession – moisture.

Does Black Skin Age at a Slower Rate than White?

We've only got to think of some 'ageless' beauties to know it's a fact. Lena Horne's skin is still as smooth as that of somebody half her age; so is Cleo Laine's. Why is this so?

Colour counts. The darker the skin, the slower the ageing process, for a variety of genetic, environmental and skin care reasons. Here we go again – the earlier you start, the better your skin will be. If you have a baby in the house, remember that.

Some people think black skin ages at a slower rate than white because it's more oily, but this is controversial. Black skin is not more oily, some doctors and some black people say, while others swear it is. Doctors answer back with: 'It appears more oily because light reflecting on it gives it a sheen white skin doesn't have.'

A spell of cold weather and one tends to agree with the doctors, for dry skin shows up in the *ashen look* that dark skin can then have.

Basically, because the black woman knows her skin so well, and believes in skin care as a natural part of life, inheriting a routine from her mother as her mother did before her, she often appears to have an ageless look. But whatever the colour, ALL skin needs the same amount

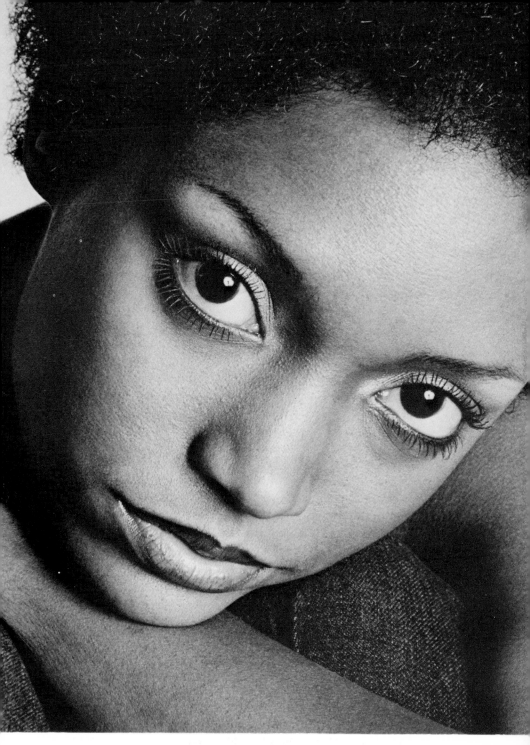

Black skin – slow to age?

of cleansing, protection and stimulation of the circulation to offset what the years can do.

WILL SKIN EVER BE RECYCLED AS GOOD AS NEW?

If you've been a good girl and stayed away from sunbathing all your life, and if you've kept your life free from stress and your nutritional intake high, the chances are you don't need to read this section – but it's fascinating just the same.

Rejuvenation isn't a word that slips off people's tongues easily these days. When Dr Niehans was alive and well, busily 'rejuvenating' the rich who flocked to his clinic in Switzerland, rumours circulated all over the world about how good and genuine his treatments were. He injected his usually celebrated patients with the embryos of unborn baby lambs, took fatigue away from the weary, replaced old lamps for new, one might say, as far as vitality and youthful vigour were concerned. Dr Niehans' work goes on today, as controversial as ever, carried out by disciples in Marbella, Spain, in Switzerland, and, to a lesser extent, in London. In America, the omnipresent watchdogs of the Food and Drug Administration preclude anything untried and untested by their medical authorities, so the treatment is not available.

In France, many women subscribe regularly to a royal jelly treatment, anointing the skin with the same nourishment that enables a grub to turn into a queen bee with a life-span of five years rather than a worker bee which lives only two months.

The miracle of the moisturizer – alleviating to a certain extent the dryness that contributes so much to looks ageing – is well over forty years old. It's time for a new miracle – but where is it?

Biochemists, dermatologists and enzymologists have been trying for decades to circumvent the sluggish stratum deep in our skin that's responsible for new cell output, to isolate the protein present in human cells responsible for skin regeneration and every metabolic process in our bodies. Enzymes, described by Professor Jevons of Manchester University as 'life's basic device', are the same complex proteins we depend on for a radiant complexion.

Various compounds have been mentioned as having a bearing on the subject; procaine – a generic term for novocaine – is the one for which the most regenerative claims have been made. The Rumanian doctor, Dr Ana Aslan, has been prescribing a buffered version at her Bucharest Geriatric Institute for years. Called Gerovital H3, it was made famous long ago by patients like General de Gaulle and Nikita Krush-chev. It is said that procaine can forestall the formation of the M.A.O. enzymes (generally found in ageing people, and responsible for the depression that often accompanies old age), and that it can also en-courage the body to produce certain hormones that spur on a more youthful attitude to life and sex.

Gerovital H3 is available here, and because of the *quality* of the case histories (rather than the *quantity* of 'rich and famous') Ana Aslan's work is also being studied by many leading U.S. scientists. However, with typical protective reticence, the U.S. medical authorities will only allow that Gerovital H3 is being investigated 'through the normal channels regarding its effect on depression'. For American bootleggers of the product (they often buy supplies in London) even this small admission gives rise to the hope that one day Gerovital may be available to everyone on or off prescription.

WHAT HAS HAPPENED TO VITAMIN E?

Scientists are too canny to commit themselves totally on the subject of the controversial vitamin E. However, it *is* known that anti-oxidants, vitamin E among them, can and do help preserve purity in such things as butter, and are also used to slow down the deterioration of leather and rubber.

When vitamin E was fed to laboratory mice, their life expectancy in some tests was increased by as much as 40 per cent. Because of the huge flash of popularity that vitamin E experienced a few years ago, as news of this type of experiment filtered through to the general pub-lic, scientists became even more wary about admitting that vitamin E plays any part, however small, in slowing down the ageing process in humans.

Nevertheless, as research continues to reveal, vitamin E cannot be disregarded. Many gerontologists take 100 units a day of vitamin E, but because so much is still unknown about its precise action, they do not necessarily recommend similar doses for their patients.

Many women have reported in surveys carried out on its use that it has benefited them, particularly when coping with the menopause. The most frequent benefits cited are: increased energy, a sense of well-being and, above all relief from hot flushes and leg cramps.

P.R. has been going strong – for 4,000 years – on the benefits of the ginseng root, and many who use it say that physicians in the West are unfairly sceptical about its use. They maintain that this plant extract can alleviate menopausal discomforts as well as many other ailments of both sexes. Prized in the Orient for centuries, Chinese and Japanese doctors often recommend ginseng because they say it can change the metabolism of the body for the better over a long period of time, helping to delay ageing of the skin, stabilize weight and calm nerves.

COSMETIC PROGRESS

Years ago the word 'colloidal' was used as a prefix to many skin-care mask-type products in an endeavour to prove that they were the result of scientific processes. Today, research and development chemists look to the mask area with optimism, many of them believing that the mask is where research will pay off and a new 'miracle' might come about. More and more products based on collagen (the protein naturally present in our skin, and responsible for its elasticity) are receiving serious attention, too.

It could be that one day we will have pharmaceutical cosmetics or pharmaceuticals for cosmetic purposes. In this way skin care would obviously be more specific and individual, because these cosmetics would have to be 'prescribed' – on prescription – for one skin at a time.

As Charles Revson, one of the greatest innovators the cosmetic world has ever known, once said to me, 'For your skin I have treatments, products that will retard age, take away poor skin tone and eradicate wrinkles – but for the woman next to you, the products may not work. To create sensational products that will produce dramatic results for everyone – that's my aim and one day it will happen.'

It didn't happen in his lifetime – but he was right. It will happen one day.

Many spectacular scientific advances have been made in other fields that have been found to have cosmetic overtones. It may be that these overtones will provide the keys to future cosmetic progress. Until then, we'll keep on hoping and must keep on cleansing, toning and moisturizing.

HANDS (AND NECK) GET THE WORST DEAL – GIVE THEM SOME HELP

Hands, like necks, are tell-tales, and often give away one's age. Why? The skin is thinner there than anywhere else on the body (except for that immediately surrounding the eyes). With few oil glands, the skin dries and 'creases' fast, while there's little flesh beneath to support moisture. In short, the hands show *every sign of wear and tear*, and they get a lot. The skin is also thin round the neck, but the neck doesn't work so hard, even though it has the hard job of fighting gravity to hold our heads up high. Also, necks can easily be hidden under turtlenecks or scarves, whereas you can only lengthen a sleeve so far if you want to hide your hands! Unfortunately hands, wrinkled or not, have to stay in view.

Can anything be done? Plenty. First, there's that underrated product, hand cream, which regularly turns up in Christmas stockings,

Hands can give the beauty game away

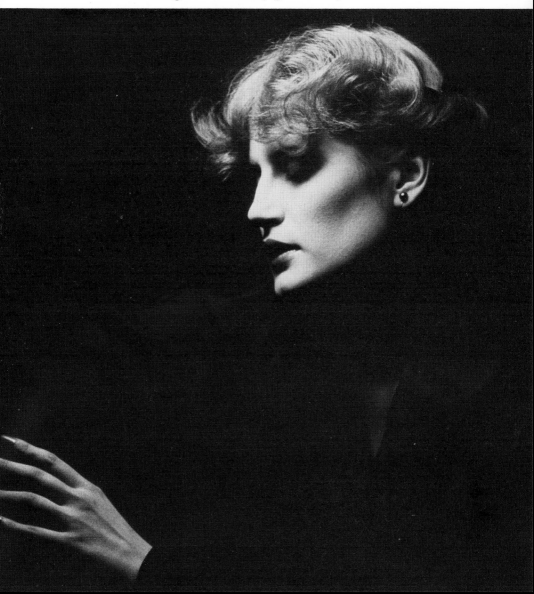

only to be put away in the bathroom cabinet and then forgotten. It's a pity, for most hand lotions (usually about 80 per cent water, 20 per cent moisturizer) at least help the skin cells *retain* any moisture around, and form a barrier against the elements outside, which can do so much harm to unprotected skin.

Some hand lotions are sticky and so even more forgettable, but recent developments have introduced polymers that don't stick, allowing the moisture to sink into thin skin and stay there, down deep.

Delicious oils from the avocado or aloe vera plant give the hands marvellous protection, while some creams claim that their ingredients can penetrate *six cells down*, which sounds useful. Six cells or one, the regular use of hand cream really does help preclude that ugly sight – chapped, wrinkled hands.

If you're too busy to remember hand cream, you can catch up in the bath. Keep the richest cream you've got on the side and smother your hands in it. Steep your hands in the warm water, hopefully laced with a rich bath oil, too. Run them through the oily water several times, in and out, in and out, until they're well saturated. You'll be amazed how much oil they soak up, because they need *all* they can get, particularly in winter.

The best hand care products feed oxygen into the pores, have anti-bacterial properties, and set out to whiten the skin as well as soothe it. *Look for the label* that spells out that *polyunsaturates*, *vitamins* and *lubricants* are inside the bottle or jar. Those ingredients mean business. Massage the lotion down each finger as if smoothing on suede gloves; again, the hands will soak it up. For any brown marks use a de-pigmenting cream; there are plenty around and they're getting better all the time (see page 36).

ONE LINE OF DEFENCE FOR THE HANDS, ANOTHER FOR THE NAILS

Nails are in the front line with bright colours.

To start, leave your nails naked for a day, then paint them with white iodine and leave on overnight to encourage growth and discourage flaking and chipping.

In their basic state nails should be pearl-like in texture and slightly pink in colour, like an oyster shell. But beautiful nails don't grow on hands without help.

The matrix is at the bottom of nature's deal, located at the nail base, showing only its top, which we call a 'moon'. Whatever natural sheen and surface you have on your nails depends on what diet is part of your life (read pages 198 – 239). The better the natural gloss, the more nourishment you're giving your body; it finds its way to the matrix and then to the nail itself *via* a myriad of tiny blood vessels.

If you feel you're eating right, yet your nails still let you down, a genetic factor could be the cause, for heredity does play its part.

Remember to moisturize your nails. They can suffer from dryness. Use a cuticle cream, protein-packed and emollient enough to reduce the dryness that makes even those with the most saintly dispositions start to ruin their resolutions, picking and pulling at their manicures. Use a cuticle jelly to make the cuticles soft and easy to push back, leaving the nails trim and elegant.

Do have a weekly manicure to help you keep any resolutions you make about your nails.

Do file your nails in one direction only, never back and forth; a sawing motion causes snags.

Don't cut cuticles. Push them back with a wooden stick.

Do avoid water at least for a few hours after a manicure.

Do use gloves for cleaning jobs (except when you clean your face).

Do dial with the end of a pencil; using a finger ruins the nail.

Do use the cushions of your fingers to pick things up.

Don't wear a frosted enamel all the time, it's too drying.

Don't overuse nail hardeners, strengtheners or nail polish removers. Touch-ups are preferable to re-dos.

Don't remove polish mid-week. If you think the colour looks murky, add another coat. If you want to switch colour, add it on top. Better to build up enamel than keep using remover on your nails.

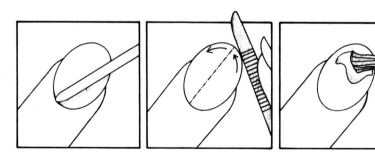

THE BEST DO-IT-YOURSELF MANICURE: scrape nail surface with a wooden stick after removing old enamel; this eliminates roughness.

Clean cuticles, then coax them back with a wooden stick impregnated with cuticle remover.

File straight across tip towards nail centre, using either an emery board or a metal file covered in diamond dust (preferred by many manicurists because although the dust gives the metal a smooth surface, it's still abrasive enough to take away snags and split edges).

On weak nails use a strengthener, applied only to nail tips. This works by penetrating and fusing the nail, helping prevent breakages and splitting, as well as encouraging nail growth to stay in place – as length.

Find a hardener that's also a coloured enamel, otherwise use two coats of polish, plus one of sealer to see the manicure through the week.

Toe nails get seen, too. Get a pedicure at least once a month or follow the same procedure as you do for your manicure. Both hands and feet should have a pick-me-up at the end of a day – a massage in and out of each toe, or along each finger, with a fragrant emulsified lotion. It can't hurt. (See page 82.)

EVERYBODY SHOULD

Thoroughly cleanse their skin at least twice a day.

Be seen by a dermatologist once a year after twenty-five – unless there are problems that need professional help before that.

Follow a regular regime of skin care treatment.

Learn how to compensate for dry or dehydrated, greasy or hydrated skin.

Avoid excessive exposure to the sun *always*.

Use a sun screen, if not a sun block, when the sun is at its height.

Watch for any allergic reaction to a product.

Avoid heavy smoking – it's not good for the skin.

Drink up to eight glasses of water a day – it's good for the skin.

Wear frequent masks according to skin type.

Stimulate the circulation by lying head down, feet high on a slanting board.

Jog, walk, run, exercise for the skin's sake.

Remember that only *neglect is ageing*.

Beauty and the Beast

ARE you proud of the way your man looks? If you're not, start analysing why not and how to start on an improvement course – for both of you. You must think of it that way because any man, however saintly his disposition, is going to take it as a personal affront if you present him with a self-improvement routine for one. 'Who me? You can't be serious.' I can almost hear his grievous cries.

If you live with a man you're probably in charge of the skin and scalp department. If that seems a strange statement just ask yourself who chooses the soap in the soap dish and the shampoo on the bathroom shelf. Do realize that his skin needs soothing, too. If you can't see him settling for a cleanser in a bottle or tube (one that needs water to activate it, less abrasive than most soaps), start looking for soaps that stress their emollient, moisturizing factors, or buy the transparent kind; they may not cleanse so deeply, but they are less alkaline and so less harsh than the average soaps.

If your man has a troubled, blemished skin try to get him to use a medicated cream that can help. Present it to him as an ointment, if he's overly sensitive. When the wind is howling outside tell him you've just heard that a sun screen can act as protection against chapped skin in bad weather, too. Be sure to use an *emollient* sun screen though, then you'll be telling the truth.

When it's time to buy presents, shop around for products that will really help him. A better shaving cream, for instance, to help keep his skin well moisturized, as well as helping the shave along.

Remember that shaving is a man's daily blessing. All over the world women come up to me to bemoan one inequality in life: 'My husband's ten, five, three, two years older than me and yet he looks ten, five, three, two years younger. It's so unfair. What can I do about it?' I used to answer jocularly, 'shave', until a sharp-tongued lady in

67

Tokyo assured me that she did, every day. The fact is that in shaving every day or twice a day a man gives himself a mild skin clean or dermabrasion treatment. Scraping off his dead skin cells along with his beard he stimulates the blood circulation in that area of the body, helping to activate the production of new cells, all giving him that slightly *fresher* edge over his maybe younger-in-years partner.

There's another built-in advantage that men have over women, connected with their facial hair. The hairs of a man's beard are stronger and spikier than a woman's 'down', as anyone can vouchsafe who has ever been in a clinch with more than one day's growth. These hairs, dermatologists tell me, act as props for a man's skin, so that it often doesn't sag so quickly as a woman's – well, certainly a woman who doesn't give her skin the proper attention. Encouraging a man to shave can mean encouraging a younger look, but there's no need for you to dot the 'i' and cross the 't' to get him to the sink. The important thing is that when he shaves, he does it with a moisturized product, so his skin is also kept well lubricated.

MAN TRAPS

Watch out for signs of a dry scalp. Those giveaway flakes on dark jackets tell the story. Keep two shampoos handy. One for no-problem days, rich in protein. The more you wash your hair, the more protein you need in the suds to build up hair body. The second shampoo should be directed towards dealing with dandruff, something that's all too easy for both males and females to get, particularly in winter when the hair and scalp often get buried without oxygen under wool and fur for long periods.

Show him you love him by massaging his scalp. This will stimulate the circulation and distribute the natural oils. All good for the hair, and he doesn't need to know that your loving care is for the sake of his looks, and not just for his morale.

Some men are still wary about the whole scent syndrome and prefer to keep the fact that they wear cologne a top secret between them and their bathroom door. Some dramatically ignore every Christmas and/or birthday present of after, before and in-between shave, insisting they can get as clean and fresh as is necessary for a man to be with good alkaline soap. It isn't true. A soap smell doesn't stay in place a minute once a nippy east wind hits the cheek, whereas a cologne or toilet water definitely does. There's no longer any sissy

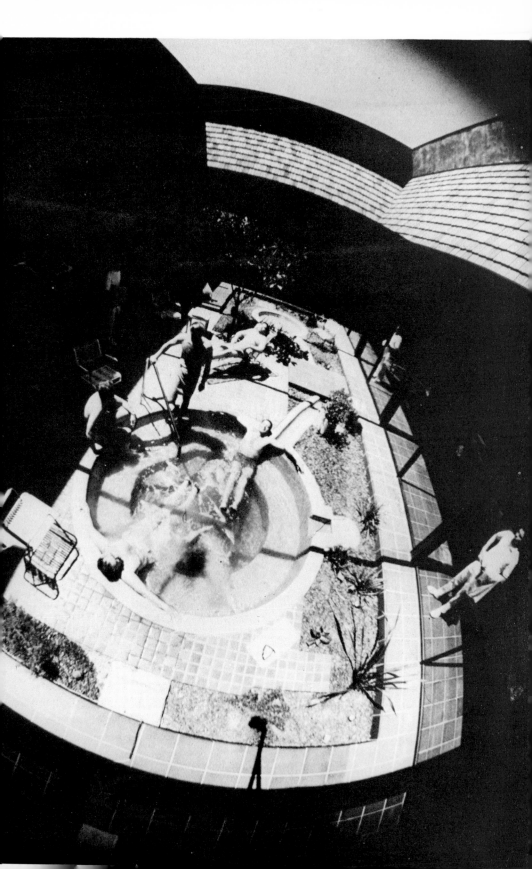

connotation about a man who wants to smell like oak or moss – or rose petals, for that matter. Sandalwood, cedar and even camphor are all good masculine smells – and I'm not referring to mothballs.

The bath or shower is the perfect place to persuade the most stubborn anti-cologne man. In this area male goodies run rampant, from Scandinavian bath salts and sauna bath rubs to he-man stuff like sportsman rubdown cream. He, like she, can be convinced it's okay if the name and the smell of the product are right. Well, so say the marketing experts.

DE-PAUNCHING

If his skin, scalp and smell are in good fettle but you feel his paunch is letting you down, check up on your cooking before you rush out to buy his and her jogging suits. Increase the roughage in your meals (see page 221). Serve more fresh fruit, and raw vegetables in the form of *crudités* before the main course, as they do in the best restaurants – raw cauliflower, asparagus, radishes, celery, carrots and spring onions. Most men love to crunch these, and they really are helpful to the digestion.

If you've been a sedentary pair, go slowly on introducing a new jogging routine before bedtime (see page 281). Work out at your own pace, increasing speed and the course s-l-o-w-l-y. Once a week will get you nowhere. Select simple stretching exercises, like toe touching and knee bending, and do them together.

Face up to it, if he's out of shape and you're not, you're still going to have to join in to guarantee results. Even if you hate the thought, suggest you take up a sport *together*. Tennis is the obvious one, but if that doesn't gain his approval swim together, dance more and certainly take long walks as often as possible. *His health is more in your hands than maybe you realize.*

MALE GROOMING

Men all over the world are already wearing bronzers to cover up dark circles beneath otherwise lustrous eyes. There are already portable wall bars that men can take with them on business trips to continue keep-fit programmes in dull hotel rooms. Although it hardly seems possible, in certain parts of the world men can order sporty eyelashes to cover up the fact that they've lost their own through playing with fire or something equally dangerous. There are men who use toning up lotions to uplift their wilting pores, others who use toning down emulsions to eradicate any possible martini flush; there are ready warmed lathers to take the edge off the early morning shaving chill, and after-shave conditioners to moisturize the cheeks, and these are just part of a whole range of products aimed at sending men out looking well nourished and well tended. In other words, wash-and-brush-up would hardly be the description given to a man's grooming programme today.

Whether you like that sort of male or not, they are still in the *minority*, particularly in this country. Remember you can be the beneficiary of the end product. Decide on how far you want him to go and then concentrate on getting him there.

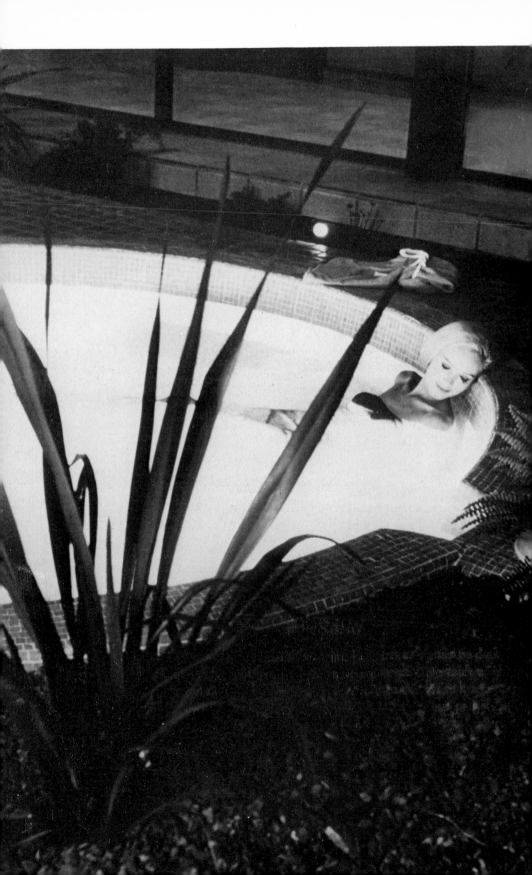

4

From the Deodorant to the Bath

AND WHAT EACH CAN DO FOR YOU

IT's no longer merely a question of whether your best friend will ever tell you. Every skin worth its epidermis has to be dressed these days, not only with treatments and make-up for the face, but with lotions and potions for the body – the choice grows daily. There's no longer anything narcissistic about bathtime beauty rites, oiling, foaming, nourishing, powdering, whooshing fragrance literally all over from top to toe. *Cleanliness isn't enough any more.*

DEODORANTS AND ANTI-PERSPIRANTS

Before I dwell on the powers and pleasures to be derived from the bathtub (which ladies from Poppaea, Empress of Rome, to Elizabeth Taylor, once Empress of Hollywood, have enjoyed), the *purpose* of the deodorant and anti-perspirant should be recorded.

Deodorant power has grown over the past few years, since research established more exactly the cause of body odour, the iniquitous B.O. or sweat. 'Not to be mentioned in refined conversation,' says the Oxford Dictionary.

Why do we sweat and why does it smell? It seems a discriminating process but it isn't. It's all part of a well run plan, as practical as the rest of the body's mechanisms.

We sweat mainly to keep cool, and it isn't the sweat that smells but what it meets with on the way out – bacteria present on the surface of everyone's skin

There are two kinds of sweat because we have two kinds of sweat

73

The bath – perfect place for beauty treatments

glands, eccrine and apocrine. The output of neither smells on its own; perspiration is, in fact, almost odourless.

You wouldn't put a deodorant or anti-perspirant all over your body where the eccrine glands are distributed – about 6,500 to the square inch (1,000 to the square centimetre), with a concentration on forehead, palms and soles. Their secretion is about 99 per cent pure water plus a few salts, and exuded from a clean, healthy young adult it even has a fairly pleasant slightly salty smell – apparently an aphrodisiac to some.

The eccrine glands mostly handle the job of keeping us cool, plus that of eliminating waste; they work round the clock, regulating the body's temperature at or near its normal level, using the evaporation of water from the skin's surface as a cooling system.

You *would* apply a deodorant or anti-perspirant to the areas where the apocrine glands are found, as these secrete not only water but also some protein and waste substances, thus providing a much better environment for bacteria to thrive on. Larger than the eccrine, the apocrine glands are restricted mainly to the underarms, the anogenital region and the nipples. Their growth, closely associated with hair follicles, is stimulated by the same hormones that cause hair growth under the arms and around the genital areas. That's why body odour is rarely a problem in children and old people, where hormone – and therefore hair – supply is less.

Stress and Sweat

Recent research has proved that body odour seems to occur more often at times of emotional stress – sweating from heat alone doesn't cause the same sort of smell or the same sort of problem. That's because it's during times of stress – fear, excitement, tension – that most apocrine sweat is secreted, – although the apocrine glands also handle some normal 'air conditioning' for the body. Merging with the eccrine sweat secretion this is all added inducement for bacteria and so odour.

Diet can affect body odour, something generally not noticed by humans, but apparent to keen-scented animals like dogs, who can distinguish vegetarian natives from meat-eating Westerners, and lions, who can spot a man a mile away when the wind is in the right direction.

In Western countries, where emotional problems are frequently countered with an annual consumption of billions of tranquillizers, the stress factor plays a significant part in producing excessive apocrine sweat.

While some products are efficacious enough to control bacterial action, and so odour for the majority, the minority who suffer from excessive perspiration problems are still waiting for a major breakthrough. Research goes on but medical opinion is divided as to whether it's a problem which can only be finally solved with nerve blocking drugs administered under medical supervision.

Vive la Différence

Many don't realize there's a considerable difference between a deodorant and an anti-perspirant.

A deodorant is formulated to mask or diminish odours, and to inhibit bacterial growth to a small extent, without affecting the flow of perspiration.

An anti-perspirant, composed of chemicals, actually *reduces* the perspiration reaching the skin's surface by partially closing the pores and inhibiting the sweat glands. The pores are not completely blocked – they couldn't and shouldn't ever be, for if they were a prickly heat rash would quickly result. The curious thing is that the physiological processes involved are still something of a medical mystery.

The advantage of using an anti-perspirant is that by checking perspiration bacterial growth is also retarded. It has less to grow and feed on.

Almost all anti-perspirants contain one or several aluminium salts, however, which means that sensitive skins can experience a slight irritation if they are used every day. Alternating between a deodorant, which has a gentler action, and an anti-perspirant is the wisest course for this type of skin. The one simple act often overlooked in choosing this sort of product is READING THE LABEL.

A friend of mine with a heavy perspiration problem (nerves are the culprit here, too) said there was nothing on the market to help her condition. When I asked her what she used and when she should use it, I learned she never read the instructions, which clearly said she should put the anti-perspirant on *before* going to bed, an early morning shower or bath wouldn't lessen its ameliorating effects. She carried out that instruction and has had no problems since.

Another fact often overlooked is that relative to shaving and getting rid of underarm hair. Hair is just another place where bacteria loves to thrive, turning the combination of apocrine and eccrine secretions and bacteria even faster into odour.

We need to sweat for our body's sake and for comfort. To

75

reduce perspiration to the minimum required for our 'air conditioning' is the goal, and our choice of product has to be based entirely on personal requirements – so, once again, *don't forget to read the label.*

Whatever the commercials imply, no product can become a substitute for cleanliness. Bathing comes first and last, with deodorants or anti-perspirants fitting neatly in the middle.

BEAUTY IN (AND OUT OF) THE BATH

Before the modern advances of science and the advent of the deodorant (Mum in 1888, Odo-Ro-No in 1914), bathing was the answer. The Hebrews believed in it, the Romans even more so, as can be evidenced today from the remains of their many elaborate bathing establishments all over Europe.

The great cover-up of body odour with fragrant oils and essences, which were used instead of cleanliness (phew!), began in the fourteenth century and lasted till the beginning of the eighteenth – all because church dogma equated nudity with lewdness, so that any public bath had to be a place of debauchery.

As the *Michelin Guide* points out, in the thirteenth century there were twenty-six public baths in Paris. Under Louis XIV only two were left – and he himself boasted that he never had a bath. The one bathtub left in the palace was thought to be so superfluous it was moved to the garden as a fountain, while Marie Antoinette bathed in a white flannel nightshirt, brainwashed since birth into believing that bathing naked was a cardinal sin.

Earlier, Queen Elizabeth I, forever emphasizing her individuality, had revealed that she bathed once a month, 'whether it was required or not'. Of course, her best friend never told *her*.

For the last 150 years the importance of regular bathing has become increasingly obvious. The only controversy left is over which has the more merit, the bath or the shower. Americans generally regard the British as a less clean race because of their anti-shower, bath-mad attitude, but whether you bath or shower the end result is the same if you use soap. You get wet and clean – for soap makes water work more efficiently, the kind you find in a jar working best of all, as it is the mildest, approximating to a cleansing cream that needs water to activate it.

Water, Water Everywhere – but Where's the Softest Kind?

The best water to bath or shower in is soft water. It allows a rich lather with less soap, and rinses off soap more easily, too.

With hard water, a thin film is likely to remain on the skin after washing, causing irritation and dryness, especially on the face. The remaining film may entrap small amounts of bacteria and dirt, hazardous to any skin that's sensitive or already a victim of acne or break-outs. Shampooing hair in hard water is a thankless task, leaving a film on the hair that dulls it, however much elbow grease went into the wash. Anyone who lives in a hard water area has to rinse harder than those in soft water areas – unless he or she invests in a water softener, a much more practical buy than many people think. You can always buy a small sink size if the large size eats up too much space and money. For beauty's sake, it's worthwhile having at least one area in the house with soft water.

Temperature also plays a big part in determining how good the water in your bath or shower is for you. Extremes of either hot or cold are bad. *Too hot* shocks the system, dries and ages the skin. *Too cold* can cause blood vessels to constrict and so reduce the blood supply to the skin – dangerous especially in the case of older people or anyone with a weak heart.

The best temperature when bathing for relaxation is pleasantly warm (from 85°F [29°C] to around 90°F [32°C]). The best atmosphere is candlelight (discovered by many people during an energy crisis and frequently kept as a good habit) or at least soft lighting, with a background of whatever music happens to send you, from Elton John to Verdi.

Apart from the restorative powers of the bath, relaxing and refreshing after a long hard day at the backgammon board, the skin is at its most receptive *underwater* when, wide awake, the pores can receive, without resistance, all manner of benefits, banishing parch at least until it's time to step out into the great outdoors again.

Bath Accompaniments

The well dressed bath these days is never without:

A loofah: the dry, rough-textured gourd that swells and softens when wet, yet sloughs off dead skin with accuracy leaving the body tingling. A natural loofah is usually about fifteen inches (38 centimetres) long, long enough to get to hard-to-reach spots on your back. Underwater massage with a loofah makes do-it-yourself leg shaping easier,

77

providing you move every day, day in, day out, with steady, firm strokes *up* towards the heart, the water pressure making the movement more meaningful.

A friction strap: usually made of hemp and blended with horsehair. This is useful for the same reason as the loofah, sloughing off dead skin, helping a do-it-yourself massage obtain results.

A body brush: the best are made of stiff, natural bristles, useful for whipping up the circulation, particularly on shoulders and back, while a natural bristle hand brush should be put to work on legs, arms and abdomen, where circulation is often sluggish.

Pumice-stone: this piece of ultra-porous volcanic lava fits into a palm easily to work away at small rough spots on ankles, elbows and heels. Don't forget to use it.

Soap and water go together as far as the body is concerned, but some soaps are better for some bodies. Greasy skin, for instance, will benefit from a glycerine-based soap, which does its cleansing job without adding any extra oil. Soap with a cucumber formulation is good for greasy skin, too.

Any super-fatted soap, rich with lanolin, cold cream, cocoa butter or coconut oil, lubricates dry skin, which needs every bath aid it can get in the way of oils, foams and milks. Submerging dry skin in a fragrant oil bath is a fast, easy way to soothe it everywhere it touches.

Super-sensitive skin has more and more to choose from in the way of fragrance-free soaps, the mild Castile or transparent kind, plus soaps with added vitamins.

Poor skin, prone to break-outs, needs medicated soap, full of anti-bacterial agents, which do their bit towards controlling infection and clearing up problem areas.

Normal skin (perfectly balanced between dry and oily) has the whole soapsud world to choose from, and can indulge any fragrant whim and enjoy a bath like nobody else. However, soap for the face – even one with 'normal 'skin – is something else again. The alkalinity present removes acid in the same way that detergents do. The natural guardian of the skin, the acid mantle, can be broken down in time if highly alkaline soap is regularly used, exposing skin to irritation – some dermatologists now believe you can 'catch cold' through your skin, if the acid mantle is displaced. If you must use soap on your face, be sure it's the mildest, most emollient one you can find.

Gels, milks and oils – produced from things as diverse as the avocado pear and the juniper plant – work on the skin by attaching

minuscule globules to receptive open pores, to get 'polished' in afterwards by the towel, soothing dry patches that may appear on the
skin's structure, often due to the onslaught of the elements. All these
products leave a light all-over aura, that can be intensified later by
wearing a perfume from the same fragrance family. They differ only
slightly. Gels will clean you as you soak; they're gentle on the skin
and don't leave a ring round the bath. Oils contribute more lubrication
than gels, while milks, rich in fats and oils, contribute still more. Bath
salts and crystals can soften water, and often add colour to lift the
weary spirit – for pampering and soaking aren't only for the sake of
the skin.

The bath has therapeutic value, too. Some women, like sculptress
Louise Nevelson, dress designer Jean Muir and actress Lyn Redgrave,
use the bath as a think-tank, the place to go when they have a particularly knotty problem to solve. Others, like Faye Dunaway, consider the
bath as part of a work-out regime and stay in fragrant, warm water
for only a few minutes, so as to perspire, then get out to work on their
bodies hard with a loofah or friction glove, finishing off by making
their bodies glossy with baby oil. Faye Dunaway's bathroom is the
room she particularly loves. It's well stocked with salts, oils, sponges
and brushes, but there are no heavily scented products. She believes
there's nothing better than the smell of clean skin following a bath.

Sonia Rykiel, the Parisian designer, treats the bath in exactly
the same way, and is out of the water in five minutes to her exercise
period, while worldwide nightclub owner Regine spends most of her
bathtime standing up, rubbing herself all over with a friction mitt,
sitting down only for a few minutes for a massage from her 'nanny' of
twenty years.

The Japanese attitude to the bath – dirty if it's used to wash in –
is accepted by author and historian Lady Antonia Fraser. She likes to
spend twenty minutes relaxing in a tub of clean, fragrant water, *after*
washing herself thoroughly under the shower. 'This is the time for
discussion with any of my children.'

Some people resort to the bath to counter a horrible day, as others
rush to a psychiatrist's couch. There are a number of tried-and-tested
homemade pick-me-up baths – from the euphoric cucumber one,
where slices are scattered on the water, and two slices are placed on the
eyelids (cooling and calming), to the oil of rosemary and wheatgerm
bath.

There are old-fashioned remedies to soothe sunburned skin – like

79

adding bicarbonate of soda or oatmeal to the water (tied in cheese-cloth so you don't clog up the drain). This sort of bath helps the feeling of burning heat to escape from the body. One tablespoonful of dry mustard in warm water eases a tired aching body but mustard or half a pound of borax won't do anything like so much for the psyche as, say, a lily-of-the-valley milk bath.

An hour spent in the bath can be good for looks, but not for books. I've never understood the habit of reading either the paper or a paperback in the bath. Soggy edges would fray my nerves, not soothe them.

Set up skin supplies on a bath tray or stool next to the bath. Include a facial mask, pumice stone, brush or comb, razor, tweezers, nail file, cuticle oil, bath oil, magnifying mirror, plenty of cotton wool and deep cleanser. Dampen the fingers and apply the deep cleanser all over the face, neck and shoulders, sliding back under the water so that a little steam opens up the pores. Clean off thoroughly with the cotton wool, then apply the mask. If your skin feels ultra dry, apply a moisturizer first, *beneath* the mask. Relax for several minutes or work on your nails with file and cuticle cream, applying the cream thoroughly around every finger. Brush or comb brows up, so you can see the natural line clearly, then tidy them up with tweezers. *Never* use scissors on your brows. Pumice all rough spots away, then apply a trace of bath oil directly to what were the rough spots. Finally, lather yourself all over with the sweetest smelling soap, shave off any superfluous hair, empty the bath, then shower away every vestige of soap and debris with a cool, direct spray. Once out of the bath, rub your body all over with bath lotion, before hugging yourself in a huge bath towel to pat yourself dry. It's a soothing experience – especially just before bed.

Bath Habits to Get into

A.M. Make up before getting into and quickly out of a tepid to warm bath. Moisture from the water softens lines, helps keep make-up looking fresh. Add a last touch of translucent powder before leaving the house to make it last still longer.

A.M. Try an algae, seaweed, sulphur or mineral bath to de-tense muscles. Each one can give an all-over pick-me-up feeling to the skin, as well as boosting morale. Stretch in the bath and try to do early morning exercises there. You have to expend more energy to do exercises in water. Moving your muscles against its force helps you make smooth, unjerky movements. Press your feet against the end of the bath, brace your arms on the sides, and slowly raise and lower your hips as many times as you can. Or brace your head on a soft bath pillow, hold the sides of the bath, raise both legs, bend the left knee slowly, then straighten. Repeat with the right.

Sitting, raise one leg, grasp calf and pull leg slowly towards you – five times each leg. Flex then relax muscles underwater. Contract buttocks for a count of five, then contract in turn your abdomen, bosom, neck and shoulders. Relax and slide your shoulders underwater for a few minutes before repeating the movements.

P.M. Just before bed, lounge in a foaming milk bath; drink your warm milk there, or hot buttered rum. Relax for ten minutes, then quickly dry yourself and get between cool, clean sheets. Lights out!

P.M. Give yourself a double cleanse in the bath, using first cleansing cream, then a skin tonic, then a light peel-off mask, ending with another pat of astringent or a freshening clean-up lotion.

Love Me, Love My Shower

For the anti-bath, love-my-shower brigade, instant energy seems to shoot out of the nozzle along with each jet of water. Certainly a shower can liven up the skin, and no area need be neglected – back of ears, nape of neck, under each foot, in between each toe (see page 287). Temperature changes can be useful to help the freshening up. Start with warm water, washing with a soap-filled mitt, then switch to tepid mid-stream and finish with cool to rinse off *thoroughly*. If you direct the jet to individual parts of your body, switching from hot to cold and back to hot again, it zips up the circulation in every area. If you have backache you can alleviate it sometimes with the shower treatment. Sit on the floor of the bath, resting your head on your knees, and let warm to hot water pour down over your back, shoulders and the nape of your neck. Three minutes of this can relax muscle tension.

After the Bath

Whether you love the relaxation of a bath or the energizing quality of a shower, or sensibly combine both – bath first, shower second – after-the-bath therapy gives you another opportunity to dress up your skin.

Moisture can be replenished with lazy strokes of *body lotion*, helping keep the skin as supple as it was meant to be. Smooth it on when you're damp and the pores are still relaxed. The fragrance lasts longer that way.

Maxi-coat yourself with *an anti-peel bath-oil spray*, leaving the skin silky and pretty.

Splash yourself all over with *a cologne version of your favourite perfume* to help the true scent last. Remember to add one touch more of the Big Strength before you leave for day or night.

Massage face, neck, shoulders and bosom with *creams that have special jobs to do*, emulsions that help the skin cells absorb 20 per cent of their water content, 'plumping out layers, diminishing the poor colour, sallowness and dullness often caused by lack of moisture.'

Some emulsions are called *isotonic*, which means they're correctly balanced to the skin's own oil and moisture content (pH), so carry out 'plumping' easily, making all the difference between facing the day looking your best or looking not-so-good.

All these body accoutrements, lotions, bath-oil sprays and splashes, not forgetting the good old standby of yesterday and today, talcum powder, are nowadays so refined that their *effect* is noticed by others, too, leaving an aura of loveliness behind via their perfume.

Quick Bath Guide

Rounding up the bath business, here's a neat guide:

For a *wake-up bath:* test with a thermometer and aim for a temperature between 70°F and 80°F (21°C and 27°C). Bath briskly, don't linger, don't forget the bath oil. Dry fast, powder well.

For a *warm-up bath:* after you've been in the snow and hail, take it above normal body temperature – about 102°F (39°C); comforting, but don't stay in long. Soap, rinse, jump out and dry vigorously with a big nubbly towel.

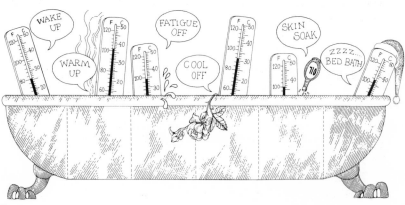

For a *fatigue relieving bath:* keep temperature at body temperature, between 98°F and 99°F (about 37°C) and soak with shoulders beneath the hot soapy water for at least fifteen minutes, finishing with a cool rinse. Blot dry, and work in body lotion all over, particularly at tense spots – shoulders, upper arms, nape of neck, ankles, calves, feet.

For a *cool-off bath* (when you're in a climate that's over 100°F (38°C) outside and humid): a cool bath will cool you down for longer than a *cold* one. Take it at about 92°F (33°C), soak for twenty to thirty minutes using a fragrant bath essence, the more floral, the less exotic the better. Blot the skin dry, then powder lavishly, so your clothes will slip on without sticking. This should cool you down for at least four to six hours. Repeat as often as you like; it isn't enervating.

For a *skin relief bath:* if you're burned, chapped or simply parched, take a warm 95°F–100°F (35°C–38°C) bath, laced well with bath oil. Run the bath at body temperature, then let warmer water trickle in as you soak – the length of the soak is important. The longer the better. Don't use soap, don't rinse, blot the skin, dry very gently and leave a slight film of oil on top for protection. No bath powder.

For a *bedtime bath:* always a good move for insomniacs, particularly if it's the day for clean linen. Turn the bed down before you turn the tap on, and have it between 98°F and 105°F (37°C and 41°C). Soap yourself before relaxing for about ten minutes, then shower in warm water, gently blot dry and powder well before rushing between those sheets. Lights out immediately. *No T.V. please.*

Water is good, it benefits all things, said the Chinese philosopher Lao-tzu, way back in the sixth century BC – and he was right. Nothing affects the body more profoundly. It's the fluid of life itself; 70 per cent of our body weight is water. More than half of most of the food we eat is water, and, best of all, *water* in all its many forms can be a great beauty tonic.

SPAS – WHERE TO GO AND WHAT HAPPENS WHEN YOU GET THERE

Not so long ago the word 'spa' meant miracle water place in the Indian language, mineral spring to the well travelled, and a place to rest and hopefully rejuvenate to most of us.

Today 'spa' suggests more a 'resort', but one where there's an emphasis on health – perfect shape and condition being aimed at via a medley of things, often the *least* important being a mineral spring on the property.

The true spas like those of Wiesbaden, Baden-Baden, Vichy and Eugénie-les-Bains still offer programmes under medical supervision, based on drinking the waters (all-day-long drinking from the fountains is actively encouraged), bathing in them and – sometimes – using the steam or water itself in specific treatments.

A recent medical study provided the following figures for people taking 'cures' annually via the waters in Europe:

Russia	6 million
Germany	1 million
France	400,000
Italy	1.5 million
Czechoslovakia	700,000

But nobody goes to Bath any more 'to take the waters'. Instead, more likely they'll go to Forest Mere in Sussex where they drink the same H_2O (decorated with a slice of lemon) that comes out of everyone's tap.

Today anyone going to a 'spa' is not thinking of drinking a daily quart of restorative water, but more likely of sauna baths, mud packs (for the body as well as for the face) and pampering in general, either at a rule-bound, totally non-permissive health and beauty establishment or at a permissive do-it-if-you-like-it beauty pleasure park.

A hundred years ago all over the world people dutifully drank and bathed in mineral waters, but more for social than for therapeutic reasons. One famous place – Hot Springs in the U.S.A. – was 'patronized' by ladies and gentlemen, not so much for the sake of their health as of their marriage 'prospects'. There was even a Billing, Wooing and Cooing Society set up there in the 1830s to lay down ground rules.

Spa life at that time was very pleasant. After rising at 8 a.m., an obligatory glass of mineral water started the day. Then came a lavish breakfast (calorie counting hadn't even been invented). Mid-morning champagne and watermelon was served, followed an hour later by a big luncheon and more mineral water. A siesta was necessary before afternoon tea; then came a concert or garden party and in the evening more mineral water, followed by supper, more champagne, and a ball or cotillion.

Such rounds of pleasure still carried on right up to the Second World War; the Duchess of Windsor, for one, remembers them well.

It seems ironic that although the meals were as lavish as banquets, with champagne served as often as mineral water, most of the figures photographed on the scene seemed as trim as her own. More proof that women did not go to spas then to lose weight!

Today, the European spas are regaining popularity *because* of their stringent rules and the emphasis on medical help. In fact, a medical check-up is a *must* before anyone is allowed to embark on what is usually a rigorous week of dieting, if not fasting, exercise sessions and all manner of baths, directed towards ridding the body of flab and/or toxins.

Once given a doctor's okay you are *supposed* to follow a programme to the *letter*, one that is generally tailor-made to force you back into condition. Yoga may be part of it (see pages 251–4), and there's plenty of rub-a-dub-dub, via a dazzling display of equipment, to deliver a variety of de-paunching routines.

Permissive or Non-Permissive: Take Your Choice

One of the first things you have to decide today when you and/or your husband decide you and/or he ought to go to a spa is just how strict you want that spa to be.

If you know you get better results on a long rein, a permissive spa would be for you. If you know you need an instructor breathing down your aching back, then it's best to put yourself fairly and squarely in the hands of people long experienced in delivering a tough, get-fit programme which includes low calorie foods, well programmed exercise and activity, and, most important of all, medical supervision.

No alcohol has to be the way of life (at least for the week[s] you're there). Anyone caught smuggling in even an airline-size martini is sent to her room or sent home without refund if unrepentant.

FAT GOING, GOING, GONE . . . Just as some people always leave the cap off the toothpaste and others always place it neatly back on, the world is divided into dieters who stick grimly to their objectives and those who see nothing peculiar about starving themselves for twenty-four hours in order to stuff themselves back 'into sanity' for the next twenty-four. There are also the 'ambiguous people', who, having paid a small fortune to come to a spa in the first place, like to cheat between rigorous work-outs and fasting routines with secret sips of gin and tonic and nibbles of cheese on toast.

I've often been asked over the years, 'Which spa should I go to for results?' My answer has evolved into what I describe as the 'auctioneer's system to spa classification,' scaling each one on a 'going, going, gone' basis.

The first two 'going' categories apply to those places that can really get fat and flab *going* – providing the participant really puts her mind to it. The 'gone' category applies to the type of spa that isn't interested in even opening its door to anyone (if indeed it has anything as formal as a door to open) who is not totally willing to obey all the house rules in an attempt to see their excess fat *gone* – forever.

EAT TO GET THIN. In the 'going, going' category is Eugénie-les-Bains, a twist and a turn away from Bordeaux in France, where Michel Guérard of the figure-conscious Guérards launched what the world now knows as '*minceur*' cooking, labelled in France as '*diététique gastronomique*'.

If the idea of a boiled egg filled with caviar instead of its own yolk appeals to you, you will like *minceur* cooking. If you like the thought of liver pounded so thin it looks as transparent as smoked salmon on the plate (it's cooked fast over a charcoal fire) you will also like Eugénie-les-Bains, where it's not only *available* but *compulsory* for lunch three times a week. With the *minceur* plan no fats are used in cooking. They are often replaced with the natural juices of plants and herbs, all of which makes every bite a triumph for our gastric juices.

People used to go to Eugénie-les-Bains only to drink and soak up the thermal waters which come bubbling out of the earth from three sources at the rate of 220,000 gallons (1 million litres) a day. Sufferers from arthritic and rheumatic complaints have been helped there over the years, both with expert underwater massage, carried out in deep thermal water tanks, and with jet sprays in special rooms, where thermal water warmed to body temperature is applied with steady pressure to afflicted areas.

Now, with the joys of Monsieur Guérard's cooking, Eugénie-les-Bains is attracting a more varied clientele, including those who want to get thin fast, but don't want to suffer while getting there. After treatment lasting eleven days (special attention is paid to treating cellulite, see page 280), obesity is on the wane for some – but Eugénie-les-Bains cannot be described as 'non-permissive', because patients on the 'cure' sit in the beautiful dining room beside those there simply for the beauty of the countryside, ordering from an à la carte menu, employing hundreds of calories to make every meal a feast.

SEAWATER SUITS YOUR BODY. One of the best presents you can give your body at any time of year is a dip in the sea, and if you can do more than dip – swim for instance – you've evolved for yourself the easiest do-it-yourself health treatment readily available. As one seer wrote, 'The human body perpetuates the characteristics of the marine environment.'

The minerals present in seawater *can* penetrate the skin, helping the body to function normally as they are absorbed into the bloodstream. An ancient word has recently been resurrected to describe a number of treatments using seawater together with modern technology to help 'cure' a number of contemporary aches and pains. Thalassotherapy is the word, involving a number of seawater treatments as well as seaweed treatments, utilizing the iodine content of seawater and the high vitamin A and D content of plankton (the minute organisms present in seawater that fish thrive on).

In the Bahamas and at Quiberon in Brittany (and other places in France) thalassotherapy treatments aim to restore balance in a disturbed system; disturbance can show itself in a number of ways – from gastro-enteritis and other stomach disorders to rheumatism, arthritis, sinus and asthma complaints. When seawater is fresh, collected straight from the sea, it contains gases that when inhaled in what is known as the 'aerosol room', together with oxygen and herbs, have already been proved to help the asthmatic.

In Brittany at Quiberon the three times Tour de France bicycle champion Louison Bobet has monopolized a small dose of the Atlantic for his customers' own use, pumping an average of 70,000 gallons (320,000 litres) of seawater daily into his seaside spa, using it for a variety of treatments to attack, among other things, excess *avoirdupois* (pounds to you and me).

The most popular treatment at the spa is the Atlantic's own Bubble Bath, where heated seawater is forced so vigorously through special pipes it literally bubbles up in what appears to be a most normal bathtub to massage any skin that gets near, vibrating and smacking all at the same time. Very relaxing, I'm told by that beautiful specimen of womanhood Catherine Deneuve, who heads for Quiberon whenever she can tear herself away from work and play in Paris and Rome.

Another treatment on the list is more arduous and some say more effective in cutting down fat deposits and firming up muscles. This is the underwater pressure massage, where seawater pours out from a fat hose just like the garden variety to 'water you down'; it is handled by an assistant who directs the water at all the places that need attack.

It's no good saying it doesn't sting – because it *does* sting. Work out at home with your own hose and you'll find I'm telling the truth. You'll also learn that the water pressure does zip up blood circulation, which we all know, don't we, is the first step to a pretty, small size.

Just as spa 'guests' are encouraged to jog after fasting in England, in France, after their water treatment, guests are introduced to gym training. There, not surprisingly, Monsieur Bobet, who made so much money from the bicycle, has a number of special models so that you can pedal more weight away, if you have the energy.

Seawater is pumped into other modern spas or clinics throughout Europe and warmed to blood temperature to lessen the shock of contact. There are low pressure seawater showers, fast hose showers of various pressures, as just described, seaweed baths, vigorous bubbling baths and underwater massage chambers where water jets of different strengths 'massage' flab more energetically than human hands could ever do.

For those learning to use their muscles again after illness or accident, there are seawater swimming pools where again immersion in the water is considered as important as the movements used there. Exercise carried out in sea air also has an extra bonus – which is why thalassotherapy spas have well equipped gyms where plenty of sea air fills the room while the gym sessions are in progress. 'Ozone is good for you' is *not* an old wives' tale.

Hydrotherapy also utilizes water, but not necessarily seawater. Again, it is warmed to body temperature first before being used on the human body. At Tegernsee, outside Munich, there is a spa much favoured by U.S. astronauts, some of whom have been there for 'true relaxation' (*not* inertia, but an alert, perceptive mind, see page 251). There, large tanks filled with warmed mountain water are used for underwater massage, jets of water attacking fatty tissue, while a trained masseur also manipulates muscles underwater.

Fresh is the key word as far as the water is concerned. When seawater is bottled, boiled or 'kept' for a few days, it 'dies' as far as its natural resources are concerned.

This obviously means we are all lucky when we get an opportunity to dip in the sea, because without really trying we then give our bodies a great pepper-up. If you swim, realize you're then exercising every one of the 600 muscles in your body, even the ones you rarely use on your face, which you will move in unusual ways as the spray and surf hit you. But more important is the effect of the water on your body. Think of the sea as a bowl of life-giving properties, with every known chemical element that's essential to human life present.

The Benefits of Mud

If water sets your teeth on edge – and some people I know can't take it without a drop of whisky – there are mud pie places in the world that have been known over the centuries to give therapeutic benefit to the overworked, underpaid, underprivileged male and female.

Salsomaggiore mud is super to soak in, for example. Just outside Milan, Italy, Salsomaggiore would be just a strange name on the map if it wasn't for its naturally heated waters and iodine-based mud. The rumour is that Sophia Loren, who had a hard time getting pregnant in the first place, regularly went to have mud baths there. As we all know, she finally achieved her greatest wish in life – to have a son. In fact, two sons!

For island lovers, Ischia off the coast of southern Italy is the best mud hole, the 'best' meaning the most comfortable and comforting, because the thermal cures, using island mud, take place in the various luxurious hotels, where you can easily wash and brush up whenever the mud gets you down.

Mud baths – the mud being of volcanic origin – draw out toxins in the skin (to clear up a spotty back, for instance) and help ward off arthritis – but DON'T cure it. Helena Rubinstein used to import vast quantities of volcanic mud from Italy into her London salon, in the 'good old days' when she ran salons in all top European cities.

Other Baths You Won't Find at Home

Apart from eating and drinking differently at the spa of your choice, you can also bath differently and specifically for the sake of your health. Here's a brief rundown on baths you can expect to find somewhere in the world and what they do for you:

Oxygen baths are great pepper-uppers for both psyche and circulation. Pure oxygen is pumped into a whirlpool bath, so a good mix of oxygen and water swirl around you; the oxygen suffuses the skin, and generally has a revitalizing effect. You will find these baths in Swiss spas, at the Grand Hotel Beau Rivage in Interlaken, for instance.

Paraffin wax baths were originally introduced into salons by Elizabeth Arden. Likened by one of her operators at the famous Maine Chance Spa in Arizona, U.S.A., to 'causing a storm in the river, causing it to overflow its banks', the wax bath *does* cause a flood of perspiration, which sweeps away a great deal of impurity from the bloodstream and skin. Beauty operators start painting you with layer after layer of soft, warm, white wax. Usually you're asked to keep your hands at your side. Then from under your chin, right down to your toes, the white wax covers everything until you are completely encased. You can be wrapped up still further with a thin layer of tin foil, totally trapping any heat that your own body may generate close to your skin. While the wax isn't uncomfortably hot, the process is a demanding one; it stimulates the heart, which is one reason no one should have a wax bath without a medical okay first. Because various oils are added to the wax, the skin afterwards looks and feels as near to silk as it will ever do.

If you think you have the controversial fat condition known as cellulite (fat trapped by water), with your skin looking like chicken skin or orange peel, dimpled and not at all dainty, wax baths, in drawing off the excess water, can be beneficial.

Vitamin baths involve many vitamins plus minerals being added to a whirlpool bath by a separate pipe; you find these baths where there's no natural mineral spring on the property. Otherwise, where there is a natural spring, you bath in water gushing out of the ground, loaded with minerals, such as iron, potassium and lithium.

Sand baths are rare, but they do exist in the East, where they are taken as part of a special beauty regime. On the island of Kyushu at Ibusuki, Japan, the sands beside Kagoshima Bay are heated by an underground stream. At low tide, health seekers are buried up to the neck in the hot sand by attendants, only to be dug up again when the tide turns. No, the results are not the same on the beach at Bognor Regis, or in Barbados for that matter.

Sauna baths, originating in Finland, are now almost commonplace – except that in Finland there is usually an ice-cold pure stream or lake outside the sauna for constant dipping between dry heat sessions, all wonderfully good for the circulation providing you're in A1 condition as far as your heart and blood pressure go. You're advised not to take a sauna or steam bath if you have diabetes or while you are under the influence of alcohol or taking drugs such as anti-coagulants, anti-histamines, hypnotics, vasoconstrictors, vasodilators, narcotics or tranquillizers.

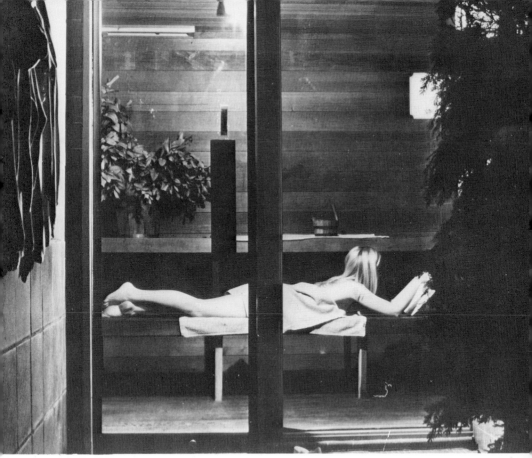

The sauna bath – great place to while away the time – and the excess pounds

You can also bath in *camomile* in Scandinavia, in *seaweed* here and in France, and in *peat moss* in Germany – all to soothe, purify and heal.

How to Succeed

If your report card isn't encouraging and the tyre round your waist – the one you promised your husband you'd lose if only he'd foot the bill at the Spa – hasn't noticeably diminished, you have to face facts: you cheated, and he will probably never cough up the cash for you to go through it all again.

I remember a former member of the Esther Williams Water Ballet who came to visit me when I ran a beauty clinic on that most magnificent ship the S.S. *France*, before she was put into mothballs.

Shy, sad and at least 16 lb (7 kg) past her prime, this former swimming champion confided in me that her husband had forcibly enrolled her on the Beauty Cruise, with the dire threat that if she didn't shape up on board she could turn into a mermaid for all he cared. Filled with fire and anger at this monster's attitude, I set out to return a superstar, one I secretly hoped would elope with the captain if he were eligible or certainly someone more worthy than the man she'd left behind on the quayside.

I became a tyrant, creeping up on my 'pupil' at mealtimes to see if she was sticking to her solitary lettuce leaf and cold chicken, conniving with the wine steward to see he delivered nothing but water to her cabin and/or table, working out with her in the ship's pool and gym for at least ninety minutes a day, insisting she sleep for an hour after lunch, *before* her ten times 'round the deck' walk, *before* the lettuce leaf dinner.

She had facials galore, learned she had a glorious bone structure, which the right use of blushers could bring into full prominence, and – because it was the beauty cruise to end all beauty cruises – dared to have a complete change of hair colour from a wizard of a French colourist.

The moral of my story is that because she had a keeper – me – someone she knew she had to answer to for results, we achieved them. At the end of the cruise, she'd lost 10 lb (4½ kg) in the right places, she loved her new make-up and hair colour (the old one had been far too dark for her skin tone – 'lighter is younger', always remember), and, most important, she had *confidence* in herself.

She promised me she'd tell her husband the rules she had to follow, so she'd never slip again! I'm sure with that sort of man as a taskmaster she never did.

Turning over the rules to someone we respect and want to answer to is one sure way of adhering to each and every one of them.

You won't *need* to go to a spa if you write down a list of rules you know you have to follow for your looks' and health's sake – and follow them. Try it for a few days after you've chosen your 'boss'. If it's your husband, make sure he realizes how vital it is that you follow the rules. Ask him not to be easy on you. If you know he always will be, choose somebody else. If they're old enough ask your children; they can be the greatest critics of all.

Write our your menus, keeping to 1,000 calories (4,000 kilojoules) a day or slightly less if you want to lose weight quickly, 1,500–2,000 (6,000–8,000 kilojoules) depending on your age if you want to maintain your weight (see calorie count, pages 232–9). Cut out alcohol, cigarettes, salt, taxis, late nights (after midnight counts as late), lifts. Double and then treble the amount of walking you do; sleep by an open window, unless the air is very polluted; try to swim at least three times a week, and if that's impossible at least do 'underwater' exercises in the bath.

Never, ever go to bed with your make-up on, and if possible give your skin a deep, deep cleanse with a mask at least twice a week, early morning if you're dry skinned, late in the day if your skin is greasy.

Make up your own regime and ask the person you respect the most to mark your report card. I'm sure you'll pass.

When Our Lips Are Sealed . . .

W E talk about our colour rinses or switches or wigs. We don't bat an eyelid when confessing to false lashes, and nowadays even a body lift or a thigh trim by the plastic surgeon's knife is discussed with hardly a qualm. However, even with our 'best friends', we rarely open our mouths to discuss the state or number of our teeth, and the less they get the more we keep our mouths tightly shut. We talk about our dentists – statistically a visit to the dentist is still the number one excuse to slip off a few hours early from work – but when it comes to admitting that our teeth are no longer home-grown, we *don't* admit it and why should we?

False teeth and real ones get more and more indistinguishable every day. Our teeth can be capped, crowned, implanted, sealed, treated with fluoride, resin-bonded and cosmetically contoured. Any moment now there will be vaccines available to build up tooth resistance to decay, as research reveals that tooth decay is no accident, but closely related to total body condition.

However, despite all this brilliant progress, more than 35 per cent of people in this country over the age of sixteen have lost all their natural teeth. In America 25 million people don't have one tooth they can call their own. The fact is that prevention rather than cure is only just catching on as a way of life to maintain our health and strength, and that goes for maintaining the health of our teeth, too.

SPARE THE BRUSH AND SPOIL THE SMILE

Take a look at your toothbrush. It may tell you something about the condition of your teeth. If it's soft and frayed, if many of the tufts are gone, if it's large and cumbersome, more than likely your teeth are in dire need of help and you probably have bleeding gums to prove it.

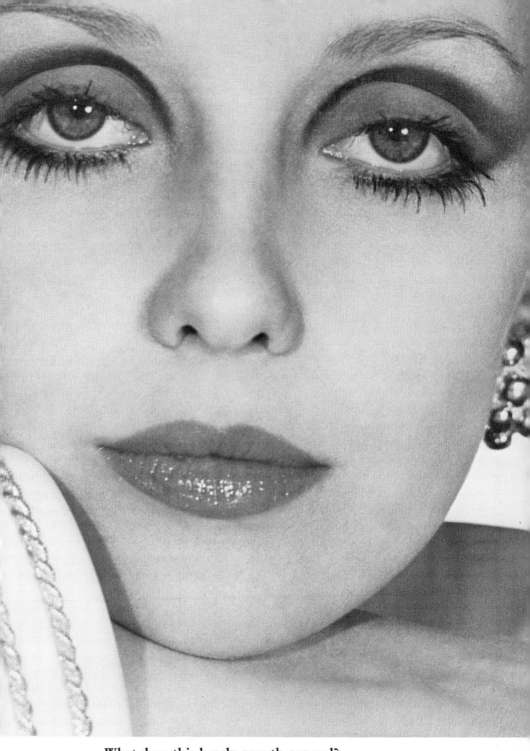

What does this lovely mouth conceal?

A frightening number of people don't own a toothbrush at all. In some families, one is shared. It seems incredible, but it's true. The simple fact has not been brought home loud and clear that inadequate cleansing is at the root of all tooth disasters. If you find your gums bleed when you clean your teeth this is the first signal that something is wrong. Bleeding is not caused by brushing healthy gums, nor by eating hard, firm foods. Healthy gums rarely bleed. Bleeding is a sign that the gums are inflamed, and if this is left uncorrected the fibres holding the teeth in their sockets can weaken and eventually cause the teeth to become loose. Bleeding frequently happens when through inadequate cleansing a sticky film builds on and between the teeth. It's called plaque and it's the greatest enemy of teeth.

Soft, sticky and, unfortunately, invisible to the naked eye, this substance, forever forming on our teeth and under our gums, turns into tartar and starts the decay that leads to eventual tooth ruination.

Plaque is actually a combination of protein material from the saliva and food particles, both of which combine and become impregnated with bacteria, building up imperceptibly to create an acid with the strength to dissolve the enamel surface of our teeth. Like many problems in life, the solution is really very simple. It begins and ends with the quality of the toothbrush because, obviously, if the 'tool' is inefficient, it affects the quality of the essential brushing. Everyone should invest in a new one every three months, and most dentists today agree that the long natural bristle brush, hard and abrasive, is not the best type for keeping the teeth in good condition. Instead, they generally recommend brushes with nylon tufts, medium to soft in texture and easily manoeuvrable.

Too large a brush tends to miss the nooks and crannies. It's also important that the brush feels comfortable in your mouth. Make sure yours is not too hard, for bristles can scratch the gums and cause small wounds, which can then easily become infected. Let the brush dry thoroughly before you use it again. Better still, work with two brushes. Natural bristles are hollow and may harbour bacteria when wet. Nylon can't, and dries more quickly anyway.

Dental sticks and/or floss are essential, too, because plaque collects in the spaces between the teeth and no brush can ferret that out. The unwaxed dental floss is more efficient that the waxed kind because it causes more friction.

If you want to find out for yourself just how much plaque you have on and around your teeth get a disclosing tablet from your nearest chemist. Made of a harmless vegetable dye, the colour clings to every vestige of plaque you have, making it horribly apparent that you have work to do.

Some dentists advocate brushing before meals instead of after, unless the patient likes to finish up with a sugary, sweet dessert (more about this later), then another brush-up is essential because a sweet tooth is still the deadliest kind to have, leading to decay if the sugary stickiness is not removed at once. Brushing before meals means food particles have less plaque to cling to, so the build-up is not so great.

More 'prevention' comes about with protection against plaque, and that means fluoride, proved to strengthen enamel against acid attack. There are two methods of using fluoride – systematically and topically. Using it systematically means taking it internally, which includes water fluoridation, an effective if indirect way of cutting down on dental disasters.

Topically applied, fluoride is more direct, easier and more effective through the systematic use of a fluoride toothpaste, proved to cut down tooth decay by up to 30 per cent. Most dentists will tell you that fluoride is the best thing that ever happened to toothpaste and teeth. Many dentists will also tell you that few patients have any idea of how to use it. Their easy tip, always brush from the gums to the tip of the tooth and start at the same spot every time, carefully working round like carrying out a regular exercise regime.

Ideally, flossing and fluoride brushing should take about seven to ten minutes after every meal. To go all out to prevent tooth decay, make the effort to clean your teeth after every meal or snack, just as you wipe your mouth or freshen your make-up. If a portable floss–and–brush-up is out of the question, at least eat a hard or fibrous food like a carrot or piece of celery. Most dentists prefer this to the toothpick which, they say, can injure the gums.

SWEET TOOTH TROUBLE

How much the consumption of sugar is related to tooth decay is still a controversial subject, but dentists the world over agree that sugar plays a big part in producing plaque.

If you think of consuming seven teaspoonfuls of sugar it makes you feel queasy, doesn't it? Yet that's how much we consume when we eat a piece of plain old apple pie or choose a water ice instead of an ice cream, thinking we've done our bodies a good turn. Sugar turns up in a lot of food, yet most of us haven't a clue as to how much sugar is buried there, not only adding to shape problems, but also definitely contributing to the number of trips we have to make to the dentist. If you think you aren't a sugar consumer because you don't take any in coffee or tea, think again. Even drinking too many soft drinks, loaded with sugar, can increase your plaque problems, so beware. Sugar not only increases the amount of plaque, but also creates enamel-penetrating acids immediately it comes into contact with the bacteria invariably present. Once natural enamel is pierced, it's so vulnerable it decays fast.

A PRETTIER PS.

Check on the colour of your teeth. If you have to admit they're more on the yellow side than the white side, stay firmly away from all coral, auburn or brown shades of lipstick. Although these are fashionable colours, they have a devastating effect on dingy teeth, making each one look more yellow. On the other hand, pink shades tend to take away the yellow effect, while unmistakable red tends to lessen the tinge of grey associated with tooth capping. Colour does count. If you're contemplating caps for your teeth, don't insist on detergent white – natural tooth colour deteriorates with age, tending towards yellow, so ultra-white caps will be too much of a contrast to live with.

6

Your Make-up

TYRANNY OR THERAPY?

HOW much notice can you or should you take of an expert's advice? How much notice, even, should you take of the do this/don't do that paragraphs that you're reading now in this book? It depends upon the expert. It depends upon the subject. As far as skin care, hair care, exercise, health and all those important matters are concerned, I hope you take a great deal of notice. The same rules apply to everyone and there's a great deal of good to be gained through observing them, at the same time following the various tips I have passed on to you to make your whole Better Looks Programme as painless and as fast as possible.

I regularly travel the world with experts in fields as varied as nutrition, yoga, hair and wig styling and, of course, make-up. I'm always intrigued to see how make-up artists mesmerize women; how every scrap of information – from the use of powder blusher above the brows for a quick 'lift' to the use of coverstick on wrinkled eyelids – is scribbled down on notepads produced from practically every handbag. Yet this kind of expert is probably the only one to take not with the proverbial pinch of salt, but with a strong dash of common sense.

Of course, there are some make-up rules which can apply to everyone, but equally there are many that cannot. Which are which? This section of the book sorts it all out for you.

Working for *Harper's Bazaar* and *Vogue* for many years I came to realize that make-up has to be 'psychiatry for the face', not tyranny but therapy. Make-up artists that I've worked with around the world may put it differently, but it still comes to the same thing. For instance, a few years back I would hear this type of remark around the studios and salons: 'I wish women didn't feel they *had* to follow this or that trend, and then get depressed out of their skulls when they find they can't wear the current look.' Nowadays, the remark is more likely to be something like this: 'Women used to be copycats, trying to look like Liv Ullmann or Doris Day – now it's easier. The pressure's off. I don't have to pretend I can get them to look like somebody else. They usually don't want to.'

Once it wasn't fashionable to be ourselves, so we didn't give ourselves a chance. Today, more health-conscious, more serious and above all *busy*, we don't want our looks to be rubber-stamped. We're using make-up to learn how to look like more beautiful versions of ourselves.

Along with the demise of the Louis Quinze salon, the little black dress for 'six o'clock' and the back-combed, honey-comb hairstyle has come a fervent desire to look 'natural' – but as pretty as possible at the same time.

We look younger than we did a decade ago, because we're able to buy better products and increasingly know more about how to use them to bring a look of youth to the skin. This encourages the development of more products along the same lines – products that improve our skin as they colour it, products that can deliver a 'beautiful' image, handled the right way.

The products we left on the shelf were eventually shelved forever. We didn't buy them because they were too heavy, too perfumed, too 'artificial'. Consumer disdain is more powerful than consumer demand.

Now we all know you can't do a good paint job on a poor canvas. The skin has to be right before make-up can do its best job, so we buy more treatment products and more of the 'conditioning' type of make-up to take care of that basic requirement first.

The leading make-up artists applaud the way things have gone – artists like Count Pablo Zappi Manzoni, discovered in a Via Veneto salon in Rome by Elizabeth Arden herself. Pablo has seen many dramatic changes in looks and attitude since then. Today he says, 'In make-up one should try to follow nature as much as possible. A woman should look clean, soft, "natural" by day, more dramatic at night, but *never* as if she is wearing on her face everything in her make-up case, even if she is.' Make no mistake about it, the 'natural look' requires talent and time, too; more talent (or practice) than the old fashioned 'made-up' face.

The idea is to look as nature should have made you look, had she been more of a designing woman, and not to attempt to change features, something many experts particularly disapprove of. Remember the old song: 'Accentuate the Positive, Eliminate the Negative?' That's the secret,

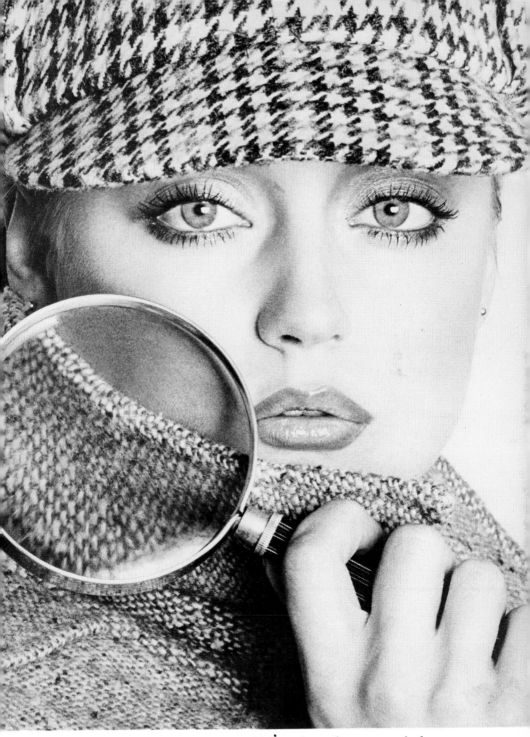

Do check your make-up with a magnifying glass when you switch locales and lights

and make-up is what you use to make it happen.

Another great artist is Paul Corène, who was 'discovered' by Helena Rubinstein and persuaded to change his mind about becoming a museum curator. He's very glad he did. Paul works all over the world, as he puts it 'to emphasize the character in a face, even if that character is illustrated best by a big nose or wide-apart eyes'. He believes a flaw can even add value, and he works to make sure it does. In other words, he works with make-up so that a big nose doesn't seem to stick out but rather to belong perfectly to that particular face.

HAIR FIRST

Before American *Vogue* introduced its contemporary *Beauty Annual* in 1973, make-up editorials frequently urged the reader to study the shape of her face and put colour on it accordingly – rouge or blusher high on the cheekbone for one shape, lower for another and so on. When I started to plan the *Annual* with Pablo and a talented hairstylist called François (then working with the most famous name in American hairdressing, Kenneth) we experimented with a different idea. We planned the hairstyle first to govern where the make-up should go on the face – because we reasoned that a hairstyle so often gives a face an entirely new shape. It worked, and it was a great idea to launch *Vogue's* new venture.

Pablo plotted his make-up *after* François had given new shape to our one model's face with each style he created. With a fringe, for instance, her face appeared smaller, shorter, wider. With another style, her face shape appeared to be elongated. All this affected the placing of the make-up, so much so that we came to the conclusion: *Your hairstyle should always come first. Make-up contouring must be plotted afterwards to obtain the best results.*

There are a few basic, easy tips that everyone can follow to accomplish a 'free and easy, pretty look,' in the shortest possible time.

BASE COAT

No top model ever wears base all over her face – only where she feels she needs it, perhaps to ensure all blemishes are covered, or to even up skin tone, particularly sallow patches. Nothing looks more fake than a one-coloured skin, for skin wasn't made that way.

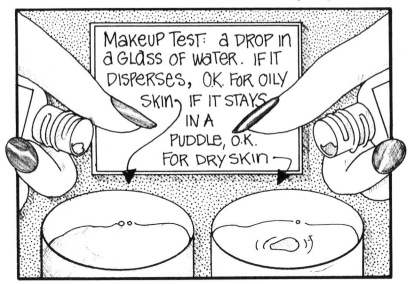

Choosing Your Base

The better the skin, the thinner the base can be. If you have a good skin choose a gel or translucent liquid that gives glow but minimum cover and lets your make-up's best asset, your naturally good skin, show through. Gels are tightening, and good for firming; extra good when the skin is lightly tanned. A translucent liquid product sometimes uses a powder formulation suspended in liquid, so it must be shaken before application. It's good for older skin because it doesn't emphasize fine lines, best applied with a sponge.

An emulsified (moisturized) make-up base is fine for dry or normal skin (dry sides, oilier centre panel) – the oils in the formula contribute a dewy look.

Today, if you can get to a top department store, it's likely you will be able to carry out some nifty self-skin-analysis with the help of a sophisticated cosmetic computer, an electronic device invented to take much of the guesswork out of choosing products.

If you can't find a friendly neighbourhood computer, test you're using the right base for your skin by dropping a drop into a glass of water. If it disperses and looks like café au lait, it's oil-in-water – water-based and right for greasy skins. If it stays put in a little puddle, it's water-in-oil – oil-based and the one for dry skin. Anyone with dry skin should always wear a moisturizer beneath her make-up to help it glide on and stay put longer.

All bases are best applied with a slightly damp sponge to remove any residue (even as it's being applied) and to ensure a smooth, even surface.

If you have something to hide – a blemish, broken capillaries or irregular features to balance – a cream or cake make-up does the best job; again, this works well if applied with a damp sponge, as this gives the smoothest finish. A cover-up product is labelled that way to show it's heavier and made with heavier waxes and ingredients. Read the label when looking for a medicated, cover-up product; the ingredients – anti-bacterial – will be listed and will have been chosen and blended to help calm problem skin, while colouring it at the same time.

For women who suffer from allergies there's more and more choice in make-up as an increasing number of cosmetics are deliberately made fragrance-free (perfume is often the allergy culprit, see page 37). This specialized type of make-up is low in common allergens – although today most make-up has as few common allergens as possible for the obvious reasons.

If you have dark circles under or lines around the eyes, touch them out with a cover-up type of product, being sure you choose one to match your skin tone as closely as possible. Too light a concealer produces a white bag instead of a dark one, just as bad!

Do's and Don'ts

Don't apply base to an area where there's fuzz – it only accentuates it. That definitely means between nostril and upper lip.

Don't create a demarcation line between face and neck – make-up and bare skin. Stop short with base application about an inch above the jawbone, then blend down from there. By the time you reach your neck, the base should have dwindled down to match the natural skin colour there.

Do practise using two shades of the same base, one darker than the other, for contour purposes. If you feel your face is too long, too wide or too round, two bases can help spell 'illusion'. Actress Vanessa Redgrave has an extra long face. She uses a shade that's fractionally darker than her basic base across her forehead just below the hairline for a fraction of an inch. She also uses the same darker shade on the tip of her chin, which tends to 'reduce' the look of length.

In the same way, actress and Las Vegas star Ann-Margret slims down her rather wide face by blending a slightly darker shade of base in a wide inverted V, up along both sides of her jawline diagonally towards her earlobes. She traces an imaginary straight line in her 'mind's eye', using her pupil for the starting point, down to her lower jaw – and this is the point on her jaw where she starts the darker colour.

Don't wear the same base year in, year out, Skin changes from season to season as I've already explained (see pages 51–58).

Don't wear the same base day and night either. Light is the catalyst, making or breaking make-up's effect.

Just as artificial light affects the way your make-up looks, so does geography. Latitude and the position of the sun are as deeply involved in the final result in the mirror as are fluorescent lighting or candle-light.

Do check with a magnifying mirror when you switch locales and lights. Take a frank look at yourself in the most telling place of all, in the 'truth light' above the clouds in a plane.

If you remember the higher the latitude, the stronger and more revealing the light, you'll know how to adjust. In New York, for instance (latitude 41), the light is more flattering than in Stockholm (latitude 59), where skins have almost a natural searchlight on them, tending to 'blue' everything, making colours more intense or spectacular depending on make-up skill.

In low latitudes near the equator (Barbados, latitude 13° Nairobi, latitude 2°), the light cast is warm, adding yellow to orange to gold tones to make-up and hair colour. This counts more than that skin-damaging tan towards making you think you look so well in the sunshine.

After dark, the best lighting to light you is incandescent, similar to the natural light you experience in low latitudes, giving you glow, as well as hiding dark circles and other facts of life. At the other end of the wattage is fluorescent lighting, which is like the light found in high latitudes, hard and revealing.

When choosing your make-up base for evening, avoid anything with a yellow note (this also applies to nail enamel – even coral can be tricky). Artificial light tends to 'yellow' everything, so it's safer to wear a base with pink undertones to warm up your skin.

Remember pink warms, blue harshens, yellow turns sallow. A degree or two lighter or darker can make all the difference to getting the maximum mileage out of your make-up.

The good news is that today's make-up is actually good for the skin. Far from enlarging the pores or creating disturbances, a good

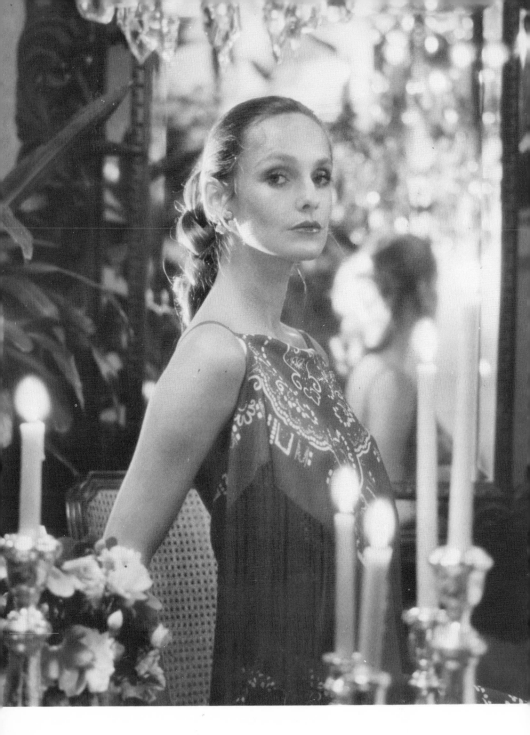

Light is the catalyst, and electric light can make or break your make-up. After dark, a new set of colours rules

base protects the skin, setting up an invisible barrier against pollution and its inherent dangers. If you use the right foundation, you're doing your skin a good turn, a healthy turn.

Special tips: Raquel Welch uses a bronze gel on cheekbones, cheeks, chin and cleavage – one more 'C'. It's captivating and spotlights her all-over tan.

CONTOUR COLOUR/ROUGE/CHEEK GEL/BLUSHER

Whatever it's called, contour colour is an increasingly vital piece of make-up equipment, appearing in as many guises as it has names – in sticks, jars, sponges, powders, pencils and tubes.

Contour colour basically highlights good 'bones' or 'invents' them for those born without.

Believe it or not, Raquel is one of those born without; she knows, however, how to use a blusher with devastating effect. I know. I've seen her apply it and 'draw' in cheekbones that just don't show up on her naked skin. Whenever there's a suspicion that good face shape exists, a contour colour can emphasize it. Above all, it adds the right blush of health when used correctly. Models and actresses use a contour product for many things – to 'hollow' their shoulder blades, to slim their calves, even, using a glossy blusher, to add a touch to fingers to give an effect of tapering, elegant length. For most of us, it's enough to know how to use it for its original purpose.

Contour colour is every bit as important to a face as eye make-up. It fights the downward force of gravity and can even 'lift' a face with its illusionary powers. Paul Corène uses a touch of pink/brown at the hairline for this purpose, plus a little under the brows for the same reason.

If you know you're heavy-handed and liable to smudge, use powder blushers (the same goes for eye shadows), easier to blend than the gel, cream or liquid varieties. If you want to *intensify* colour, apply with a slightly damp sponge.

To add warmth to your foundation colour, brush contour colour over the high points of the face – cheekbones, chin, forehead, and even the tip of your nose. For definite contouring (affecting shape with effects of light and shade) use under chin, on the forehead, in cheek hollows, and along jaw-line.

If you feel happy with cheek colour, NEVER suck in your cheeks or make 'puffed out' cheeks to see where to apply it. Remember, the key word is NATURAL. Smile broadly to see where to get the most natural effect and apply colour upwards 'stroking your smile'.

Don't bring colour too far up the sides of the face towards the eyes – too near beside or below and cheek colour can take sparkle away from the eyes. Too near the nose, it can make a nose appear larger.

There's a difference between a glossy and a matt blusher: the former adds lustre and emphasis to the face (because gloss is also a highlight) without adding too much additional colour; the latter gives generous colour and can warm up and/or even diminish any area it touches.

Anything light – glowing – *emphasizes* by leaving a larger impression, while a matt, flat shade will absorb light to diminish size. If the matt shade is dark, it can also *conceal*. Some make-up artists use more than one colour blusher and even more than one glosser all to redefine a face shape, aided and abetted as already explained with a supporting hairstyle.

To streamline a round face, for instance, use a warm matt colour over the brow bone out and up to the temples, from the chin in a wide inverted V to the earlobe. Use a lighter but still noticeable colour on the cheekbone (when you smile you see your 'bones' more clearly), and a gloss or highlight on the forehead and under the eyes.

To 'shorten' a long face use a warm terra cotta or copper shade (which most resembles the colour of our own blood) on the temples, and just below the hairline, a lighter shade on the cheekbones and under the chin, and a highlight (glossy blusher) on the forehead.

At night cheek colour is vital. There should be plenty of it. To avoid calling attention to any facial lines or under-eye circles, a warm chestnut-red cream rouge can be blended lower than usual on the cheek and more to the side. Colour used on the fattest part of the cheek is not becoming at night.

If you're a blonde or fair, try a bright pink stick (applied with a damp sponge) over base (which should match your skin tone as closely as possible), then, after a light touch of translucent powder to set make-up, use the *same* pink in a powder blusher product on cheeks, under brows, down the nose and on the throat down to the hollow. For 'mousy blondes', all coral blushers help bring life to the skin.

If you're a brunette with warm colouring, try a bronze cheek colour during the day, a gold one at night.

Gold works perfectly for a *true redhead* too, day or night, so do all shades of terra cotta – the most versatile 'natural' looking colour of all;

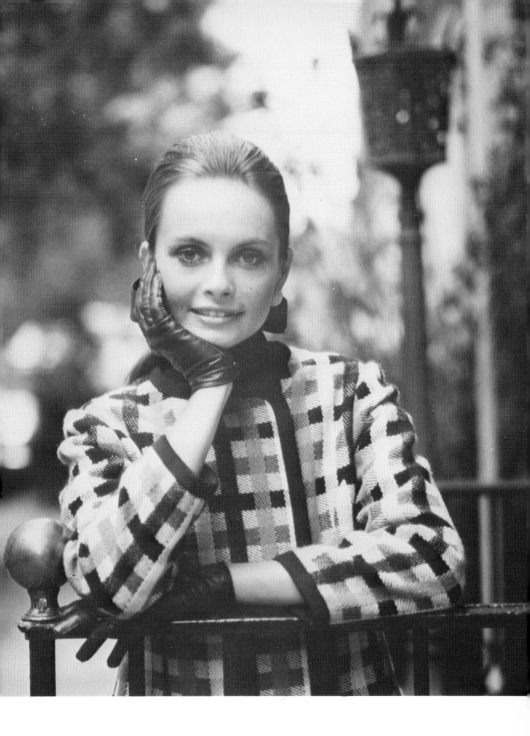

Smile to see where the natural 'apples' of your cheeks are, then apply colour dead centre to get the most natural effect it does wonders, neutralizing too much natural red in the skin, just as peach reduces the 'blue' tinge of an older skin.

Never rub in contour colour; always pat it on first, then gently blend. Practise your blending, then you can begin to mix two or three colours together, blending one into the other for extra shading and vibrancy.

The merest touch of rouge at the corners of the eyes gives the eyes more emphasis, while if you wear glasses a touch of blusher *above* the brows can help give the eyes more life and sparkle.

The contour colour that lasts longest and stays looking freshest is the cream variety. The brush-on blusher works wonders as a finishing touch, but for staying power (even underwater) a cream formula leads the field.

Special tips: Model and great American beauty Betsy Theodora-copulos uses a coral blusher stick on cheeks, forehead and earlobes to spread the warmth of her personality. Bianca Jagger draws stripes with a bronze contour stick under her cheekbones, then blends them together on her cheeks with other little stripes of orange and pink. A quick dot of bronze blended on her chin she feels also gives a healthy look.

EYE MAKE-UP

Once a woman would have chosen to take her lipstick in answer to that old desert island question. Today, if she had only one choice, it would probably be her eye shadow or, if she is a model, perhaps her 'contour colour' – to be worn on her eyes just as much as on her 'contours'.

Eye make-up is a personal matter, but experimentation is the key. The amount of colour and where to put it varies from face to face, so, though copying Angela Rippon or Catherine Deneuve may seem a lovely idea, you won't know until you've tried it on yourself.

Easy tips: Matt and glow (or gloss), dark and light, produce different effects, matt making smaller, glow making larger. A woman may choose a *frosted* green (glow) shadow to match her green to hazel eyes. Because it is a frosted colour, it will emphasize her already large eyelids. If she chose a *matt* green, she would still have large lids but they would not look so prominent. The matt green would make one notice her lovely green eyes rather than her green eye make-up.

Eye make-up *can* be matched to eye colour, but it isn't a crime if

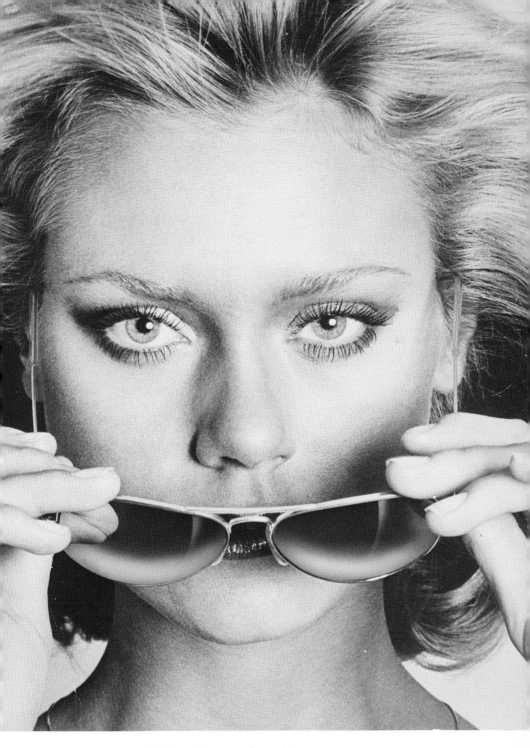

Today, the eyes have it

you don't. There are so many shades to try, and, to reiterate, experimentation is all-important. You don't know what you're missing until you've tried it.

Work it out for yourself: if you haven't much 'lid', use a light or frosted colour to emphasize what little you have. If your eyes tend to protrude, use dark colours and highlight with a spot of *white* under the brow to bring the brow bone into prominence. Not everyone should wear frosted or pearly eye shadows – particularly not those with fine lines on or around the eyes.

Eye shadow (whoever thought of the name goes to the top of the class) comes in cream, liquid or powder form, and all give best results when applied with a brush or spatula. Your finger is too large to make the initial application. Of course, you should *blend* with your fingers.

Cream shadow gives a moist, soft look, but is apt to smear and smudge unless you have a very practised hand.

Powder shadow is longer lasting and easier to apply.

Liquid shadow is lighter but still long lasting if put on with care.

To prevent shadow 'creasing' on the lid, delicately pat eyelid skin with a non-alcohol toner first to make sure there's no natural oil or perspiration lurking there. Use powder shadow rather than cream and 'set' it by dusting over lightly with translucent powder.

When it comes to *liquid or cake eye liners* (not used so much since the introduction of the easy, soft eye pencil), both need practice. Lines should *never* be the object, rather a soft blur which can be achieved by simply dotting or dashing tiny lines along the lid, as close as possible to the top lashes – all adding a luxuriant look to the lashes, a smoky look to the entire eye. Cake liner is easier to use than liquid and lasts longer if the brush is dipped in hot rather than cold water.

Mascara is vital, and for best results should be painted on each lash separately, working from the root up, using only the wand tip. For bottom lashes it's best to work *down* with tip used vertically. Everyone should put mascara on looking down into a mirror, coating first the topside, then the underside of each lash. Regular stimulation of the lashes helps them grow.

If you're timid about eye make-up, start slowly and try only the most subtle effects, stroking on colour with the applicator, gently stretching eyelid skin away from the nose to colour only over the eyeball. Always stroke shadow *up* towards the crease or brow and avoid moving beyond eye shape unless you're experienced.

Try to use a liner just on the lash line to create an effect of lushness

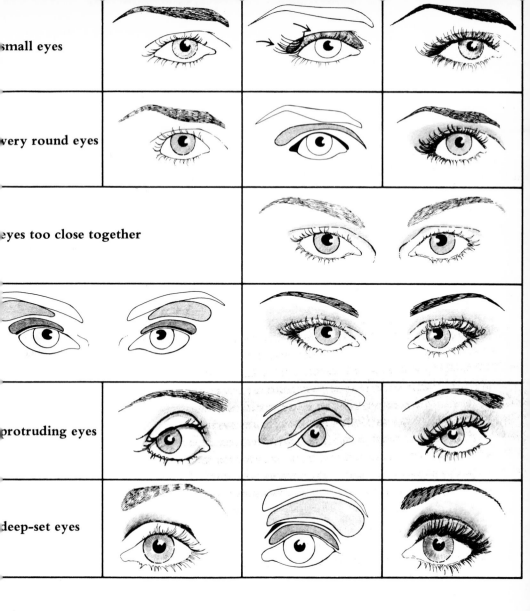

small eyes		
very round eyes		
eyes too close together		
protruding eyes		
deep-set eyes		

and thickness. Use a colour deeper than your natural eye colour, yet still in relation to it. Hold the brush parallel and for softness break or blur the line you make, stopping at eye corners. Once again: *never* draw a straight 'line', it's too harsh.

For small eyes, use a bright shadow close to the upper lashes, blending it out very slightly at the outer corner. On outer upper lashes use a lash-lengthening mascara or a small swatch of false lashes.

For very round eyes, apply shadow only *above* the crease towards the brow tip. Use liner above top lashes, thickening it slightly at outer corners, sweeping it slightly upwards. Use mascara more heavily on outer lashes.

For eyes too close together, blend eye shadow so that it is *deeper* on the *far side of the lids* away from the nose to give an impression of width. Using a light base beneath the brows also gives an illusion of width, as does liner dotted close to the upper lashes, starting about a third of the way along to the outer corners. Eyebrows could be slightly thinner towards the nose to give more 'space', too.

For eyes that protrude, dark shadow should be applied over the entire upper lid, blended up to the brows.

For eyes that are deep set, a light shadow should be used on the upper lids all the way to the brows. Not everyone should wear liner – particularly not those with tiny 'lids' and deep-set eyes.

False Eyelashes

If you want to try false lashes, use a trick from another make-up maestro. He instructs his customers this way:

> Hold lashes in an outstretched hand and think of them as a plane coming in to land. Bring hand in slowly, steadily at eye level to 'land' lashes in place. It's extraordinary, but this movement makes putting lashes on easier than if you crouch over a mirror, using little movements.
>
> Of course, first you must apply adhesive to the lashes – and some may even need trimming as they tend to be made extra long to suit all eye shapes. Adhesive should be applied with a toothpick *sparingly*. You should aim to 'land' your lashes on the centre of the natural lash line, gently pressing them into an arc shape and into place with fingertips.

Individual lashes *can* be put on at home, but, except in the case of professional models, look better when an expert is in control.

If you hate false lashes (which most models rely on for 'instant plus'), curl your own with a lash curler, available at most good chemists, remembering to apply lots of mascara once they're curled.

Special Eye Tricks from the Stars

An easy way to ensure eye make-up comes out looking pretty and 'natural' (key word) starts with a dotted line of soft brown pencil applied beneath the bottom lashes, lightly 'smudged' with fingertips until almost invisible. You'll be surprised to see how this immediately

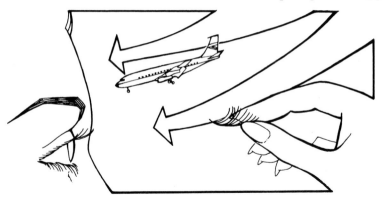

How to put on false eyelashes

makes the eyes appear fuller, prettier. Continue by lining the upper lid from corner to corner in the same way, keeping to the shape of the top lash line with the pencil, being careful not to extend the 'line' beyond eye shape. Stop before the last lash to make the eyes look wide open.

If your hand is shaky, start from the inner corner of the eye to the centre, then from the outer corner in to meet it, then softly 'blur' together.

If you prefer to use eye liner instead of pencil, start by gently pulling your eyelid taut at the outer corner and work from the inner one, keeping as close as possible to the lash line. Use small strokes, and make sure before you begin that your brush has no loose ends and has a fine, small but not sharp point. The right equipment is all important.

Shadow should start at the inner corner of the eye, keeping close to the top lashes, and should not be carried above the crease or fanned out towards the brow. Cover the lid with a soft brown or grey colour – it suits most colourings – or something you *know* suits you, then blend a little white in under the brows. Again this 'opens up' the eyes and makes them look 'smiling'.

You can never use too much mascara, and rich dark brown can be prettier than black for day, except for the really black-haired senorita. The cake variety gives a particularly lush look, providing you let each coat dry, building up the lashes to look thick and beautiful.

At night, retrace your steps, using *eye make-up that is stronger, more dominant.* Use a frosted pastel shadow in place of the grey, either blending the colour up towards the outer corner of the brow in a diagonal shape, or adding a slightly lighter colour at the crease to move towards the brow.

One trick is to use dark brown cake eye liner diluted with a lot of water; this creates a light brown 'wash', which can be brushed all over between crease and brow, giving a more delicate effect than that achieved with cream or powder. A touch of gold beneath the brow delivers a gala note finishing with lashings of black mascara, better for all colourings at night – even the light blondes.

Special tips: Sandra Linter, one of the few top *female* make-up artists, is an integral part of many magazine photo sessions, making up many of the models you see on the fashion and beauty pages. Sandra is an innovator, believing that brunettes should wear dark plum and aubergine shadows for day, bronzes and deep golds at night, while blondes should go for auburn or rose tones on the eyes. She says redheads can get away with 'the whole metallurgic bit – from copper to bronze to gold' – but not yet to tin. Redheads with pale lashes need plenty of mascara and liner; they can wear yellow shadows, particularly the frosted variety, although most other colourings shouldn't try it.

The Importance of the Eyebrow

A clean light brow is essential if eye make-up is to get off to a good start – and the most 'natural' looking brow is the answer, with no straggly ends.

The brow shape you were born with may not be the best 'natural' shape for you. The eyebrows count a lot where eye make-up is concerned, so consult an expert about yours if you can or, if not, try the pencil trick to determine whether you have the perfect eyebrow for your face.

Look in the mirror and hold a pencil perfectly straight and vertical in front of your face so that one end touches your nostril. The other end (if held correctly) is where your brow should begin. To check where your brow should end hold the pencil out diagonally at 45° from the nostril to the brow. Where the pencil points is where your brow should end.

To check brow curve, look dead straight into the mirror; the highest point of your brow should be directly above your pupil.

Don't draw harsh lines on your eyebrows. Use short, close together strokes with a soft brown or grey pencil if you need to 'lengthen' them. *Don't* tweezer brows from above. *Don't* cut them with scissors or tweezer the wrong way; follow the way each hair grows.

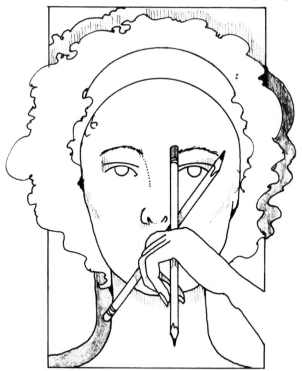

THE BEST NATURAL FINISH – POWDER

Powder is with us again – better than ever. It is often encapsulated, with all sorts of moisturized benefits 'encapsuled' within each tiny grain. These break invisibly on the skin as the powder is applied, adding a dewiness instead of a 'powdered' look to make-up, as well as carrying out powder's usual job: setting make-up in place.

Because pigmented powders tend to change colour when in contact with some skin oils (oh, the horrors of that faint orange moustache as touch-up follows touch-up in the dark at the theatre), a better touch-up choice is the transparent kind, unchanged by the skin's oils, giving instant luminosity. Powder should always be one or two tones lighter than your base.

Cotton wool makes the best applicator (because powder puffs for some reason hardly ever get changed – just get dingier and dingier) helping the powder cling without smudging the colour beneath. Powder is best used lavishly, then brushed off with a fine sable brush.

117

This enables make-up to stay intact all day, when even if perspiration and skin oil shine through they don't spoil anything.

To touch up too often, even with translucent powder, takes away make-up's fresh edge. Far better to blot with a tissue, or if possible to give the face a quick spray with water, literally to freshen up. Skin is always thirsty, especially in cities.

Powder has the added advantage of reflecting light, so that tiny lines become less visible, which means that at night it really comes into its own. It doesn't matter if your skin is dry. Powder today is generally moisturized. (Look at the label!)

Pressed powder is a neat portable idea, but when base is incorporated with powder it should be left at home on the dressing table, as obviously it's no good for touch-ups. An accumulation of base and powder looks stale and certainly doesn't help the health of the skin. Pressed powders without base are meant to be taken along on the trip for touch-ups when you need them.

To go gala all the way, a pearly or frosted powder gives a superb luminous effect, especially when blusher is pearly, too. To correct too much ruddiness in the complexion, choose powder that's pale green; it works like a charm (or a pale green moisturizer also controls excess natural colour).

When you really want your make-up to last round the clock – on that still-too-long flight to Australia, for instance – *press* in your powder (the encapsulated kind is perfect) with a slight twisting movement rather than just casually brushing it on. This *presses* home the fact it's meant to stay and stay – unless you happen to cry. The chemical composition of tears is a sure annihilator of any make-up, pressed in or otherwise.

HOW TO MAKE YOUR LIPS SEDUCTIVE

Lipstick is a very important accessory and likely to stay that way. The mouth is a very seductive part of the face and extra colour there proves it.

Whether you like a creamy, opaque, translucent or pearly lipstick, working with a brush is key. The most *lasting* way of colouring lips is to use an opaque stick first, then cover that with a pearly colour or gloss.

If you like pale lip colours, cover the whole mouth with one shade, but add a gloss or darker shade in the *middle of the mouth only*. It's sexy.

If you like dark colours, line lips with a dark shade, using a brighter one to fill in and gloss the middle of the mouth. That's sexy, too.

For a bright, *vivid* mouth, fill lips with the *brightest* colour, then coat with gloss to soften. Do remember, though, that if teeth are less than bright and white, an overly bright lipstick will draw attention to that fact. Far better to stick to pink shades.

Sometimes you might put lipstick colour *over* gloss instead of the other way around – starting from the centre, put it on the inside edge of upper and lower lips, as if you were sucking a red lollipop. Start

A lip brush is the key to making better lip shape

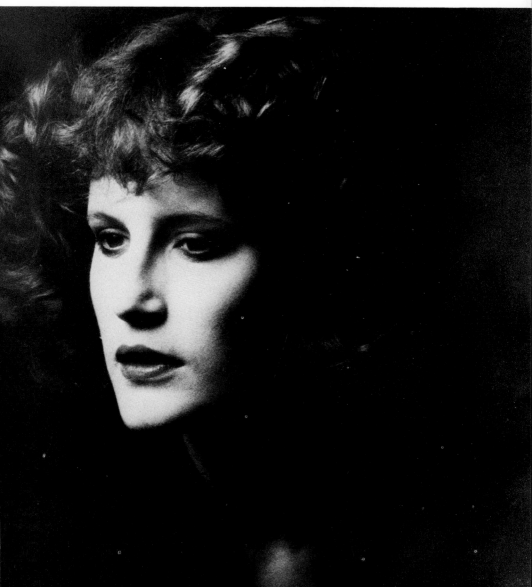

with a little, then add as much colour as you like to intensify. If handled correctly, the colour blends, so no hard edges are noticeable.

A lip liner is useful, and if you use a pencil it's child's play to outline the lips, thus preventing smudging or seepage of colour into the fine lines that can develop around the mouth. If you're an apprentice with a lip brush, pencils are easier to handle and practise with – until you graduate to a brush.

The reason a brush is so key is simple. It can follow mouth contour or, if contour isn't all it should be, invent a new one for you without any strange blurred lines or smudges.

For a soft, pretty mouth, coat lips with lip balm (winter and summer), let set, then wipe off; flaky unwanted skin goes, too. Next, outline the mouth with a pale lip colour. Ideally you need a brush for this so that the 'highlight' appears around the rim to make the mouth fuller, richer. The final appealing touch: a bright, transparent colour in the middle of the mouth, plus another coat of shimmering gloss on top.

Simple Tips

If your face is small, don't exaggerate your mouth. Remember to keep the highest points of the upper lip (the 'cupid's bow') within the area defined by the outer edges of your nostrils. Make sure lower lip is not fuller than upper lip at the corners – the mouth should have fullness in the middle.

If your face is large, outline mouth on the outer rim of the natural mouth with bright colour and use only gloss inside.

If your face is long, keep width in the mouth from corner to corner rather than having any fullness from top to bottom. Avoid any indent or 'bow' on the top lip.

If your jawline is heavy, paint mouth wide with more colour in the middle than at the sides.

If your lips are too thin, round upper lip and make middle indentation shallow. Extend upper lip slightly out beyond natural corners, then bring lower lip up and out to meet corners of the new upper outline.

If your lips are too thick, outline mouth *inside* natural shape. Use a darker shade on top lip, lighter on the bottom.

Mouth too sad? Use a bright colour and accentuate 'bow', slightly extending colour up and out on lower lip. Use a touch of gloss dead centre in the upper lip.

Special tip: Mary Tyler Moore sprays mouth colour with an atomized mineral water to keep a moist look through the day.

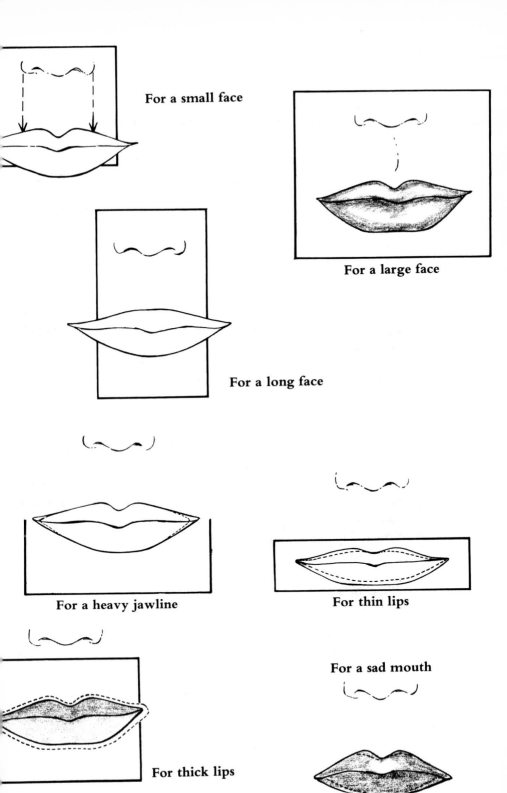

For a small face

For a large face

For a long face

For a heavy jawline

For thin lips

For thick lips

For a sad mouth

COLOURS FOR THE BLACK SKIN

Make-up has to be special for the black skin, because black skin is special. There are thirty-five variations of basic shadings in make-up colours for black skin, only twelve for white.

Bases and powders formulated for white skin are often no good for black, because some of the ingredients used can turn dark skins grey, while other ingredient substances like umber can turn black skin unnaturally red or yellow.

The solution was a long time coming, but finally cosmetics for black women are arriving on the scene – created by black women who know exactly what is needed.

Because black women have a natural bronze note to their skin, they don't really *need* much foundation, but their skin *does* need a lot of care, particularly in winter, when their skin should wear an 'overcoat' of moisturizer to stop it turning grey from the cold. In summer a sun block often is necessary to prevent uneven dark patches developing.

To even up skin tone (the black woman's main problem), a deep bronze gel is often the best answer, plus a tan powder brushed over the middle of the face, between the brows and around the nose and mouth – to take away any grey notes. Bright red cream rouge isn't only useful for the cheek area, but for above the brows and on the forehead too, all adding a 'big glow', something the black girl can get away with.

Eye make-up has to be bold and imaginative to live up to that exotic skin colour. The black girl can wear the most vivid turquoise, emerald and grass green liners, with gold-flecked bronze and beige shadows under the brow *and* lightly under the eyes – all to reflect the vivid pupils that most black women have.

Lips look better out of the conventional bright reds and into transparent chestnuts or coppers, softened with pink gloss and out-lined in auburn, or glossed over with the black woman's favourite (the dermatologist's favourite, too), petroleum jelly followed by a touch of bronze gel on top. It sounds sticky, but it can look terrific.

Beverly Johnson is a top model with light black skin who outlooks most models away from the camera because she is so outstandingly beautiful. (Many models, top and otherwise, as I may have inferred, aren't beautiful at all in real life; the camera 'creates' beauty through the magic of its lens.)

Because most black women – like white – have dry skin (not, as is erroneously thought, oily, see page 58), Beverly is a great user of moisturizer, carefully and lavishly applying a plant-based moisturizer from the bosom up to her forehead before a touch of make-up goes on.

A regular trick she uses is to apply stark white highlighter on the eyelids, under the eye area, on the bridge of the nose and over the upper lip – all to 'lift' areas she feels need it. Beverly brushes on a soft brown shadow to widen her brows and eye shape, drawing a line from the inside corner of the eye, along the lower lid half in white, half in brown.

She likes to use lipstick for paint jobs other than her lips. On her eyes particularly she likes to apply a plum lipstick all over the lids, then on the forehead, cheek and chin, blending colour here outwards to the ear lobes on both sides to decrease the width of her chin.

'Using a powder on top of a cream stops colour fading' is her belief (in common with other models). After working for ten hours a day for weeks on end in the world's major studios, she should know.

Another regular trick: she always whisks transparent powder *all over her face* except her eyelids to give a 'put together' look.

Special tip: After her mascara has dried, Beverly Johnson curls her lashes with an eyelash curler, then adds a touch of very dark red (almost brown) *lip gloss* to the tips of the lashes to dramatize a beautiful glossy look.

This is the way Beverly likes to make up – which she has to do six days out of seven, often several times a day for each photographic session. Some of her tips will apply to you, some not, for the question of 'how to make up' is not one that can have a simple, rubber-stamped answer. Apart from the fact that new ideas, new colours and new methods of application arrive every day, every one of us has to discover how best to *adapt* those new ideas for ourselves.

But make-up can improve everyone – and practice *does* make perfect.

For Women at Work - 2

HOW TO BE NOTICED WITHOUT BEING NOTICEABLE

MARY WELLS is considered to be the highest paid woman in the business world. She earns considerably more than £200,000 a year as head of her own advertising agency, and, believe me, it has little if anything to do with the fact that she's a natural blonde, weighs around 8 stone (51 kg) and has naturally cheerful, neat features, which means she looks pretty without really trying. Something Mary told me long ago stuck in my head as being real words of wisdom, not only for the woman wanting to compete with a man for a top job but for all working girls. 'I don't want to look glamorous, or even particularly chic, but it's vital that I look well,' she told me. 'My clients are top executives of leading corporations so I mustn't look tired when I feel tired, which is often. You could say I have to look 'up' all the time. Men want a woman in business to be – and look – feminine, but in my case it's equally important they forget what I look like after a while to concentrate on the business on hand.' To me the key words there are *'forget what I look like'*. In business it's important for a woman to forget what she looks like, providing she knows she looks – to repeat Mary once again – 'well', and also immaculately clean and tidy.

To wear anything to the office which makes you feel uncomfortable, that forces you to fidget, isn't only distracting to you but also to other people. A hairstyle that needs combs to hold it in place, for instance, is a hairstyle that's going to need attention all day long, as the combs invariably loosen in the hair, particularly if your job means you use your hands. That movement travels right up to the combs, which means you have to touch your hair constantly to keep it in place, so activating the scalp's sebaceous glands, increasing oil output,

124

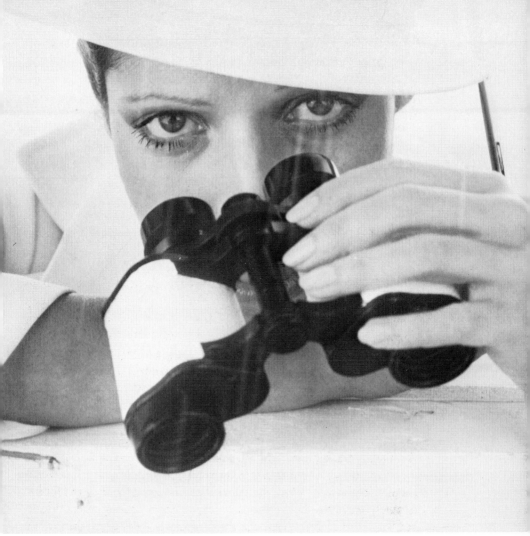

Annie Lambert photographed by Helena Rubinstein

and leading to greasier, stragglier hair – if nothing else – by the end of the day.

I believe if a woman has found 'her look' – one she feels suits her perfectly and one she feels comfortable with – she should stick with it. It makes the whole performance of facing the day easier and faster, and that goes for after six o'clock, too, when accessorizing the look with flowers, scent and a stronger make-up application is also easy, fast and fun.

Nature gave us all potential. It's up to us to use it well. We may have mousy hair and skin but a perfect shape and good legs. Then a good haircut is the first thing to aim for, followed by a dash of henna to bring out some brightness (seen to advantage under office lighting). Sallow skin needs a pink tone base to eradicate the 'yellow', while a good shape never needs to be 'eradicated', hiding under bulky, loose clothes – instead stick to tailored, fitted dresses, tops and skirts.

If a shapely figure with good legs is precisely the reverse of your situation, concentrate on diminishing the large impression you may make by wearing matching skirts, stockings and shoes. Choose dark colours and make sure your clothes fit well. If your top is hefty, wear a dark colour there, too; dark diminishes, 'light' emphasizes in fashion as well as in make-up.

Use make-up predominantly to look 'well,' not wayward or sexy. That means a *subtle* use of blusher on cheekbones and briefly beneath the hairline. Concentrate on feeling comfortable, then it's much easier to be alert. Never experiment with fashion or face at the office.

THE ALL-PURPOSE FACE – FROM WORK TO PLAY

The face you take to work is going to look better with make-up. All faces do except for most of those under twenty. The key make-up questions are: 'how much is too much', and 'how can one apply it so that it lasts throughout an eight-hour centrally heated or air-conditioned day?'

Smeared, tired make-up is guaranteed to make you look – well, tired, not fresh. Believe it or not, some men interpret this as, 'She won't be able to give a clear lucid answer or opinion today.' I know. I've heard them say so about female colleagues who were looking considerably less than their best.

First things first. To help make-up stay looking fresh for long hours, the skin has to receive it at the right time – when it's scrupulously clean and totally clear of all dead cell build-up (which can mix with make-up without you ever knowing it, putting the proverbial 'fly in the ointment'). The skin should also be cool in temperature and sufficiently moisturized to protect it from whatever elements may be raging outside and inside.

Few people have time to apply a mask in the morning, but the regular use of a mask does keep dead cell build-up *down*. The mask is the most efficient cleanser available, and if you know you're going out straight from the office it's a good idea to apply one early in the morning to wear in the bath or shower before making up for the big day ahead.

If the night before was a big one and your eyes are showing it, don't just cross your fingers and hope for the best. One cure for puffy, out-too-late eyes is an easily made eye pack of boric acid powder, water and cotton wool. Dissolve a quarter of a teaspoon of boric acid powder in a pint ($\frac{1}{2}$ litre) of boiling water. When cool, soak cotton wool thoroughly in the mixture and place the 'pack' across your eyes for as long as you can spare. Don't throw the residue away. Keep it in the fridge for later that night when you can reapply another pack. Another antidote is even simpler. Use sliced raw potatoes to reduce puffiness and any sign of strain before you put on your eye shadow.

Help make-up stay intact by being sure to use a toner (also called an astringent, a refresher, a skin balm and other fanciful names), after that thorough morning cleanse. This will not only guarantee that all old make-up and skin cell debris is cleared away, but it will cool the skin temperature down, an important factor in keeping a fresh look for a long time. Soak a little cotton wool in toner and take it with you to the office in a waterproof container. Whenever you feel hot and bothered, gently pat the cotton wool over your face without disturbing your make-up, again reducing skin temperature. If you forget to take the toner with you to the office, at least pat your face gently with ordinary water before you leave, if you're going out on a date. I do mean 'pat'. I'm not suggesting that you try to wipe away your day-time make-up. You haven't time for that. Although, obviously, if you can find time to re-do your make-up it is the best idea, both for your skin's sake and to make you feel fresher for the evening ahead.

The moisturizer really does create the perfect surface for all make-up, as well as offering the protection you need, rain or shine. If one drink sends a bright pink flush straight across your face, wear a moisturizer that's tinted pale green. It takes all pink notes out at the right level – *before* you put on your make-up – and it's helpful in keeping any extra pink down where it belongs – in the bloodstream.

A cream base is one that's known for its staying power and it stays even longer when applied with a damp sponge. The same goes for a liquid or cream eye shadow.

All women who work should use waterproof mascara. Originally created by Helena Rubinstein for the Esther Williams' water ballet, it is practical not only for swimmers but for all women who blink or rub their eyes.

Portable items to take to the office to help your make-up stay put are: a coverstick matched to your skin tone (for quick touch-ups in

127

areas that tend to shine – around the nose and chin), pressed powder, blusher (particularly if you're going out straight from the office, when you will need more colour to combat the lighting), lipstick and perfume. Take dark and light eye make-up along, too, plus a transparent gloss.

Use eye make-up sparingly during the day at the office, but reapply before going out, using a light colour under the brow to highlight and 'open up' your eyes, the darker shade on the 'crease' at the point where the eyelid begins to cover the eyeball. Blend the darker shade up to and into the lighter shade. If your eyes are small, extend colour in a smoky way up and out towards the temple. If you've taken time with your mascara in the morning it should last easily for twelve hours. Remember to apply looking *down* into a mirror, first on the underside, then on the topside, two coats on top.

To add life to your appearance without overdoing the colour, use the transparent gloss on brows, lips and cheekbones – it's useful all day, in fact, to add shine – for nothing looks worse at the office than overbright colours. Frankly, they look awful everywhere except at a fancy dress party – if you go as a puppet or a doll.

Use dark blue pencil along the rim of the lower lids to make the white of your eyes gleam and to deliver the *true* colour of your eyes, particularly if the colour happens to be brown.

Eye drops will refresh eyes that have been hard at it all day, studying a balance of payments sheet. Use a drop of wych-hazel on your brush or comb to freshen up your scalp. Better still, if your hairstyle is a movable one (it should be these days) bend from the waist to send a rush of blood to the scalp, giving it the best tonic in the world.

Brush up your brows – it looks younger. Splash cologne inside your elbows, behind your knees and at your temples. Change your tights and heel height, too, if you can – all this will keep you in top gear until the party's over.

Not Giving into a Frame-up

DOROTHY PARKER never had a make-up lesson in her life, which could be one reason why she wrote that immortal phrase 'Men seldom make passes at girls who wear glasses.' It hasn't rung true for ages – or certainly not since stars and starlets took to wearing dark glasses, which gave them such chic that thousands of fans started going around looking like mysterious owls, too. Whether

The shape of these glasses balances the jawline and draws attention to the eyes. The top line of frame gently contours the brow, creating a sense of harmony and proportion.

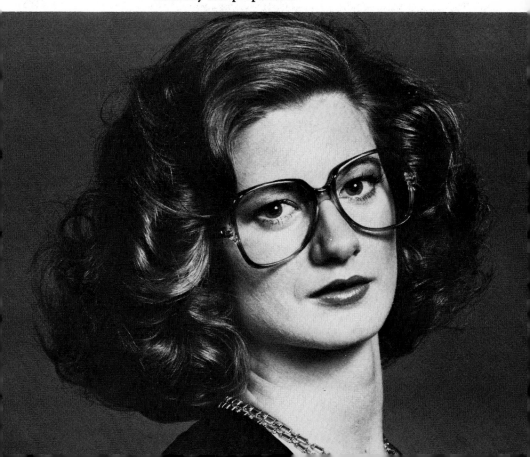

they're dark or light, round or square, glasses can add something to a look these days, but there's still a lot of guidance needed re the eye make-up to go beneath the specs.

Just as many women with weight problems tend to be negative about new fashions, so women who wear glasses often ignore the benefits of eye make-up. 'Who, me?' they will ask in stunned disbelief, blinking their often large unpainted lids – and being unpainted of course makes them look larger. 'Why should I bother? My glasses cover my eyes anyway.' Unfortunately, in most cases, the lenses of the glasses emphasize every facet of the eyes beneath and no part of the face looks more naked than the eye part without make-up.

For starters, many lenses throw a spotlight in the direction of the little fine lines which can appear around the eyes. Girls who wear glasses should definitely apply a concealer or coverstick to blot them out of sight. It's not a bad idea to use a coverstick over wrinkled eyelids, too. This not only hides lines, but gives an excellent base for the eye make-up to follow. It's important to choose the right colour cover-up. It usually comes in fair, medium or dark tones and the most common mistake is to choose one that's too light, so the wearer ends up with a white bag instead of a dark bag. Just as bad.

Eye make-up should be subtle; a gel, cream or liquid shadow is softer and prettier under glass than the powdered variety.

EYE MAKE-UP FOR THE SHORT-SIGHTED

If you are short-sighted your glasses will probably be concave, thinner in the centre and thicker at the periphery, giving the effect of diminishing and rounding out the eye. The more short-sighted you are, the more this effect will be accentuated, so it's important that the frames should be thin, to lessen the effect of the thick glass around the border. The lenses themselves should be the non-reflecting kind.

To 'correct' the impression of short-sightedness with eye make-up, it's important to enlarge the eye area, and to build up lustre (often taken away by glasses). This means using definite colours; if you have blue eyes, use anything in the russet to brown class, while brown eyes are peppier with slate blue or dark green. No pastels for the short-sighted. Eye make-up should cover the lid entirely, with a little shadow traced with spatula or sponge applicator beneath the bottom lashes – all this to 'open' up the eyes, so giving the impression of size. Highlight should be applied along the eye crease and above, concentrating a spotlight of light colour (at night it could be frosted for extra luminosity) just above the pupil, blending out and up towards the brow. Eyes should be lightly outlined with black, brown or grey pencil, and before applying mascara (black in most cases, except for the ash blonde who should stick to dark brown or blue) the lashes should be curled – again to 'open' up the eyes.

Practice makes eyelash curling very easy. It's important to hold the curler on the lashes firmly once, not twice, as there should be no fidgeting about, otherwise lashes can weaken and break. Eyelash curling is good for all girls who wear glasses, as it keeps the lashes from beating themselves to death against the lenses.

To accentuate the iris, a touch of black or grey pencil could be traced along the bottom lid, just above the lower lashes – this trick works for all except very small, deep-set eyes.

All women who wear glasses should use mascara lavishly, and unless the lids are very tiny – or even 'non-existent' – liner should be drawn just above the top lashes in a very thin, smoky line; in fact you shouldn't really draw a line at all, but instead create a gentle blur. This gives the impression of thickening the lashes, besides creating a natural frame for the eyes. A few false lashes can help the short-sighted; as their glasses do tend to make the eyes look smaller, the whole approach to eye make-up has to be to make the eyes look larger.

And it isn't only eye make-up that has to be considered. Equal time and attention has to be given to the mouth, painting it more widely and handsomely in order not to be out of balance. Your hair-style may need extra care, too, particularly if a fairly severe style is being worn. With glasses, there's no doubt about it, you have to emphasize femininity, which may mean an altogether softer look for hair as well as make-up.

EYE MAKE-UP FOR THE LONG-SIGHTED

Hypermetropes or long-sighted people usually wear convex lenses, the reverse of those worn by the short-sighted, being thick in the centre and thinner on the outside. These glasses tend to make the eyes look larger – and the defects around the eye area look larger, too. Long-sightedness is not generally considered a defect in the eye structure, but rather a slow-down in close vision (occurring around the mid-forties to fifties). Concealer stick is a must here, around the thin skin eye area, matched as closely as possible to skin tone. Eye shadow should again be subtle, the size of the eyelid being taken into consideration before a final choice of colour is made. Too light a shade and the eyelid can loom out from behind the glasses like the head-lights of a car. If the eye make-up is too glossy this will also emphasize the size of the lid – something to be avoided. A matt 'quiet' shade is the one to aim for – soft brown, apricot, grey – matched by a very soft, thin pencil line, drawn as close as possible to the top lashes to tone down any dilated look, which the long-sighted type of glasses can project. At night dotting then blending a white or light pink high-lighter vertically down from the brow to the root of the top lashes helps the eyes to glow. In fact, this gives great *élan* to evening eyes, glasses or no glasses.

When the lenses are clear, a touch of the main colour eye shadow around and under the outer eye corners can make the natural colour of the eyes appear more dominant. When the lenses are tinted, you have to make sure eye make-up can cope. Use a touch of frosted or pearly shadow just beneath the eye and emphasize the eyelid crease with a touch of white.

DARK GLASSES

When it comes to sunglasses for those who have to wear glasses any-way to help their vision along, the colour of the lens is of great im-portance. The most protective lenses against ultra-violet and infra-red light are always dark green, brown or anything in the grey family from light to smoky grey. Photo sensor lenses, which change gradually from light to dark when exposed to bright sunlight, also give adequate protection. However, most opticians seem to prefer to prescribe a darker lens for their patients. Apparently, the yellow lenses seen on beaches all over do not work so well, according to the experts I know; they say they have been designed more for sports wear or driving in fog. The most important thing, if you wear glasses as a general rule, is to ensure that the sun variety help and don't hinder your sight.

NEW WAY TO FACE SHAPE

Cosmesis is a new science that some might say is attempting to 'pull the wool over your eyes'. I guarantee that it isn't. It uses spectacle frames as the latest way to 'contour' facial appearance. When spectacle frames join with make-up to 'contour' face shape and features, I've

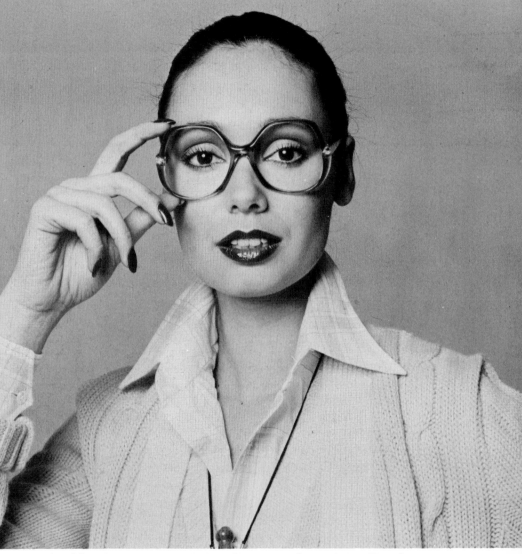

seen with my own eyes miraculous transformations. Based on Leonardo da Vinci's theory that the perfect face shape is oval (and so perfectly proportioned), cosmesis works to attain the best proportion possible through fitting the right frames to the right face.

Personality can diminish or highlight shape and features, but in general we tend to remember the features that are outstanding – like a big nose for example. But what makes a nose too big? What is it too big for? On somebody else's face it might be too small. Proportion is

133

Soft, round, elegant frames lending fullness and soft definition to the face

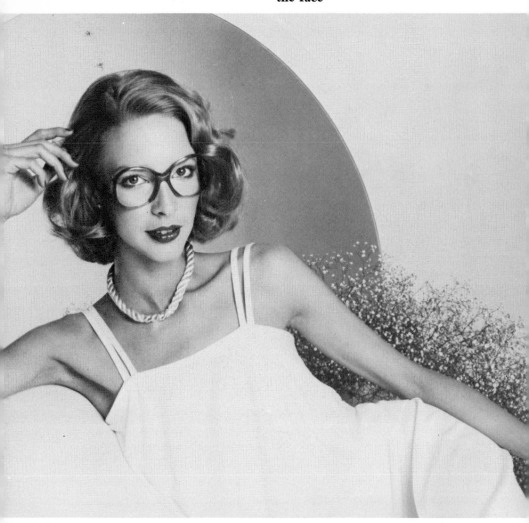

the key, and if you don't have to wear glasses you can still apply cosmesis to sunglass frames, using them as an extra adjunct to all your make-up tricks.

Face shape is obviously the first consideration. When we look at two similar shapes together they tend to emphasize each other. For example, when we look at a cube by itself, with nothing to interact with, it isn't particularly noticeable. When we look at two cubes side by side, one gets an intensified feeling of squareness. If, instead of a cube, you look at a sphere beside a cube, the two shapes de-emphasize each other. The eye doesn't receive a strong message of either roundness or squareness.

When this principle is applied to face shape and spectacle frames, it's equally effective. A round face will look much rounder in round frames – the two shapes emphasize each other – whereas a frame with straight lines will de-emphasize facial roundness. The same is true of a square face shape with predominantly straight lines. A square-shaped frame with straight lines will make a square face look squarer, and harder. Round frames will de-emphasize the face shape and soften it, too.

When face shape is more triangular or heart-shaped, with a wide cheek area tapering to an almost pointed chin, cosmesis can 'reduce' the width of the upper part of the face by using dark colour frames that expose as little skin as possible at the temples, made in a heavy material and fitting closely to the head, with the top of the frame covering the eyebrows.

All eyebrows should always be covered by the frame. If brows appear over the top of frames, it can look peculiar to say the least, giving the wearer a permanently surprised look. It's best to get brow and frame on the same even keel, but if that's not possible the frame must cover the brow, which incidentally should be 'well tailored', brushed smooth with no straggly little hairs spoiling the line.

With a long face, dark-coloured frames are essential to give an impression of 'reduced' length, although if the glasses are too small it won't work, even if the frames are jet black! Frames with vertical straight lines should be avoided, as the overall impression of the face is already vertical. Instead, all focus has to be horizontal, with rounded lines, thicker at the top and bottom than at the sides.

Frames like this narrow a large, square face, too, providing the frames extend below the cheekbones, so 'shortening' and 'narrowing' by breaking the distance between jaw and cheek.

Colour, Size and Weight are Motivating Factors

Just as we use light and dark make-up to bring forward or diminish certain aspects of the face, so light or dark frames will make an enormous difference to the way your entire face looks.

A big face must face up to its size, for instance, and make sure glasses are in similar perspective, bold, important. No colourless, rimless specs for this face. But a large face will look less large if a dark

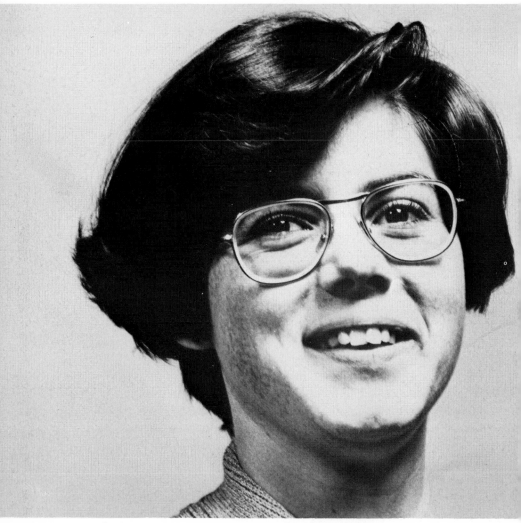

frame is used, concentrating colour at the centre, on the bridge and top wires. If, instead, a frame not much darker than skin colour is chosen, it won't 'diminish' anything.

The weight of the frame is just as important as its colour. If you have a petite round face and sensibly choose a frame with straight lines to de-emphasize the roundness, the straight lines won't help if they're delivered in a thick, heavy material. Instead of looking less round, you could end up looking drowned.

On the other hand, if a dark-coloured frame is chosen to reduce

136

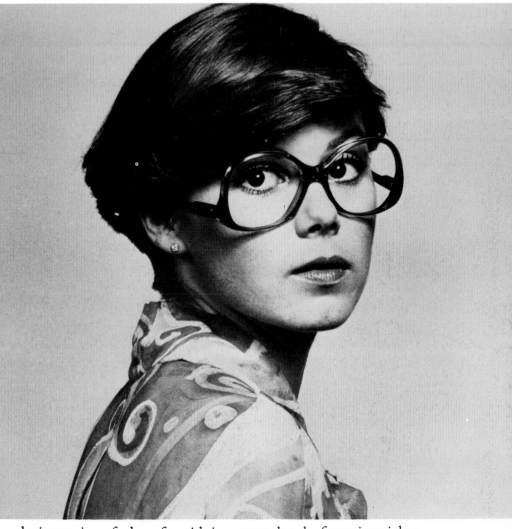

the impression of a long face, it's important that the frame is weighty enough to look important. Too thin a material and you'll have gone 'underboard'. There's not enough dark colour there to 'contour' with cosmesis.

When eyes seem too far apart, a neat trick used for aeons is to use a dark eye shadow on the part of the lid nearest the nose. Mrs Onassis applies her eye make-up this way, for obvious reasons. Girls who wear glasses and whose eyes also seem too far apart can capitalize on this make-up trick by choosing frames with a low, thick, dark-

137

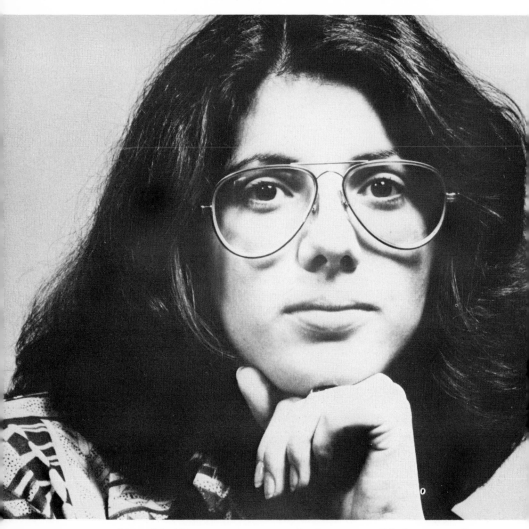

coloured bridge covering as much skin as possible between the eyes, thus 'reducing' distance.

Cosmesis doesn't work quite so well for eyes that are too close together, but one way to create an illusion of space is to choose two-toned frames, neutral at the bridge, darkening towards the sidebars. Then, the impression of space can be further emphasized with make-up – using a light shadow near the nose, concentrating a darker colour at the outer corners.

You can also create the illusion of space by leaving the part of the

After – the new frames give the face uplift, creating a sense of
harmony between the hair, the lips and the eyes

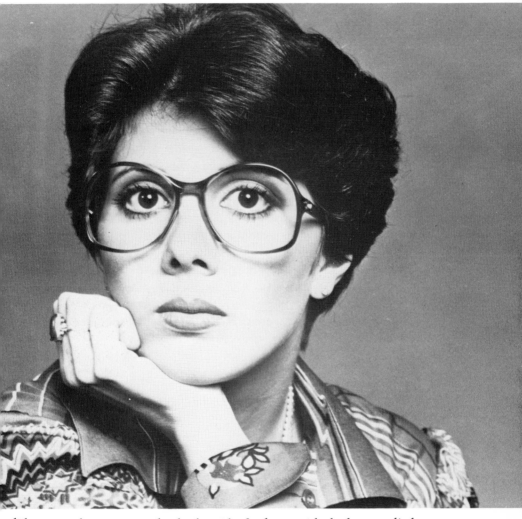

lid nearest the nose completely devoid of colour, with shadow applied
only at the other end of the lid. Lashes can help – you can either use
more mascara on the outer lashes than on the inner ones, or apply a
few extra false lashes only at the outer corners.

It's vital for girls with close-set eyes who wear glasses to avoid
reducing distance, easy to do when wearing glasses. Select a frame with
a very, very thin, high and light-coloured or transparent bridge and
you're playing safe.

To reduce the impression of a long/or large nose the frame should

139

be fitted with a low, dark-coloured bridge, concealing as much skin on the nose as possible.

A wide nose can appear to be slimmed down if the bridge is darker than the side bars and also if dark contour make-up colour is blended down both sides of the nose – *blended* being the operative word.

A tiny nose should wear frames where the bridge sits high up.

When a face is altogether too short, a roundish frame can be the answer, stopping short above the cheekbone, extra wide at mid frame.

Narrow forehead? Wear an oval shape.

Disappearing chin? Go in for a geometric shape – not too alarming – to draw other people's eyes away from your deficiency – for an unusual shape frame can help a problem that maybe only you are aware of.

If you want eyes to be directed to the top half of your face, choose frames with upswept upper wires. If that part of your face is already wide, however, forget it.

If you want eyes to focus on the lower part of your face, look for an elongated oval shape, with a slight point at outer lower corners. All this works with sunglasses, too, a fact that's often overlooked. The important thing to remember is that optical illusions do exist.

Colour Cosmesis

The colour of the frames you choose has to relate to your skin tone. If your skin is on the sallow side, it's asking for the jaundiced look if you wear green, brown or yellow frames. Following the reverse principle (round with straight – straight with round), the best colour to choose is the one not already present in your skin. For the sallow, all the pinks and warm colours work well, while the pink type of skin should avoid all blues, reds and pinks, choosing instead cool browns, greens and ambers.

Think of your type, too. If you're a cool, Scandinavian type, emphasize that coolness with cool-coloured frames, taking into account your skin tone and hair colouring, then aiming for the right colour frame in a *pale* version.

If you have warm, tawny hair, and a beige to golden skin, choose a warm-coloured frame, to emphasize your tawniness.

If you think of yourself as 'mousy' this is your chance to have a hey-day. You can play the field with many different colour frames, all to your advantage.

For black skin, warm brown or red-toned frames are excellent, while clear, bright-coloured frames from green to red to yellow can also be super. Any dark skin should avoid grey, black or metallic frames, as they don't help the look of the skin one little bit.

Think about using different frames at night, the thinner the better unless you have a facial fault you want to correct with cosmesis, which can mean that a heavy material is essential.

If you're pale-skinned with pale-coloured hair, choose a silver frame for night with slightly blue tinted lenses, so your make-up can capitalize on the medley of blue, silver and pearly tones. Behind glasses, eyes can have special radiance at night if you use deep grey to pearly tones of eye make-up with a touch of white pencil. Blend deep grey or charcoal away until it's only 'smoke' at brow level, then trace around the eye, whatever its shape, with white or grey pencil. If your eyes are very round, use a charcoal pencil or a trace of Indian kohl just above the lower lashes to make them a more interesting almond shape.

A golden girl can also wear this silver-grey-white eye package, combining spectacle frames with complementary eye make-up. In fact, it looks great on any skin that's glowing with health and vitality.

Whatever coloured frames are chosen it's vital they make sense with your natural colouring. Bizarre unusual colours can look comic, except possibly on the beach. Don't attempt to match frames to the clothes hanging in the wardrobe. This can look 'jokey'.

The best results come from choosing shades that really go with the colour scheme nature gave you, green frame matching green eye-shadow matching green dress matching green shoes – it doesn't necessarily work, because at the very least it looks *unnatural*.

Fit – Must be Fine

Fit is just as important as performance. Take time over the choice of new frames because the slightest slippage and you won't *feel* you can see any better, only that you have a face accessory you could well do without. Never choose a set of frames because you like the way they look on a friend. Each to her own – in this area, as in many others. Anything less than an excellent fit is not only a nuisance, but an incentive towards extra forehead wrinkling.

Try on as many frames as possible before making a final selection. Look at yourself in a full-length mirror as well as a small one. It's the same idea as when you stand up so that your hairdresser can get your head in true perspective with the rest of your body. Proportion is all important. When frames are too large or too small, they often spoil an otherwise terrific, well put together appearance.

As a matter of fact, like shoes, glasses frames can be fickle, for glasses can stretch. Don't try to pull and tug them back into shape. Take them back to the optician where special equipment can remould frames to fit like new again. Never be in a rush when you're getting a new pair of glasses. You'll regret it if you are.

GETTING IN CONTACT

If you should wear glasses but can't stand the idea, how about giving Leonardo da Vinci's idea a chance and investing in a pair of contact lenses? Yes, Leonardo was the first recorded person to think of adding 'a seeing eye disc' to a poor seeing eye, but nobody did much about it till the late nineteenth century.

Today, contact lenses are getting better and better all the time, developing at a faster rate than glasses, so if you're a level-headed type you may find contacts able to transform your sight without changing your looks one iota.

Hard or soft, you can take your pick, and if you don't know one from another I'll elucidate. (Another type of lens commonly described as 'gas-permeable' is in the works, too – more about that later.)

The two types now differ basically in the way each allows the eyes to receive essential nutrients for their health. Because there aren't any blood vessels on the surface of the cornea (responsible in other areas of the body both for delivering oxygen and for unloading carbon dioxide), the eyes depend upon the tear ducts and tear flow for their 'delivery' and 'disposal' needs. The way the hard type of lens ensures the eye is not cut off from this crucial service is by using a curved shape which is cut so as to leave part of the cornea exposed.

Ophthalmists don't always agree about which type of lens is best, but there seems to be a leaning towards the hard type; they are generally easier to care for, and some say they offer better vision than the soft lenses which can bend with usage, so that performance is impaired.

The reason for advocating the use of soft lenses is a persuasive one, however. Soft lenses *are* easier to get used to; in fact, they don't need 'adjustment,' as hard lenses do, and so can be slipped in and out according to the wearer's mood and/or lifestyle.

Because the soft lens is water-absorbent, the eyes have no fluid problems. Oxygen can reach the cornea directly through the lens and/or from the tear fluid beneath. But the soft lens is soft because it absorbs water from its environment. This means it can also absorb anything else in sight – chemicals, drugs, any nearby bacteria. Therefore, it can become contaminated easily. Luckily, normal tears contain an active substance, called lysozyme, that's a pretty good bacteria killer. *In other words, our own tears continually wash away contamination.*

When a person has a complete lack of success with hard lenses, it can often be attributed to the wearer's own tear production. Certain corneas have 'dry spots'. These are areas on the cornea where the tear film breaks, and they produce discomfort when a hard contact lens is applied. In fact, both hard and soft lenses very much depend on the normality of tear production, but a person with 'dry spots' usually ends up with soft lenses – because the hard variety simply hurt too much.

Soft lenses tend to be larger than the hard kind, possibly giving a wider range of vision. However, because the lens is physically soft it 'wraps' itself around the cornea, which means if there's a certain amount of astigmatism – and most people have some – it's transmitted to the lens, so that the wearer's vision also has that defect.

Soft or hard, it's vital the wearer is fitted with expert help. Usually, if hard lenses are chosen, a warning is given that it may take a couple of weeks or so to become acclimatized. If it takes any longer, it's a good idea to re-check with your optician. Most allow two or three weeks for a patient to become used to wearing them for fourteen hours at a stretch. This can be a big bore, the reason for so many happy cries of approval over the introduction of soft lenses, which need no acclimatization.

But what you may win on the roundabouts, you can lose on the swings, because as soft lenses can so easily become contaminated, cleansing has to be very thorough indeed. Unlike the quick cleanse and rinse of the hard variety, with soft lenses it's wise to sterilize occasionally in boiling water to prevent infection.

The Future for Contacts

The latest concept concerns a continuous-wear soft type of lens, allowing the best possible inflow of oxygen – the constant kind – to reach the cornea.

Developed in this country, the extremely thin lens is so thin you can't remove it – or perhaps it would be more accurate to say that you can remove it but you can't put it back because it dissolves like a piece of tissue paper. Future continuous-wear lenses – commonly described as gas-permeable – are made of silicone polymer, which allows sufficient oxygen penetration and has great potential as an 'intermediate' between soft and hard, a boon as any contact lens wearer will already know. This kind of lens is only now becoming available to the public, ask your optician if you're interested.

Make-up on Contact

Do put in lenses before applying eye make-up. Guesswork doesn't pay.

Use pencils, crayons or cinnamon/brown colour blushers for eye shadow. All of these are less likely to flake into the eyes than powder shadow and they don't smear like the cream variety.

Use a water-soluble mascara, so if particles drop into the eyes they will dissolve quickly with no irritation. Never use lash-lengthening mascara, which has tiny fibres that can easily get into the eyes.

Don't line the inside of the eyes. This can be disastrous.

Always remove lenses before taking off eye make-up, but be sure to use an eye make-up remover. The area around the eyes is delicate and vulnerable and doesn't take kindly to being rubbed and pulled. Special eye make-up remover precludes all this and helps preclude the tiny lines which nobody needs.

LOOKING AFTER YOUR EYES

There are many people who don't seem to be able to get by without their 'dodge 'em' glasses, big, dark affairs that are not needed 'ophthalmically' but are worn to hide behind, often literally. There seems no let-up to the dark glasses phase, even though opticians are always pointing out that dark glasses may lead to the wearers *needing* real spectacles, because they're forever straining their eyes, reading, writing, looking through a dark haze of their own making.

Even when we don't favour blinkers, many of us continually ill treat our eyes through poor lighting. A poorly placed lamp will cause a shadow or a glare that our eyes have to live with night in and night out, and according to statistics we frequently work, read and write with too little light.

Too much contrast between light and dark areas in a room can also be bad for the eyes – while watching T.V. in the dark is apparently outrageous.

If you like to do a lot of close work (and that refers to needlework just as much as to working out profit and loss sheets), remember to lift your eyes occasionally to look around the room. That's a refreshing exercise for the eyes.

Mother wasn't kidding when she recommended carrots for 'seeing in the dark'. Keep carrots on the menu for the sake of your eyes. They're full of vitamin A, and this vitamin is known to be particularly valuable to the eyes. Perhaps I should say invaluable. Butter is a natural source of vitamin A, so are milk, dark green leafy vegetables like spinach and kale, and all yellow fruits and vegetables (which means sweet potatoes and squash). Add liver, kidneys, sweetbreads and brains, if you can face them, and you'll be getting a monumental supply of vitamin A, all for the good of your eyes (not to mention your skin, see page 218).

The most important tip of all is to take notice of little signals like inexplicable dull headaches coming out of nowhere, days when you find you have to squint, days when things seem blurred and you even have sudden attacks of nausea. All this means you should see an eye doctor. Many people never realize they need an eye test because an imbalance of the eye muscles is not always easily detected. The symptoms just described mean help is probably needed, for the body is signalling it wants help.

If you wear contact lenses don't forget to wear sunglasses when the sun is strong; your eyes need extra protection from extra bright rays. Don't use lash-building mascaras – stick to the water-soluble kind. Keep finger-nails short to prevent scratching eyes or soft contact lenses. Keep the fumes of nail varnish remover or any permanent wave solution away from lenses. Never rub your eyes – blot them if you're trying to rub perspiration away. Except with the 'permanent' kind, described previously, just arriving on the scene, never wear contact lenses while you're sleeping and never, never wet lenses with saliva – bacteria can cause eye infection fast.

9

Hair

OUR BEST NATURAL ASSET WITH A LITTLE CARE

O U R hair can be our most reliable asset, if we give it the loving care it deserves. It doesn't 'break out', as the skin does when our plans go awry. It doesn't sag like the body when age catches up with our muscles (and our willpower). Hair's tensile strength is just incredible. You wouldn't wear a skirt or dress every day for years and years and expect it to stay in good shape – yet hair, whipped by the wind, polluted by the atmosphere, dried by the sun, is expected to recover fully after only one shampoo and set.

My name for the good hair stylists I know all over the world is 'hairdressers with a conscience'. They believe, as I do, that women make too many demands on their hair without giving it enough attention.

'You shouldn't demand from your hair more than it can do,' says top London hairdresser Michael Rasser of Michaeljohn. (He is the favourite hairdresser of many of the 'Royals', including Princess Anne and Princess Alexandra.) Michael can transform anyone's looks for the better, but he will not deliver any hairstyle on demand if he doesn't think the hair can achieve it – however illustrious the client. His attitude is gaining ground because of the most valid reason in the world – *hair health*, the most persuasive selling concept in hairdressing today. Now, condition comes before style, cut and colour; in fact, the hair's condition is the motivating basis for the style – uncontrived, untortured, unfettered, free.

How did it happen? Because the bouffant backcombed jobs of the sixties toppled as soon as the new, easy, carefree clothes came along, accompanied by the more 'natural' look in make-up.

The *fibre* is what counts, as more and more women realize – from

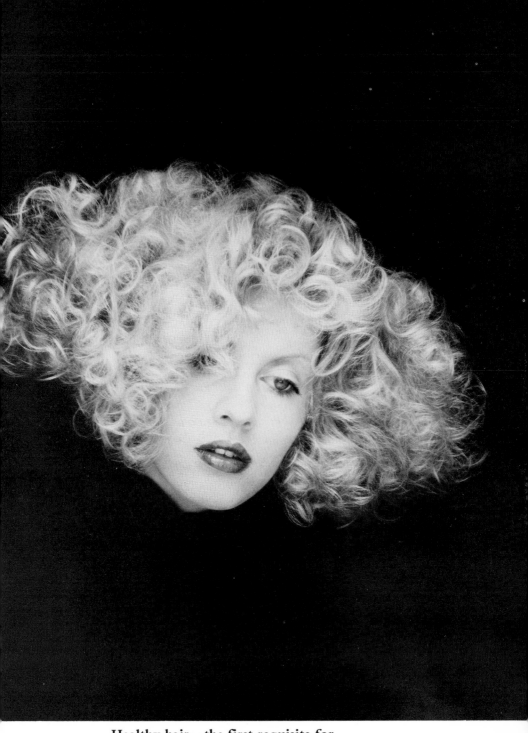

**Healthy hair – the first requisite for
any style today**

Each hair follicle has a muscle, and it is this muscle that causes our hair to stand on end when we're scared to death

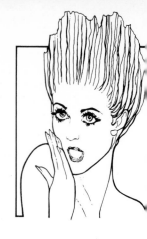

Cher, who wears hers thick and straight to the small of her back, to H.M. the Queen, who hasn't changed her style in over twenty-five years, to Princess Margaret, who cuts and grows, cuts and grows, more or less according to fashion, but who wouldn't dream of going without regular hair-condition check-ups and treatments.

HOW YOUR HAIR GROWS

Hair isn't called a crop for nothing. Hair *is* a crop, as dependent upon the food you eat for its structure and well-being as is sugar cane upon rain and sun. Sugar cane has to worry about the soil in which it is planted. You have to worry about the state of your follicles, 100,000 of them – slightly more for blondes, less for redheads – from which every hair on your head emanates. Poor follicles and your hair will be poor, and this will show in a variety of miserable ways.

How your hair looks right this minute also depends on the sort of hair your great-grandmama had, for heredity plays a big part.

Today more and more dermatologists and trichologists (who only study the hair and scalp) ascribe women's hair condition also to the way women think, pointing out links with the emotions, extra responsibilities, stress – all factors, they say, in how much shine and bounce your hair has or hasn't.

All of us, male or female, start out at birth with a full complement of follicles; each one has a blood supply and a muscle. It's this muscle that causes our hair to 'stand on end' and our skin to pucker into 'goose pimples' whenever we're scared to death – a primitive defence mechanism inherited from our hairy ancestors who, just like frightened animals, increased their bulk significantly whenever their fur stood on end! Each follicle produces one hair, which grows upward from an area called the papilla, where the hair bulb and root are located.

Unlike some mammals, our hair follicles follow a cycle independently of each other. While some hairs are growing, others are falling out, and it's not abnormal to lose up to a hundred hairs a day. Whether your hair grows quickly or not again depends on your ancestors.

The usual lifespan of a single hair is in the region of three to four years, and its life is divided into three stages:

1 *the anagen,* the growing stage; it takes a hair about three years to reach full growth;

2 *the catagen,* the regression period, which lasts about two weeks; then

3 *the telogen,* the last stage, when the follicle becomes dormant for about three months before the hair falls out, to be replaced immediately by an anagen – growing stage – hair, growing on average about half an inch ($1\frac{1}{4}$ cm) a month.

On the scalp, the growing stage is long and the resting stage short;

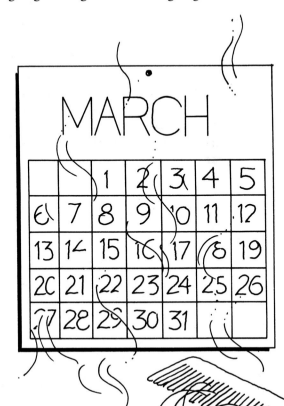

For climatic reasons more hairs are shed in March and April than at any other time of the year

90 per cent of the hair is growing, while 10 per cent is resting, a situation that is fortunately reversed on the body.

This three-stage cycle operates for each of the 100,000 hair follicles about fifteen to twenty times before it starts to slow down and mal-function, having the same limited capacity to regenerate as any of our other body processes. This is the law of ageing, whether we like it or not, though it can differ dramatically from individual to individual, according to genes and hormones, and depends most of all on *how much care we give ourselves.*

Although the follicles act independently, they are affected by outside stimuli, so for climatic reasons more hairs are shed in March and April than at any other time, the lowest amount in July, one reason why those hairdressers with a conscience I mentioned like to deter their clients from having their hair cut at that time – good hair-dressers like to see hair at its best, i.e., at its fullest, with less hair being shed.

HAIR LOSS

How to keep your hair has become as controversial as how to keep your cool. Hair loss can be temporary ('reversible', as the dermatolo-gists put it) or permanent. If it is temporary it means the follicle is still alive, so there's hope of a new hair.

A number of things can be responsible for the warning signal of more hair left behind on the brush than there should be.

The innocent-looking ponytail can – and frequently does – produce a temporary spot baldness, providing medical terminology with a new label, 'traction alopecia', acquired when the prolonged pulling back of hair into one position causes inflammation on or below the surface of the scalp, invisible to the naked eye. If the ponytail is worn constantly, the inflammation eventually hinders normal hair growth. The injured hair gives up the struggle and breaks off, perhaps

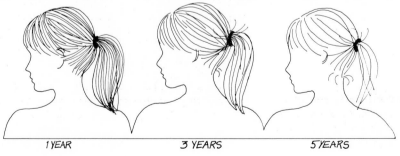

| 1 YEAR | 3 YEARS | 5 YEARS |

to be replaced during the next cycle, perhaps not. If breakage is continual, the hair bulb and papilla, on which the hair is lodged, shrink, dry up, and stop manufacture of new hair. Sometimes a new hair breaks through, but it will be thinner in texture, dull and brittle. The reason why the ponytail is a potential hazard to hair health is that its success as a style depends on the degree of *tightness* that can be achieved with ribbon, barrette, or, worst of all, elastic band. *The strain on the hair can be intolerable.*

After studying twenty-four cases of traction alopecia, an eminent dermatologist reported in *The Archives of Dermatology*, 'Once the ponytail was abandoned in favour of a more relaxed hairdo, there was complete regrowth of scalp hair in every case except two. In these two instances, there was some return of new hair, but after six months the remaining bald spots on the sides and back were taken to be permanent.'

Scary, to say the least, so beware of too much traction – even when you use heated rollers. Curling the hair up too tightly too often is harmful to its health.

Continuous hair straightening, over-vigorous brushing, excessive intake of vitamin A supplements, over-bleaching, over-perming – over-*anything* that isn't a natural way of life for the hair is harmful, too, and means *hair damage*. Statistics show that the greatest damage to hair we inflict on ourselves.

THE PILL IS A PILL

The effect of the pill on hair (and skin, see page 36) is still under investigation. A few years back a series of medical papers was released relating to women who had taken the pill over a long period of time and who felt their hair had thinned as a consequence. After further observation, the papers divulged, however, that hair loss was greater a month or so after they stopped taking it.

A parallel was drawn between those women on, then off the pill, and women who experience sudden hair loss *after* having a baby, the reasoning being that just as pregnancy increases production of the hormone oestrogen, helping to prevent baldness, so the pill, using oestrogen, also keeps hormone levels high. In other words, the women were wrong to blame the pill. Hair had thinned *after* they had stopped taking it.

When pregnancy is over or the pill is abandoned, usually the hair cycle eventually returns to normal, but curiously *begins* by rapidly producing the telogen and last phase of the hair cycle when hair is shed.

If you take drugs or any medicine, then suffer from hair loss, the two things could be related. If you feel the problem warrants a visit to a dermatologist, even your aspirin intake should be recorded – it could have a bearing on the matter.

WOMEN ARE LOSING MORE HAIR

You may be able to blame the amount of hair you lose on your grandparents – for heredity has a long reach. Your parents may have had thick heads of hair, their parents may not – and it could be *their* unwanted 'hair loss genes' that have been passed on to you.

Age is another factor in hair loss – age and the menopause, when women start to produce less of the female hormone but go on producing the same amount of the male hormone, about two-thirds the amount men do. Because the hormonal balance is disturbed, some women find themselves losing hair faster.

Hair loss among women is on the increase, that fact dermatologists have noted over the past decade – ten times as many cases being the conservative estimate.

A group of research doctors have an explanation for this, based on their theory that *women are making more of the male hormone since they assumed male attitudes, responsibilities, and tensions under the banner of women's liberation.* More androgen, says one dermatologist, and more women will suffer from 'the hitherto mainly masculine privilege of baldness'.

The normal ratio of hormones in a woman's body is one part androgen (male hormone) to eight parts oestrogen (female hormone), the oestrogen giving her fine skin and a high resistance to hair loss (only 5 per cent of women ever go bald).

As one of the prime believers in the women's lib theory explained, 'Once that ratio is disturbed, the genetic force takes over. In the case of the woman making excessive androgen, it means the male side of the family tree dominates. If her father or grandfather had a disposition towards baldness, the rate of her hair fallout can surpass the normal rate of regrowth or replacement.'

Not every dermatologist goes along with this theory, but it is generally agreed that extra *stress* results in an extra output of androgen, which in turn affects the hair follicles, causing a noticeable change in the hair cycle.

What Can Be Done about Hair Loss?

There is cautious optimism about counteracting the bald facts of life – eventually for both sexes. Patients who suffer from premature hair loss are likely to be given a thorough examination on their first visit to a trichologist. This includes a thyroid test, kidney, calcium, enzyme and liver studies, plus, in the case of female patients, an Oestrogen Maturation Index (commonly called E.M.I.), a vaginal smear which tells whether the body is secreting enough oestrogen.

A scalp injection aimed at breaking the genetic tie that may develop when a woman produces excess androgen is in the experimental stage. So is an anti-androgen pill to neutralize excessive male hormone output, without producing the reverse effect of extreme femininity.

The medically approved method of hair transplantation is forging ahead, although the situation isn't easy – donor hair is sparse (currently, hair has to come from the patient), while baldness is extensive. The method involves transferring small circular scalp plugs from an area where hair flourishes to an area where it doesn't. Some patients have responded well, others only fairly well, but transplantation can be a viable proposition if it is helped along by monthly injections of small amounts of steroid into the transplanted sites.

Research is also going on involving transplants from a healthy scalp to an ailing one, hoping for the day when this kind of treatment can be successfully carried out on any two people with the same colour and type of hair.

The Egyptians wrote that they had a sure cure for hair loss: 'Rub into the scalp a mixture of equal parts of crocodile, lion, hippopotamus and serpent fat.' Unfortunately, there's still no modern product any more effective in *curing* baldness, BUT, according to many in that field of research, the cure is now only years away, not decades.

HELP YOUR HAIR YOURSELF

What you eat affects the way your hair looks and feels. There's a simple reason: for each hair growing out of your scalp, there's a blood supply feeding the papilla, the blood providing the energy to produce that hair. The success of the output – the difference between a poor and a strong hair – depends on whether your diet is nutritious or not.

According to the most recent research, for the papilla to manufacture perfectly healthy hairs at least 3½ oz (100 grams) of protein should be a daily part of your diet. Another nutrient for beautiful hair:

yeast pills (vitamin B). The no-no's include excess sugar, salt and animal fats.

If you have baby-fine, impossible-to-set hair, your hair bulb may not be getting the right sustenance. Add more protein (fish, chicken, lean meat) to your diet for starters.

Once hair becomes visible on the surface of the scalp, it's an appendage, not fed by anything internally, commonly referred to as '*dead*', and totally dependent for its looks and condition on its environment, and on the lotions and potions we decide to apply to it.

First requisite: a healthy diet to grow healthy hair.

Second requisite: protection for the hair against an environment that can take away its healthy qualities through exposure to pollution, salt water, chlorinated water, air conditioning, steam heat, and too much sun.

The important thing is to match your hair products to your hair type and to its behaviour. Choose your shampoo with as much care as you choose your eye make-up and think of a conditioner as an essential part of your own personal hair care programme.

Positively pH

This little symbol, as I've already explained (see page 27), means hydrogen potential. It's mentioned more and more in relation to hair care products these days because pH is the measurement used to determine the hair's level of acidity vs. alkalinity.

New hair has a *normal* pH – between 4.0 and 6.0 – which means it's mildly acidic, good looking, and *naturally* shiny, showing the minimum of structural damage.

Maintaining that acid mantle – through the right choice of products and correct hair handling – is advantageous, because a contracted (acidic) cuticle reflects light (producing the natural shine mentioned) and also provides 35 per cent of hair's elastic strength.

Many hair preparations that can change colour, add curl (permanents), or take curl away (straighteners), and some shampoos, are highly alkaline, falling into the 7.0 to 10.0 pH range — some are even higher.

With continued use of these high pH products, the hair itself will reach a higher pH, becoming more alkaline and more porous. Instead of lying flat and close to the hair shaft, the cuticle scales open and expand to leave the inner structure more vulnerable. The hair then swells when any moisture is applied; it tends to feel 'spongy' and is really prone to damage.

To illustrate the point, I only have to tell you that drain cleaners are able to *dissolve* clogging hair in the pipes completely when their pH level is *above* the 'safe' range (over 10).

This would imply that non-alkaline products with a low pH are the ones to buy for your hair health's sake.

As far as shampoos are concerned, however, the truth is that you need some alkali in order to *cleanse* well, so the ideal shampoo cleanses hair with alkaline compounds, then adds acid factors to rid the hair of dull residue and lower pH to 'normal'. This is what our grandmothers used to do when they used vinegar or lemon rinses 'to bring the shine back' following soap shampoos. In fact, without probably knowing, they were 'replacing the acid mantle'.

Next time you buy a shampoo, check out its pH, if you can, now you know it's important.

Feed Your Hair

As electronic radioactive studies have proved, hair *can* absorb protein, and likes and needs it, too, for its health and strength. Choose shampoos and conditioners with protein or collagen (a good source of protein) built in. You can be sure they're good for your hair.

Do You Know Your Hair Type

Dry or greasy? Between the two? Doctors aren't too sure our self-analysis is always (a) correct and (b) helpful. They point out that subjective observations are frequently impossible to substantiate, as fine, thin hair often shows signs of greasiness faster than coarse, thick hair, although both could accurately be described as 'greasy'.

The condition of your scalp relates directly to the health and look of your hair, and although scalp skin is similar to skin on the rest of the body, the glandular secretions are more profuse, allowing sebum from the sebaceous glands to cover both scalp and hair.

Greasy Hair

Natural oils are vital for hair and scalp protection, and the aqueous sebum which comes from our sweat gland is normal and functional. Greasy hair simply means *too much* oil is secreted, and this combines with bacteria to produce problems.

There's the problem of dandruff, for example – a term often erroneously used to describe a multitude of scalp ills. When a doctor delivers the more forbidding but accurate description of 'seborrhoeic dermatitis,' it means there's inflammation around the oil glands of the papilla or base of the hair, causing itchiness, redness, scaliness and white flakiness. It can be kept under control with products containing tars, zinc or sulphur, but after a period of time a sufferer can build up resistance to one product, so should switch to another.

Psoriasis is sometimes mistaken for dandruff but it's a far more serious state of affairs. The actual *cells* of the scalp turn over more rapidly than normal, the scalp becoming encrusted and blocked. Psoriasis definitely needs medical help.

HOW TO COPE WITH GREASY HAIR. Never brush it, only comb it with a wide-toothed comb.

Never wear a wool or fur beret or close fitting hat; this aggravates the condition, giving bacteria more encouragement to breed in the cosy, warm atmosphere. In winter wear a silk scarf. Real silk is protein and can keep you amazingly warm.

Ozone is good for greasy hair. Dip it in sea water as often as you can.

Backcomb roots to allow as much air as possible to penetrate the scalp.

Don't shampoo too often. Overwashing promotes greasiness. Don't be dictated to by your hair, washing it according to how you think it looks. Establish a hair control programme. Wash every three days and at the same hour of the day if you can.

Use only lukewarm water. Hot water activates the already over-active sebaceous glands. Only one lathering, but lots of rinses.

Choose products specially formulated to curb or at least control the amount of sebum released, mild, soapless, herbal-based shampoos.

Avoid tight curling with either heated rollers or pins.

Avoid effervescent drinks, a high carbohydrate intake, cheese, nuts, egg yolk and fats.

Eat more spinach (vitamin E), watercress (iron), egg white and fruit and drink plenty of skimmed milk.

Between shampoos wipe your scalp with cotton soaked in a clear medicated lotion if you feel itchy. Wych-hazel or an astringent formulated for *greasy skin* will do nicely.

Towel-dry rather than blow-dry if you can. If you can't always use the blow dryer on 'low'.

Once a week massage your scalp, gently rotating the skin. Start at the back, then repeat at sides, on crown and on forehead. Then 'walk' fingertips (not nails) over the scalp, making small circles with your fingers at each location, until you've covered all the ground. An anti-dandruff preparation can be applied as you massage, but hair should then be combed through and shampooed.

Use a non-oil-based conditioner (read the labels!) or a pack of refined clay that coats the hair, helping give it body and become less porous. If it isn't too fragile, greasy hair can benefit from henna, which coats the hair lightly to give it body. As most varieties of henna also give colour, it should only be used three times a year, otherwise the colour build-up can produce too harsh an effect. A vinegar rinse is also good for greasy hair.

Dry Hair

Dry hair signifies a poor oil supply from the scalp and a lack of moisture in the hair. As the norm for hair is only 3 per cent moisture to 97 per cent protein, it can't afford to lose one drop.

If the hair is dry, the skin is probably dry, too – or hair can become dry from lack of care. Too many treatments and permanents, too much tinting or bleaching, shampoos that over-cleanse and strip the hair of its natural oils – all these things can dry hair and spoil it. Too much sun, wind (particularly hitting the hair in an open car) and overheated air are harmful, too. It means hair will be hard to manage, flyaway, super-charged with electricity.

Your hair is telling you it needs help from *you*.

HOW TO COPE WITH DRY HAIR. Use a shampoo incorporating lanolin or other fats designed to remove dirt but not natural oils. Pure Castile soaps have a high oil content, so are good for dry types.

Use only the mildest shampoos, and a big sponge for washing; this is gentler than fingers on the hair, better able to flood it with water.

Brush, but only with natural bristles, never nylon, and only for a short while each evening to distribute the natural oils evenly through-out the scalp. Brushing also boosts circulation by 'massaging' the scalp. Forget about 100 strokes a night, however, positively bad for thin, fine or damaged hair.

Match bristle to hair type, soft for soft, stiffer for thick.

Brush by bending over, up and out from the nape. Again, this is a good circulation booster.

Never brush hair when wet. It stretches, then breaks.

Oil hair the night before a salon visit. Try mink oil, it's good.

Use a trace of hair conditioning cream between shampoos to calm flyaway ends and add shine and lustre, coating the hair with a water-soluble barrier so offering some protection from the elements, which are especially harmful to dry, brittle hair.

Use a conditioner regularly after a shampoo. Conditioners help make the hair cuticle (outer layer) smooth and manageable, and neutralize any excess alkaline residue left over from shampoos.

Conditioning – replacing moisture – gives the hair shine, adds various humectants and decreases split ends by reducing friction between one hair and its neighbour.

For extra benefit, use conditioners that aim for deeper penetration of the scalp, aided and abetted by heat to dilate the cuticle and set off chemical action.

A head massage with warmed baby oil can be helpful to thin hair.

Plastic wrap – the kind you keep in the kitchen – is a useful ploy. Wrap it round hair saturated with baby oil or conditioner and secure with kirby grips. Create more heat by covering your hair 'parcel' with a shower cap or thick towel. Stay that way overnight if you can. Rinse thoroughly in the morning and dry with moderate heat.

To contain flyaway hair, use a setting lotion that deposits chemical resins on the hair, making it easy to separate strands, then to hold the hair in position when combed. Some setting lotions give body by externally coating the hair shaft, adding a 'plumping' effect.

If your hair is particularly brittle, easily breaking, it can signify a lack of protein in your diet. Add protein two ways – topically, choosing an appropriate product, and internally, eating more good class protein, meat, eggs, green-leafed vegetables and vitamin B – in supplement form as well as in natural foods (grains).

Avoid spices, alcohol and too much carbohydrate.

Damaged Hair

When the hair is damaged, the parting often gives the first clue, even before poor hair begins to show. The scalp looks grey and dingy, or unnaturally pink from irritation. An expert can *feel* when a scalp is not well. It feels 'tight' from poor circulation, no elasticity, no movement.

Hair that refuses to take colour or perms or falls out of shape in minutes may also have your diet to thank for it. The wrong, low-nutrition diet means the hair bulb is not receiving the nutrients it needs to produce lovely hair; it then atrophies, causing improper formation of the hair cuticle, weakening the hair shaft and leading to easy breakage or, at the very least, hair with no stamina.

Even premature grey can be caused by a missing link in the nutritional network – for grey is simply a sign of poor pigment supply in the cortex.

HOW TO COPE WITH DAMAGED HAIR. First, whatever programme you decide on – under expert supervision at a salon or at home – it has to be followed faithfully. Damaged hair is *sick* hair and the patient won't recover if treatment is slapdash.

Intensive conditioning has to be the long-term part of the programme, but first the hair should be trimmed. Damage is most noticeable at the ends, where the oldest hairs are.

Instead of a trim, a much shorter look all over may be a faster route to healthy hair renewal – getting rid of all the old, weak hair to replace it with a sharp, new look – and a new start.

For new hair to be healthy, it's vital to have plenty of blood rushing to the scalp – and an expert shoulder and head massage is one way to achieve this. Knotted shoulder and neck muscles (which the majority of city dwellers have, see page 255), cut off the blood flow to the scalp. The capillaries constrict, the oil glands go haywire, and you could say the scalp comes down with a virus. When the scalp is smothered under layers of foreign material, it means the hair growth cycle is interrupted or blocked.

After consultation, many trichologists set about solving hair problems with a stupendous head, neck and shoulder massage which lasts for about fifteen minutes. Then (depending on the problem) the scalp may need exfoliation, with a formula containing many vitamin concentrates and organic substances. This is also massaged into the hair, with a miniature bristle brush, the polyunsaturated and water-soluble formula reaching into the follicles, where bacteria can cause a load of trouble. The finale can be a session under an electrically heated cap, the heat enabling the special solution to go as deep as it can. Often the patient is advised to keep the solution on for a few hours, washing it out later at home with a mild – preferably baby – camomile or herbal shampoo.

Regular conditioners are necessary to continue this good work, especially to bolster the hair's protein content; this binds moisture in the hair shaft, reviving damaged hair by smoothing down rough, chipped surfaces.

Never rub damaged hair vigorously – or, for that matter, any hair; it snarls it unnecessarily. Instead, blot and pat, and dry on a *low* heat, never on a high one

HOW TO AVOID HAIR DAMAGE. Avoid going bare-headed in cold weather – hair can have the 'shivers', too. Each hair shaft contains a speck of water, which is a speedy conductor of heat or cold. Outdoors on a freezing day, the hair can get chilled, chapped; when you go inside to a heated (often over-heated) room, the sudden change shocks the hair, disrupts its moisture balance still further. Wearing a hat or scarf prevents all this trauma, and maintains a good supply of blood and nutrients to the scalp by keeping it warm.

Hair should be covered on hot days, too. It may not show sunburn the way skin does, but hair can be 'burned'.

A daily headstand does wonders for your circulation, which in turn benefits hair, scalp and skin. Remember, your blood flow is your beauty flow (see page 254).

If the hair is *really* hurt and so looks terrible, never dream of trying to cover it up with a new colour, a new perm. It can only cause more harm, perhaps the irreversible kind.

Never colour and perm your hair the same week – there should be at least two weeks between.

Avoid excessive quantities of vitamins A and D (sun), both capable of causing dry scalp symptoms and inflamed hair follicles, leading to eventual hair loss.

Change your parting periodically to expose another section of your scalp.

Do give your hair a chance to hang free once a week at least.

HAIR BOOSTERS

The beautiful Baroness von Thyssen (Denise) has 36-inch-long blonde hair that she washes regularly twice a week wherever she is, a lengthy three-hour job. She believes her hair might not be so beautiful if she didn't give it a tremendous amount of attention – and she may be right. Extra long hair is weak hair, because it has obviously been around quite a few years.

To ensure it always looks and feels its silky best, this young baroness relies on three hair experts, each of whom she visits several times a year: Philip Kingsley in London, Kenneth in New York, and – the one she sees most frequently – Mademoiselle Mad in Paris. In

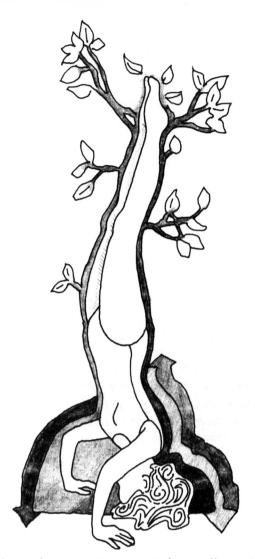

her salon on the Faubourg St. Honoré Mademoiselle Mad concocts all her own brews, treating the heads of many Paris-based beauties like La Baronne de Rothschild and Madame David Rothschild.

To build up hair strength, Mademoiselle Mad recommends her clients take intravenous or intramuscular shots of Bépanthène (panthenol) for twelve days every six months. The Baroness von Thyssen has been taking this advice for years for the best reason possible: she finds it improves her hair out of all recognition.

Why? Bépanthène is said to donate pantothenic acid, B_5, to the body and B_5 is known as the anti-stress vitamin.

A lack of pantothenic acid can lead to seborrhoea, even hair loss, breaking nails, and poor digestion, so, conversely, it would appear that an extra dose can give the hair (and nails) new strength and growth.

Other vitamins from the vitamin B family, it is said, can affect hair colour. I know many prematurely grey women who take – with varying success – a complex supplement of vitamin B that supplies 50 milligrams of each component, all in an endeavour to restore pigment to the cortex and so eradicate grey from the head. For when pigment runs out of the cortex altogether hair colour is obviously white. You can find vitamin B in natural foods, too, such as oysters, liver, broccoli, crab, mushrooms and skimmed milk.

There are other 'secret weapons' to guard against hair damage: the high frequency 'ray-gun', for example, which fitted out with different attachments, 'exercises' each hair by sending a burst of ultra-violet light through it. The hair is 'raked' with this special 'ray-gun', and so is the scalp, sending a delicious tingle right through the body.

EXPERT RULES FOR HAIR CARE AT HOME

Whip shampoo up, diluting with a little water; use an egg beater if you don't have a blender. This ensures the hair is not 'traumatized' with too much weight from the lather.

Rinse hair first with warm water, then wash with whipped-up shampoo. Rinse again thoroughly.

Blot and pat dry, never rub vigorously.

Dry hair immediately after it's shampooed. If it's allowed to dry too slowly, the slow evaporation causes loss of natural moisture retention in the hair, resulting in a lifeless, dry look. Excessive heat must also be avoided for the same reason.

Brush hair only when absolutely dry, never when wet.

Never brush dirty hair – it can spread bacteria on the scalp.

Wash every two to three days if you live in the city, three to five in the country.

Watch your diet. Build hair strength by eating nutritiously – good protein, vitamin C and food containing all members of the vitamin B family (whole grains).

Keep hair pruned like a plant. Trim every six weeks.

Always wash hair gently, like washing tights.

Use only brushes with natural bristle – boar is best.

Do change your style occasionally to give hair a change, which is also a rest.

The Experts Say . . .

Don't curl hair too tightly with hot rollers, or too tightly with *anything*.

Don't use any broken equipment – it can scratch the scalp, break the hair.

Don't use an elastic band for your coiffure. Always use a covered band.

Don't use a sizzling hot drier.

Don't over-sunburn, over-tease, over-spray, over-perm, over-colour.

Don't forget a 6-inch (15-cm) strand of hair is about a year old at its end, and has been through a minimum of fifty-two shampoos and sets and perhaps 2,000 combings.

Don't ignore split ends or they will continue up the hair shaft.

Don't use dry shampoos more than once a month at the most. They should really be for emergencies only.

Don't use just any shampoo if your hair's coloured. Look for those that are specially formulated to clean coloured hair.

Don't wait for hair damage before you use *conditioners*.

How Conditioners Work

The basic job of the conditioner is to detangle, unsnarl, reduce frizz and make smooth, with anti-static ingredients that calm down flyaway hair; it also adds *body*, and so life and vitality, to the hair.

Some conditioners smooth down the platelets on the cuticle, fill in lost patches of body, and seal split ends.

For fine, limp, colour-treated hair and hair abused through too much wear and tear (even over-shampooing) use protein conditioners. The protein coats the hair and is absorbed by it, and each strand actually becomes thicker as well as more springy. Protein is, in any case, a key ingredient in any conditioner for any type of hair. By adding body, it obviously adds *life* to any style, straight or curly, long or short.

The 'instant' kind of conditioner usually relates to one that can set hair as well, helping hair hold shape and curl, as well as depositing protein on the shaft to 'plump out' hair strands.

Corrective conditioners encourage hair to hold moisture and soften hair that's dry and brittle to make it more supple and resistant to breaking.

THE BEST SEX SYMBOL – YOUR HAIR

When master builder William Levitt extended his yacht *La Belle Simone* (one of the largest privately owned yachts in the world) by fifteen feet (4½ metres), it didn't cause any comment.

When La Belle Simone herself, his dashing French wife after whom the yacht is named, cut 15 inches (38 cm) off her then almost waist-length dark hair, it made the papers, caused remarks everywhere she went – and took ten years off her looks.

Alexandre of Paris, possibly the most famous manipulator of a pair of scissors in the world, did the job, and Simone was so delighted she went back the next day to ask for another inch off.

For Simone the cut was a risk that came off. She was right to think of it as a risk, for cutting very long hair very short is certain to bring about a transformation, one that demands another set of rules to follow for maintenance – and perhaps even a new make-up, too (see page 99 and following).

For a few years we had to grit our teeth, as the males in the family played early Samson, growing their hair to prove their strength, or to prove their will anyway – son *v.* mother, son *v.* father, son *v.* girlfriend.

That long-haired revolt is old hat now. Male hair styles have settled down more or less at the shoulder line for the revolutionaries, up back around the ears for those fed up with all the care a lengthy head of hair requires.

The women's revolt pre-dated the men's by about fifty years, in that short-lived scuffle of the 1920s when women 'won the right' to wear their hair 'bobbed' and their skirts short – both attempts to emphasize female emancipation.

Unlike men, however, women have been yo-yoing about their hair length ever since – varying from the long, long (way past the shoulders) to the short, short (introduced by Vidal Sassoon's first geometric cut of the early 1960s), and back to long again. Now, thank heavens, length is more a matter of individual opinion, and most women want to find a style they can cope with themselves. No one wants to spend hours in a beauty salon any more.

When the test of a good set was its staying power, a salon visit took at least two or three hours. One expected to emerge with hair combed and lacquered to the crisp consistency of candy-floss, and had every hope of living with this rigid headgear for at least three or four

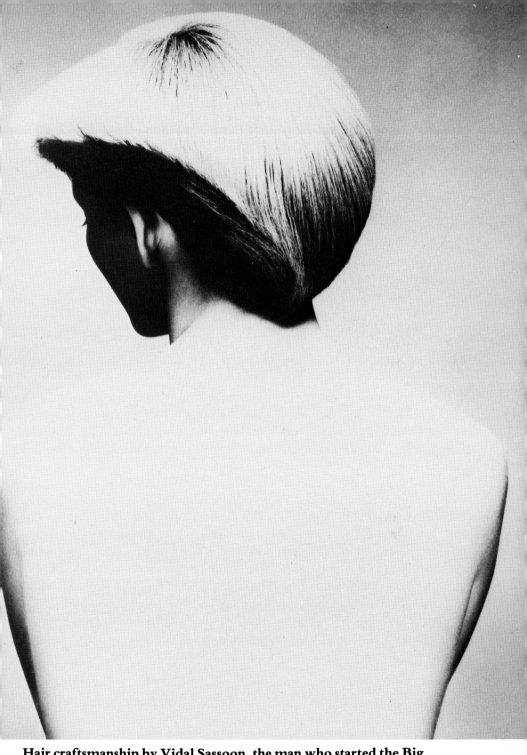

**Hair craftsmanship by Vidal Sassoon, the man who started the Big
Shear**

days before a teetering collapse necessitated another trip to the salon to hold up the remains.

That tortuous and tortured type of styling, hiding a multitude of sins, is out forever – and Vidal Sassoon can take a lot of the credit. He swept into the hair headlines in 1963 when he delivered what was considered a revolutionary idea – a cut that was longer in front than at the back. He designed it for a Mary Quant fashion show, it was picked up by French designer Emmanuelle Khanh for her Paris models, and soon women everywhere were having themselves shorn like so many chic sheep.

Nowadays, Vidal hardly ever holds a pair of scissors in his hands – more likely an airline ticket as he zips from one continent to another, watching over his empire of shops – but, like all top stylists, he firmly believes that only beautiful hair can make beautiful styles. Releasing his first hair care products in 1974, he said, 'A basic haircut can't fall properly or reflect its precision unless the hair has natural sheen and flexibility. It certainly won't hold any given shape without elasticity and tensile strength.'

Now that *style* is sublimated to *condition*, hair stylists have to be on their mettle. They often have better material to work with, but, because the style shows off the hair, the calibre of their work is shown off clearly too.

To start where I came in, length is important, not because of what fashion decrees, but because the length chosen supplies the hair shape (not the style). The busier the woman, the more she veers these days to what can only be called *a perfect length of hair* – one she can easily set herself after a shampoo and conditioner.

There Isn't a Set Length like an Army Regulation

The perfect length of hair *for you* depends on a number of things. Everything a top stylist takes into consideration, you should and can take into consideration yourself when tackling the job of finding the right length and style.

When a new client comes into a salon, a good stylist will mentally note height, shape, proportion of head to body and the way she walks. When she sits down, he will study face shape, head shape and bone structure.

Next, if he really knows his rattail comb, he will ask a few questions to establish the sort of style that will work best with her lifestyle, environment, climate and so on.

Frequently a new client is sitting in his chair because she has either (a) read about his work or seen his styles in a magazine or (b) admired a girlfriend's new style and found out the name of the stylist responsible.

But what the new client has in mind and what is *possible* may be two totally different things. 'You can't fight nature', says Vidal Sassoon, for maybe the ten-thousandth time in his life. 'When you do, clients get disappointed when the result doesn't fit the mental picture they have of themselves.'

The best stylists – those 'hairdressers with a conscience' I mentioned earlier – never attempt the impossible. They will cut, style, colour and comb out only according to the ability of the hair to perform. Once the initial meeting has taken place and the stylist knows the texture of the hair, the way it grows out of the scalp, the way it falls around the head, the experienced operator will 'produce' with no more worries – except possibly when he has to explain to a determined client why the style she wants isn't possible, why the style he suggests instead is better for her.

Dina Azzolini of Milan, one of the best cutters in the business, puts it this way:

Obviously, haircutting and styling must fit a customer's personality, which goes beyond prettiness. The style *has* to work with her life. If she lives on a farm and gets up at 6 a.m. every day, she will want her hair to work one way. If she's an actress in the theatre, who sleeps till noon and works till 1 a.m., she will need something else. Psychological research is the best part of my work – my shop in Milan can't be compared to the conventional expensive hairdressing salon. You can come here from 9 a.m. to 7.30 p.m. to relax, lunch, bath, take a massage, buy something from the boutique, and *discuss your hair* – even if this isn't the day you want to do anything about it.

New Looks for Old

The beguiling thought of a new image creeps into every woman's mind from time to time, hence the big snip that Mrs Levitt gambled on and won, the long curly postiche that Princess Margaret used to pin to her natural crown, waiting for her own hair to grow to that same length (alas, it never did quite make it – hair growth varies a great deal from person to person, see page 148), and the total change in Barbra Streisand's looks ever since, at boyfriend Jon Peters' insistence (an ex-hair-stylist himself), she grew her hair and crimped it

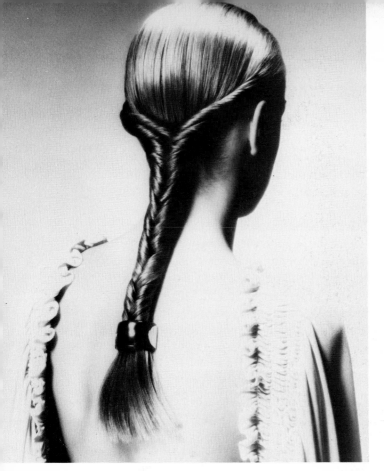

The 'Pony Plait' by
Michael of
Michaeljohn

COURTESY MICHAELJOHN

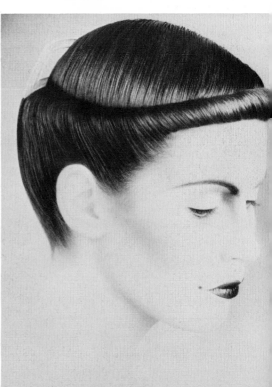

'The Roll' by
Robert of
Michaeljohn

COURTESY MICHAELJOHN

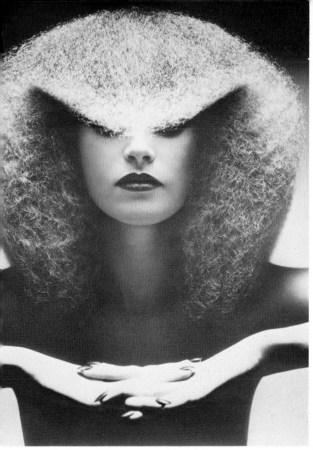

'Star Wars' – the perm of the future, by Robert of Michaeljohn

COURTESY MICHAELJOHN

The maxi-bob by Michaeljohn
COURTESY MICHAELJOHN

The 'Twist' by Robert of Michaeljohn
COURTESY MICHAELJOHN

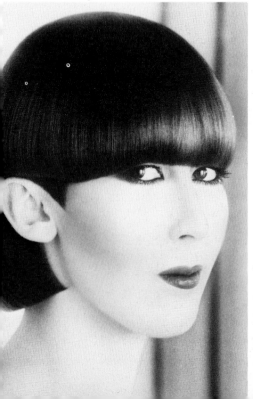

all over. Hair can make or break our looks – whatever clothes we put on our backs.

A good haircut is the easiest route to a new image. Skilful cutting can make thin hair appear thicker, limp hair bouncier, thick hair more manageable, and very long hair more graceful and contemporary looking.

Hair all one length is the easiest to have, taking less time to maintain because it's easier to handle. If you want it graduated, then the best graduation is found in the new dimensional cutting, where working to a chosen perimeter the hair is graduated only by $\frac{1}{64}$ inch (0.4 mm) all around the head. Here, as length grows so does shape. Out-of-shape does not happen.

A blunt cut is still the safest cut, however, for it leaves a firm, steady 'all-the-way-round' look, easily washed and blown dry, then worn as it falls, depending on the way each hair springs out of the scalp. One variation, carried out on very fine hair, involves lightly feathering the underneath hair so the outer layer turns under naturally. It looks like a blunt cut but the ends are more flexible. This is a job which calls for a professional. Don't try it yourself.

Hair cut with a razor often exposes too much of the inner hair shaft, allowing valuable protein and moisture to escape. This is bad,

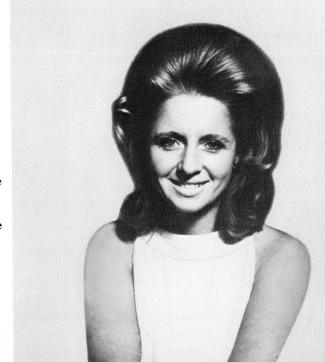

Remember the back-combed bouffant? The author had one in the mid-sixties

for remember the weakest part of your hair is at its ends, the *only* part not protected by the outer cuticle. The razor is a no-no.

How to Be Your Own Expert

When the hairstylist takes that first look at you in the mirror, if he's good he'll be trying to visualize you *without your hair*, trying to find 'your outline' whether it's oval, square or diamond.

If there's no expert near at hand, you can still work out a new style for yourself, one you can ask your local stylist to carry out with no fears of making a mistake.

If you have an *oval face*, you're lucky: you can wear almost any style, including the 'not-for-everyone' side parting, layered look with waves on both sides, hair tips lifted up with a hairpin to be light and fluffy.

Realize that a *round face* looks less round with a centre parting, hair gently falling across forehead and cheek bones, diminishing width, pinned back beneath ear lobes, covering ear tops, spiralling out in two bunches on both sides, behind the ears, lying close to the neck. This shape makes the top of the face look smaller than the bottom.

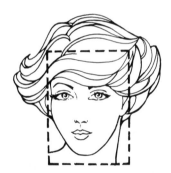 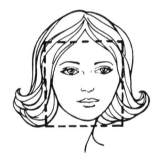

A *long face* can look prettier if a delicate fringe trails over the forehead and hair is combed out *wider* at the top than the bottom, pinned back just below the ears to fall gently, 'up' or 'under', just above the shoulders.

A *square face* needs a hairstyle to 'round' and soften it, with ends flipping up on both sides, and just the suggestion of a centre parting. To break up hard angles, hair should be combed smoothly close to the head at the temples, brushing gently over the cheekbones.

If face shape is short and fat, hair should be worn *high* above the ears, close and flat at the sides to brush over cheekbones and temples.

If your nose is large, try a curly or smooth ponytail occasionally to divert the eye with hair massed at the back of the head, pinned high to fall to midneck. Length at the back of the head brings the nose into proportion. Don't wear a ponytail every day – it can lead to 'spot' baldness (see page 150). Conversely, a fringe helps a *small nose* look more important.

If your neck is short, the hair should have height on top, being worn close to the head at back and sides to add a sense of length. Hair pulled back to create space behind the ears is 'neck-lengthening'.

If your jaw juts out, strands of hair curling on to the face below the ears, following the jawline to just below the eyes, takes away the jutting effect.

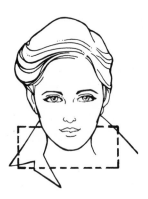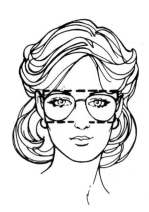

For *girls who wear glasses* an away-from-the-face style, with hair lifted at the crown and full over the ears, can look great. Hairstyles must never be too severe or too fluffy for girls with glasses; earrings should be part of the picture.

Hair swept up on top of the head adds length to any face.

Hair brought out in wings on either side of the ears adds width.

Hair brushed back, away from the face, or worn flat close to the head, makes a face appear larger.

Hair brushed over forehead and across cheeks makes a face appear smaller.

Hair massed on the crown or at the back of the crown takes away the impression of a small chin.

Hair massed low in a knot on the nape 'modifies' a long neck.

Check Your Cut against Your Hair Type

A cut must have *shape, fullness and movement*, all easily obtained if hair is healthy, straight or curly.

Really straight hair lies close to the head, and often obstinately refuses to stay back or away from the face after it's been shampooed, dried, and even set. Its natural movement is *down* and *forward* – the sort of hair that has to have a good cut to behave! The straighter the hair, the less it should be thinned out, for every bit of thickness helps hair have natural curve at the ends, while the added weight helps keep the cut's shape.

Although a layered cut takes a lot of maintenance, it looks great on straight hair, cut while wet, moulded to head shape. After the hair has been set in rollers and dried, each 'curl' is trimmed individually as it's combed out so each layer knows its place, and measures about 2½ inches (6¼ cm) long, except at the nape, where the hair is tapered to an inch (2½ cm) or less.

A fringe goes well with a layered cut, either the full deep kind or a soft half fringe. A wide face looks especially good with half fringe and layered look, both 'cutting down' face width, while a long face is 'shortened' with a deep fringe swept over to one side or the other. On a high forehead, a fringe looks best if it's long and wispy, while a low forehead should keep to the shortest fringe of all, hair merely breaking

The author with a snappy, businesslike short cut as woman's editor of the *Evening Standard* in 1960, and a new look for *Harper's Bazaar* in 1970

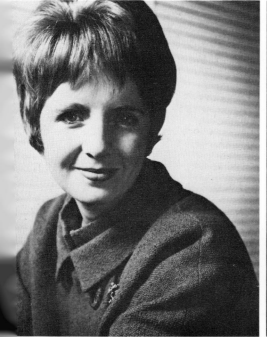
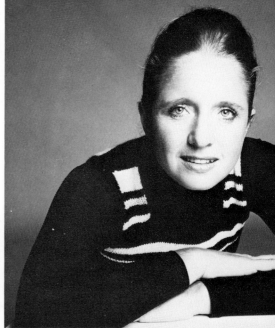

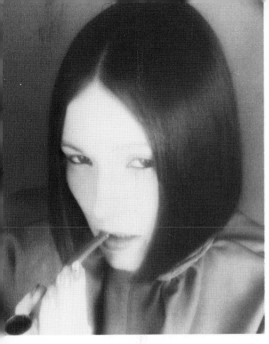

Really straight hair is the sort that needs a good cut, because it will benefit so much from it

in what look like natural tendrils (lightly permed on straight hair), leaving remainder of the hair straight but curving up or under.

Perming no longer needs to be applied to the whole head. Now it's a matter of 'perming in the right places', often only to add body and bounce, not curl. Today's perms bear little resemblance to the permanent waves of yesterday that concentrated on delivering what the consumer thought she wanted, a baked, immovable unlovely head of hair!

Naturally curly hair or hair that takes perms well can be groomed and maintained more easily than straight because curl adds life to hair.

Curly hairs needs a *blunt cut* to bring out maximum curl and good direction.

A wide face looks especially good with bangs and a layered look

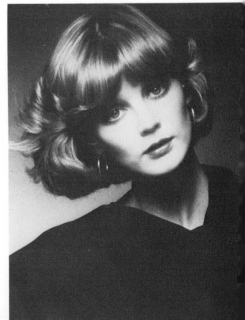

If hair is excessively curly, it should be kept one length, tapered at the ends. If cut *too short*, however, coarse, curly hair can end up looking like a brush; if left even a fraction *too long*, it can be unwieldy.

For the easiest handling, use a setting lotion on curly hair, combed through while the hair is wet, before setting it on the largest size rollers. When the hair is dry and curlers are out, two brushes are better than one for brushing the hair *flat* all round the head, holding hair in place, brushing until a real wave pattern emerges, but one that's controlled by its session with the setting lotion.

The only way to avoid over-curliness with perms, home variety or salon, is to ensure that the hair is in tip-top condition before the event, and if you are 'doing-it-yourself' follow the instructions to the letter!

If a natural over-abundance of curls is getting you down, straightening is one answer, using a method that's similar to perming. Perming softens hair until it relaxes to take on the new shape applied to it, when a neutralizer *fixes* in the new shape, until the hair grows out. Straightening works the same way – except that when suitably softened it's set to be *straight*, then neutralized into that position.

Fine hair is harder to straighten than coarse – unfortunately, fine hair has more problems whichever way you look at it. However good the straightening agent, in damp weather a little frizz can rise to the fore, in which case that old standby, a hard-hold setting lotion, has to go into action.

Although straightening lasts as long as perming (depending on how fast the hair grows), the problem of new growth is more tricky

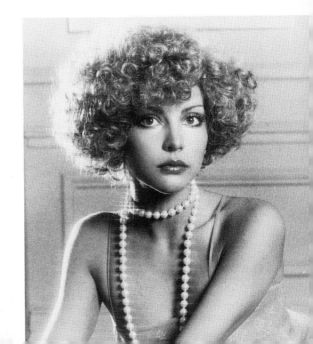

If hair is excessively curly, it should be kept to one length, only tapered at the ends – or would you rather wear a wig?

to deal with. A growing out permanent stays curly at the ends – where curl is needed most! A straightened head of hair grows in curly near the scalp – where curl is needed least.

Very curly hair doesn't work so well if blown dry. It's best set conventionally with rollers, followed by root lifting with a curling iron to get the maximum kinks out.

Sometimes there will be curl in some parts of the hair and not in others, or the stylist may decide to take curl out of one place and put it in another, using a blow dryer to 'brush out' natural curl, producing a smooth surface, putting curl in with a curling iron only at the ends.

If you find the style you like to wear doesn't stay, however hard you work, and your hair is in good condition, it could be you're working *against* nature and so fighting the way your hair wants to go. It's always easier, as Vidal says, to go with nature.

If you're letting your hair grow, a basic blunt cut, chin length at front, a little longer at back, can be maintained easily and inexpensively, as it only needs a slight trim about once every six weeks, the shape growing only into a longer version of itself. The best blunt cut starts at the nape, then works around to the front on both sides.

Beauty editors are fond of wearing this look themselves for two reaons: time and money. A layered cut is the costliest, in time and money, needing reshaping and cutting often. Another minus: it isn't easy to set oneself – mostly needs professional help.

If you feel you need extra height – and most people do, few being able to get away with just a flat crown – backcombing *without* teasing ('teasing' means the wrong sort of backcombing) is necessary. This means hair is combed only at the roots, where it's new and strong and where it isn't so visible, hair being smoothed over the backcombing to give a light, airy look. Later, the backcombing must be combed out, not brushed or tugged. Take each strand one at a time and work back through the length of the strand, inch by inch, until the comb moves freely. Brushing, backcombing, tugging and pulling, only breaks the hair.

The no-set, blow-dry style depends more on hair condition for its good looks than any other. When the hair looks like a cap of shining silk, cut sensationally, it puts any elaborate style in the shade – but the shine must be one of *health*. The no-set, blow-dry style works best when front hair is short enough to be lifted by hand drying, holding its shape with plenty of thickness at the back. Hand drying, using only moderate heat, can produce a look of vibrant, moving hair.

MODELS' HAIR TAKES A BEATING. Models often have thin, flyaway hair, because it's overworked hair that often has to put up with four changes of style a day, involving hot rollers, combs and plenty of hairspray.

To compensate for this wear and tear, most professional models shampoo their hair every two days with a protein-rich conditioning shampoo. When their hair is really in trouble, they use homemade rinses of rosemary and stinging nettle tea to strengthen it and build 'body'.

Because they 'live' with hot rollers during their working lives, most models would never dream of using them when they don't have to, preferring instead to set hair while damp on a myriad of very small curlers or even rag-curls, then sitting under an infra-red lamp for a very s-l-o-w drying session. Hot rollers should never be used every day by anyone.

The Comb-out

The transition between set and finished look obviously depends on who is behind the hair and the rollers. Practice makes perfect, and if you follow these rules for using heated rollers, devised by David Canyon, one of the best and fastest comb-out experts in New York, you'll get maximum results:

1 Don't move around while using rollers. Sit tight instead for the ten minutes necessary, five to curl and five to comb out. Once the hot rollers are installed, the heat lasts about five minutes, all that's necessary to put in curl.

2 Choose roller size according to hair type. Hair that's coloured absorbs heat faster than uncoloured hair, so the largest rollers should be used here to avoid an overtight curl. Fine hair also curls more easily than heavy, thick hair, so again use the largest size.

3 Divide hair into sections, pinning it out of the way.

4 Start curling on the left-hand side in clockwise direction (unless you're left-handed, when you should start on the right).

5 Hold section of hair straight up from the root and angle it sharply towards the face. Start winding roller in hair as if winding up a ribbon, being sure to keep the same angle to the face.

6 Use three large rollers on top; when unpinned these will give extra volume to any style. Still angle out every piece of hair towards the face before winding. Don't have straggly ends. Use the smallest rollers at the nape.

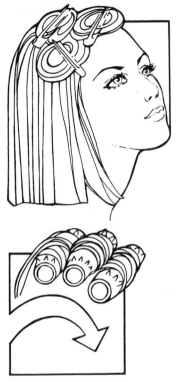
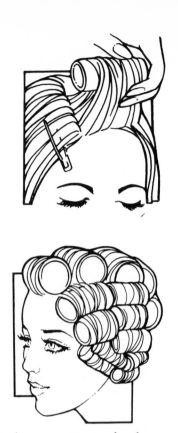

7 Unwinding is as important as winding up. Do it slowly to avoid snarling.

8 Brush out all over with a bristle brush.

9 Backcomb with a fine-tooth comb near roots. When hair is very thick, you can backcomb the ends, too. Use hands. Brush and comb to smooth, and place hair in position.

10 Don't use hot rollers every day. They dry hair and dirty it fast, because direct heat on the scalp attracts oil to the surface, which in turn attracts pollutants.

If you get good results curling your hair with hot rollers, you must check ends frequently. You will probably have to trim more often than usual.

Don't use heavy hair sprays in an attempt to keep your comb-out going strong in humid weather. It makes the hair droop all the more. Do as they do in humid Rio. Use only vegetal products or, if possible, no spray at all – it's too heavy for the hair to bear in a humid atmosphere.

For the comb-out following a shampoo and set at home with

ordinary non-heated curlers, keep drier on moderate heat while you carefully remove curlers. Let hair rest for a minute before brushing. Brushing actually helps the set last, not the reverse, and takes away any marks the rollers may have made.

Section hair according to the style you're after. If you want the ends to flip up, place a hand firmly over bottom half of hair and brush hair up around it. If you want it to turn under, place hand *under* bottom hair and brush down and around in a curve. Spray hair lightly, lifting side hair with brush, fluff it down around brush, then spray again to hold.

THE UNAPPRECIATED ACCESSORY

One way to see if a new style is going to suit you is to practise first with test-tube hair – with a wig. The wig has come a long way from the heavy, unventilated 'hard hat' of the past – worn mostly for cover-up reasons by those with poor hair, or, alas, no hair to speak of. Now wigs are fashion accessories, easy, pretty and *practical* to wear – once you get into the habit.

Getting into it is the problem. Wigs are still not appreciated for the contribution they could make, because most women fail to realize how very useful they can be.

A wig won't bite. You can comb it, brush it, trust it – almost as much as your own hair. You can cut it if it's too long, curl it if it's too straight, and, with some fibres, even change its colour – although there's hardly any point to that, and a certain amount of lustre may be lost.

One wig manufacturer (a woman) puts it this way – 'A wig is one way you can be released from the burden of coping with your own hair every day.' That's the way Arlene Dahl feels about wigs. Eva Gabor, Carol Channing and Carol Burnett, too – all of whom whisk into a wig in no time at all.

When you go wig shopping for the first time, always look at the base to check it's well sewn and – even more important – well ventilated. It should look quite lacy, and weigh no more than three ounces in your hand and on your head.

Wigs made from real hair, ironically, gave them the 'difficult' reputation in the first place. No wonder. To cope with *somebody else's hair* on your head when you can't cope with your own doesn't seem to make sense.

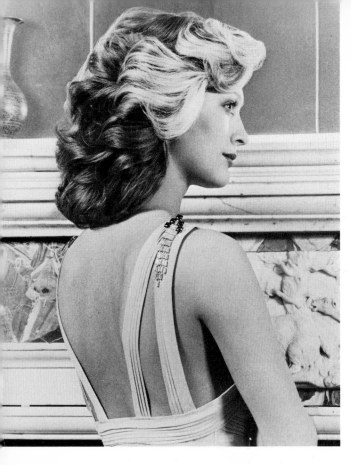

Quick change – from dark to light, from smooth to wavy – with the latest wig

Take *time* choosing a wig – just as you would when choosing a dress, because perfect *fit* is all important, leading to the day when you wear a wig so naturally you forget you have it on. If you're always thinking, 'I'm wearing a wig', it's a sure giveaway. For the more you think about it, the more you'll touch it, fuss with it, and eventually spoil it.

Unless you're contemplating a total colour change and want to experiment with a wig in the new colour first, choosing one close to your own colour, maybe one shade darker or lighter, makes more sense. Remember, wigs *are* part of fashion, *not* fancy dress.

When you try one on, don't be surprised if it doesn't fit 100 per cent – unless it's custom-made, an unnecessary expense today.

In most cases you'll have to maximize or minimize your own hair, *maximizing* by pinning hair into a knot or chignon on top of your head, *minimizing* by combing hair down completely flat around your head, the ends pinned into flat 'rings' at the ends. If you have to do too much 'minimizing', the wig is too tight. Too much 'maximizing', it's too big. Choose again.

180

If you're timid about the whole idea, yet know it would help your life, try one with a full or half fringe or a hairline that curls over your own, so there's no need to use any of your own hair in front. When you're more practised, for a totally natural look, curl about 1½ inches (3¼ cm) of your own hair in front into a roller; this will completely merge with your 'test tube' hair, providing you've chosen one in your own colour!

Put all wigs on front to back, like putting on a bathing cap. Pull it down on both sides at ear level, wiggling it into position, using large hairpins to pin it *securely* on the crown, on both sides, above the ears and at centre back. *Security is everything.*

If you're using some of your own hair, take out front roller and brush your own hair over the wig's hairline. Use a metal brush (no static) to add finishing touches, but above all *don't be afraid to pull, to move the wig about into the shape and mood you want.*

Shake your head when it's on; gesticulate as you normally do to see that it moves when you move, effortlessly.

Wigs Need Care, Too

Wigs don't need as much washing as your own hair, but they do need washing at least after every ten to fifteen wearings. Swish through gentle warm suds, rinse, shake out. Today's wig dries as quickly as a pair of tights but, unlike tights, it's made to return to its original shape.

Never brush or comb a wet wig – it can stretch the fibre out of shape. When dry, use a wide-toothed comb to get the most natural looking result.

Don't squash it while it's drying. Hang it on a doorknob or anywhere where air circulates, but not too near direct heat.

The best hairstylists plead, 'Don't ask too much of your hair.' I say don't ask too much of your wig either. It's been designed to do an efficient job, so doesn't need endless teasing – although cutting and shaping the right way can't do any harm.

Some advantages of wigs over real hair:

They don't droop in damp or humid conditions.

They don't get sticky with pollution (the fibre is non-absorbent and non-porous).

They don't fade or oxidize in the sun and change colour.

They don't get brittle in the cold.

They don't lose their hairs (unless you pull them out), get thinner or duller, or go grey.

They don't take hours to wash and dry, however long the style.

Wigs can transform looks for the better in the shortest time, providing (1) the choice is right for head shape, skin tone and proportion and (2) plenty of practice is given to putting them on – not just twenty minutes before the big evening, but regularly every day.

Once it's second nature to wear a wig, you'll appreciate that a wig can be the most useful accessory you own.

DOES SHE OR DOESN'T SHE COLOUR HER HAIR?

Does Anybody Care Anymore?

A colour change for hair is no longer a secret. On the contrary, exchanging colourists' names is a fairly common trade, while wearing a Michaeljohn colour is as significant as wearing a Michaeljohn cut. Marinella, who heads the Michaeljohn colouring department, plays colour Merlin to a number of famous ladies, who look as if they were born beautifully blonde or brunette, so skilfully does she match hair shade to skin shade. Following the late-seventies' emphasis on 'natural looking hair' Marinella likes to leave clients' hair colour as natural looking as possible.

Women may chat about their new 'lights' or 'brights', but men still rarely mention theirs, although the number of men colouring their hair increases every year.

However, despite the colossal increase both in expertise and in the range of products available in the past decade, there's still a huge number of women out there who don't *touch* the colour of their hair, whether it's the colour of yesterday's floor mop or the neglected family silver. In Britain, the highest percentage of haircolouring is carried out in the South while disinterest is at its height in Scotland. In the U.S., the highest percentage of coloured heads appear in California – where you'd think the sun would be doing it naturally – while disinterest is at its height in New England.

Where Your Natural Colour Comes From

Your natural hair colour depends on two pigments: melanin (black-brown) and pheomelanin (red-orange-yellow). These pigments are found in the cortex of the hair (see page 148), and the amount you have of either – handed down from your ancestors, along with your genes – determines the colour you write down on your passport.

As we grow up, the cortex thickens: our hair colour appears deeper because pigment concentration is greater. This explains why so many ash-blonde babies change into medium-brown-haired teenagers (commonly known as mousy). It's because the pigment becomes more concentrated as the years go by. When a baby stays ash blonde, it's because there's so little pigment in the cortex, only a small amount of concentation is possible.

The enzyme responsible for the production of pigment starts to decrease in the body after forty, which explains every grey hair on your head – just a lack of new pigment.

Hiding grey was the first – and is still the major – reason for colouring hair. Next in line comes the urge so many women have to go blonde, or at least to *lighten* their hair.

There's still a subtle sexual reason for wanting to be blonde. As many brunettes know, it's continually stressed that the blonde has more fun, and not only by Anita Loos, who wrote a book on the subject! Whoever heard of a true blonde wanting to change to brunette? It's a much easier colouring job, but it just doesn't happen – unless the lady's a spy!

Two Routes to Colouring not Three

Although hair-colouring companies tell you there are three sorts of colouring products, temporary, semi-permanent and permanent – there are essentially only two; those that wash out and those that don't. The wash-out variety includes those products labelled as temporary or semi-permanent, the temporary washing out with the first shampoo, the semi-permanent washing out more slowly – colour actually seeping away with each wash, and often completely out after six or seven shampoos, particularly if the shampoo used isn't the kind specially formulated for 'hair that's coloured'.

Wash-outs

Wash-out products *coat* hair, as make-up coats skin. They don't contain peroxide (an oxide containing a large proportion of oxygen), so in no way can they alter the *basic colour* of hair. But, depending on the colour you were born with, they *can* considerably *enhance* it, adding 'lights' and lustre, making the hair *look* more beautiful, because new shine gives a suggestion of *texture*.

RINSES. *If your hair is naturally light to medium brown*, you can have a lot of fun with temporary products (usually called rinses). You can highlight, darken, tone down any red notes or add red.

If your hair is dark, rinses don't have much impact, except to leave a fleeting touch of red if you choose a bright-red rinse. They can add a suggestion of brightness, however, bringing out your own lurking highlights.

THE REASON FOR USING A SEMI-PERMANENT. Semi-permanent products give a more intense effect than temporary ones if you want a more intense or different effect. They contain organic derivatives (as do the 'permanent real-colour-change tints') but no peroxide, so they can't *lighten* colour, but they can brighten, darken or blend in grey far more substantially than rinses.

The colour in semi-permanents also coats hair, but the film on the cortex 'grabs' hold more firmly than the temporary efforts.

If you've never touched your hair colour and it's nondescript, even drab, it's time to start. Using a semi-permanent product is one way you can appreciate how a real colour change would affect your looks. The built-in safety valve is that, if you don't like it, you know you're only a few shampoos away from returning to your natural colour.

Today this type of product usually offers side benefits. Packed with conditioners, it's easily applied, either by being shampooed in or foamed on to clean hair.

A lotion semi-permanent is concentrated to give stronger colour than the more popular sprayed on version, which is full of air, and acts as an oxidizing agent, so that mixing is eliminated.

For the best results first time around, stay within your own natural hair-colour range, and choose either from warm colours (all with a touch of red) if that's your hair type, or cool colours (no red at all) if your hair tone is pale. Don't disregard your skin tone either. Too great a contrast between skin and hair looks unnatural, which is the reason it's safe to advise everyone to go lighter as they get older, *never* darker. Skin tone fades so even on the once naturally raven-haired, an overly dark colour can look unnatural and harsh.

One-Step Big Time

Hair-colour language is confusing, although the companies do their best to translate the technicalities. Their problem is a familiar one to all manufacturers – the customer doesn't read the instructions – or certainly not carefully enough. Yet it's not only *sensible* to do so when contemplating a colour change for the hair, it's *essential*.

Using a permanent hair colour rather than a temporary one is, for instance, as different as borrowing from buying, because using a permanent product means you've made a commitment to your hair, one that involves constant maintenance.

A one-step permanent product (also known as a single process) can colour or lighten hair. You can darken it to any shade you want, but you can only lighten it to a certain degree, depending on the colour you already are.

A one-step permanent colour job, as the name implies, can't be removed with a shampoo. With this process, hair colour is really changed. The outer cuticle, which we see, is softened with chemical ingredients so that the new colour can penetrate right through to nature's paintbox, the cortex, where new colour is deposited to merge with whatever natural pigment is already there.

Once natural pigment is removed to make hair lighter, or tinted to make hair darker and different, the natural colour will never return to the treated hair. Only new growth emerging at the roots will change the picture, bringing back the natural pigmentation. The hair has to be constantly lightened or tinted if you want to stay with your new look, so obviously maintenance is key, something to be considered before you make the move.

All processes described as 'permanent' work in an alkaline medium, 'unlocking' the hair cuticle in order to let the new colour in, a neutralizer then 'shutting' it tight to keep it in. This means colour seepage can occur through the use of highly alkaline shampoos. They can't remove colour, but they can subtly change it, which is not what you had in mind. This is the main reason it's wise for those who colour their hair to use products, shampoos and conditioners specially formulated to maintain colour. Read the labels.

HOW TO CHOOSE THE RIGHT COLOURS FOR YOU. The colours shown on the product charts relate to how they appear on white hair which is why they're printed on white paper to show the shade in the truest way – with no colour interference.

Unless your hair *is* the colour of white paper – unlikely – you must take into account the fact that the colour you select on the chart will obviously be affected by the hair colour you already have. A red tint, for instance, on medium-brown hair will result in reddish-brown hair, not true flaming red (who wants it?); on a blonde, it will achieve a lighter red; on a dark brunette, it will be less apparent. Bear all this in mind when you study the colours and work out the possible effect your own colour will have, diluting the colour you choose or strengthening it.

Don't automatically choose the colour you remember you once were. As already mentioned, skin tone fades as the years go by, so hair colour should never be in too much contrast. Very dark shades are ageing for the over-forties. As Alexandre of Paris says: 'Lighter *is* younger.' If you were raven-haired at twenty, be content with chestnut at forty-five, even butterscotch at sixty. That way you won't have to regret the past.

WHAT TO BEWARE! All permanent hair-colour products contain peroxide or a similar substitute mixed with aniline derivative dyes – and that means strong chemicals, strong enough to penetrate the hair shaft in order to make a definite colour switch. For this reason, a patch test to check on possible skin sensitivity is paramount.

A patch test means mixing the colour chosen with a developer and applying a tiny drop behind the ear. It should be left there for twenty-four hours before hair is to be coloured. If any irritation at all develops, the message is clear: Don't use the preparation. It's a warning you're allergic to it.

Rubber or plastic gloves are included in do-it-yourself hair-colouring kits. They're there to be used, to protect fingernails which, like hair, are made of keratin, so can absorb the colour you want your hair to be – not the object of the exercise.

Obviously, any do-it-yourself hair colouring needs great care. Every label should be read and totally understood. Mishaps are costly. You can't wipe them away as you wipe away the wrong colour lipstick.

HAIR COLOUR SCARE. The effect on health by all hair colouring products is obviously a very important issue. Recently in the U.S., consumer attention has been drawn to reports that certain hair dye ingredients produced positive results in tests on bacteria and high dose feeding of animals. On the basis of these results, various scientists announced their conclusions: that these materials might be carcinogenic or mutagenic in humans. Although it was qualified by statements such as 'attempts to make quantitative correlations between the amount of activity in our test and carcinogenic or mutagenic potency for humans is certainly premature', the disclosures set alarm bells ringing from coast to coast, not only in the companies producing hair colouring products, but also among the millions of Americans colouring their hair on a regular basis.

In Britain, in answer to a parliamentary query on the subject on 29 June 1976, John Fraser, Minister of Prices and Consumer Protection, stated 'studies in the United States of America and the United Kingdom have shown mutagenic effects in some hair dyes. But long term carcinogenicity tests have so far produced no evidence that these dyes produce cancer. Further studies are being carried out and I am keeping the matter under review in consultation with the government's medical advisors. In the meantime, I do not consider there is any need to refer this matter to the Medical Commission.'

In an article in December of the same year, Professor G. D. Harndan of the University of Birmingham stated, 'it must be made clear there is no evidence of carcinogenicity of hair dyes in human beings'.

Naturally, however, there is consumer concern, but to put the matter in the right perspective it must be pointed out that the report to cause the latest (and most loudly expressed) concern was one in which rats and mice were apparently fed massive doses of one hair dye ingredient at a level equivalent to a woman drinking 25 bottles of hair dye a day every day of her life. On the basis of this, it is obviously difficult to reach conclusions.

On the other hand, the hair colouring industry on both sides of the Atlantic, has sponsored five studies in which animals were painted with hair dyes containing this same controversial ingredient throughout their lifetime without producing cancer. Four important studies – conducted by the American Cancer Society, and scientists at Oxford, Toronto and Yale Universities – show no difference between cancer rates among people heavily exposed to hair dyes and those who are not. Of particular interest to note is a thirteen-year study, still being conducted, which shows no difference in cancer mortality between a group of 5,000 hairdressers and that of a matched group of non-hairdressers. These results are important to pass on because they represent *human* experience – one step beyond animal studies. This, together with a sixty-year-old history of safe use of hair colour by millions of women (plus the daily applications of skin painting on animals), continue to confirm the safety of hair dyes.

Everyone knows it's 'better to be safe than sorry', but it's equally important to know the exact facts. Then it's up to the individual concerned to decide for her or himself the step she or he wants to take – to colour or not to colour.

Blonde Fever

Thousands of women still decide to go 'blonde' each year. This increases the overall number of women who colour their hair, but it also includes a great many who, after colouring their hair for years, feel the first urge to go the whole blonde route.

Going blonde all the way is easy if you can number yourself in the light-brown to mid-brown haired family. If, however, you're a jet-haired swinger, who feels she's a delicate Dresden doll at heart, it isn't easy, although it's possible. (I don't recommend it. Think of your skin tone – and reflect long and hard. Better still, study yourself in a blonde wig.)

DOUBLE THE PROCESS FOR THE BIG COLOUR CHANGE. Jet black hair that wants to be pale blonde has to travel through *seven stages of lightening:* from black down to dark brown, to brown, to red, to red-gold, then gold, yellow, and finally to pale, almost white yellow. The one-step colour process just described can't cope with this exercise. This is where the two-step (or double) permanent colouring process enters the picture.

The first half of the double process is to make dark hair light, which really means, as already described, that the hair loses its natural colour, the one present in the cortex.

During the second half of the process a toner is applied – and it is the toner that gives the hair exactly the shade of blonde required, whether it's the amber variety, strawberry, or even a silver of Siamese cat subtlety.

A toner can only do its job properly and produce the colour you've really set your heart on when the hair is paler than the toner chosen. Then, when new hair starts breaking through, the lightener then the toner only need to be applied to the roots.

This sort of operation *can* be carried out at home – there are products that achieve a double-process job superbly – but where there's any doubt (about hair condition, about the ability to achieve exactly the colour required) expert advice is the answer. *Your hair deserves it.*

Hair colouring at home often falls down in this advanced category because the right timing is not observed. *As with everything in life, timing here is all-important.* Double-process permanent colour application is a delicate matter, balanced between timing, mixing, and colour choice.

When the lightening part of the process takes place – on dry, ultraclean hair – the more time allowed to elapse, the paler the hair can become.

If not enough time is given to this major step, the toner can't produce the colour required because it gets added to the hair at the wrong stage of lightening – say at gold instead of yellow. The lightening operation also has another function: to make the hair sufficiently porous for a toner to operate properly.

As porous hair is weak hair, it needs *constant conditioning* – something that has to be stressed for hair that regularly goes through a colouring process. For example, while a medium to light brown-haired person needs to leave on a lightener for a minimum of thirty to forty-five minutes (that includes the grey or white-haired, too), a dark brunette may have to lighten twice to reach the right stage of light and correct porosity. As there has to be twenty-four hours at least between each lightening trip, that means a very lengthy time-consuming job – something all brunettes should consider before making the final decision.

Expert help shouldn't be ignored if hands aren't that steady – for lighteners vary in strength. If you're light-haired, you need only a mild one. If you're very dark, the strongest version has to be used.

There are a multitude of colours to choose from, but a pro can make sure you immediately pick the right one for your colouring and so avoid costly mistakes. Another good reason for going to a colour pro for all this is that he or she will keep a record, just like a doctor, of what exactly has been put on your hair and for how long. On your 'record', it will also state exactly how long it takes for your hair to achieve the right degree of lightness, and it will also include any notes on the texture and strength of your hair that need to be remembered. All this obviously makes life easier – but then if you're diligent, you can always keep an exact record yourself. In this area, it *has* to be exact.

Witches with Colour

Hair colouring really comes into its own in the beauty salon, where customers tend to be as loyal to their colourist as they are to their doctor or dentist.

Faye Dunaway, for instance, wouldn't dream of letting anyone but colourist Rosemary keep her pale blonde looking exactly the same pale blonde around the clock, which means Rosemary, living and working in New York, often has to make the three-thousand-mile trip to California to maintain Faye's colour, when she can't get away from the film set.

Marinella, at the leading Michaeljohn Salon in London, is known to be another witch with colour. She has been master-minding the hair colour changes of the stars for quite a while, too, and was the one to introduce Gayle Hunnicut to an auburn life (one-step permanent process). Her favourite idea involves picking a natural highlight from the client's original hair colour, then incorporating highlights of that colour over the tinted base. Where a complete colour change is required, the client's skin and eye colouring are used as a guide in selecting the appropriate shade. Marinella also likes to highlight either with a bleach or tint to give a burnished tortoiseshell effect. This method of hair colouring with highlights alone leaves no distinct demarcation line when the tint grows out.

There's also a growing popularity for the use of henna on both sides of the Atlantic. This is not surprising, in view of the controversy over the safety of hair dyes (see page 186), for henna is a natural product with the colour coming from the henna plant, which makes it a vegetable dye. White henna only provides a shine and adds body, while the more generally known red covers grey, but again, the depth of the colour depends on the length of time it stays on the hair. Marinella mixes coffee with red henna for Rula Lenska, the 'Rock Follies' star, to give the effect of heavy highlighting, so that her hair appears to be a myriad of colours.

The most important thing all colour experts take pains to avoid is a 'solid' look of colour for, just as skin is never one colour, neither is hair. Anything to the contrary looks harsh, unnatural and desperately old-fashioned. Vidal Sassoon likes to use hair colour – often red henna – to define his superb haircuts. He makes hair appear more tapered through the delicate use of henna, the colour tapering away at the hair's edge, sharply defining the cut.

At Jingles in London, henna is also used for hair health. It is mixed in a super wax treatment conditioner, so that the vegetable dye adds strength and body throughout the head, as well as a burnished glow. This is particularly good for natural blondes or redheads.

How much colour, how often, and what to mix with what is

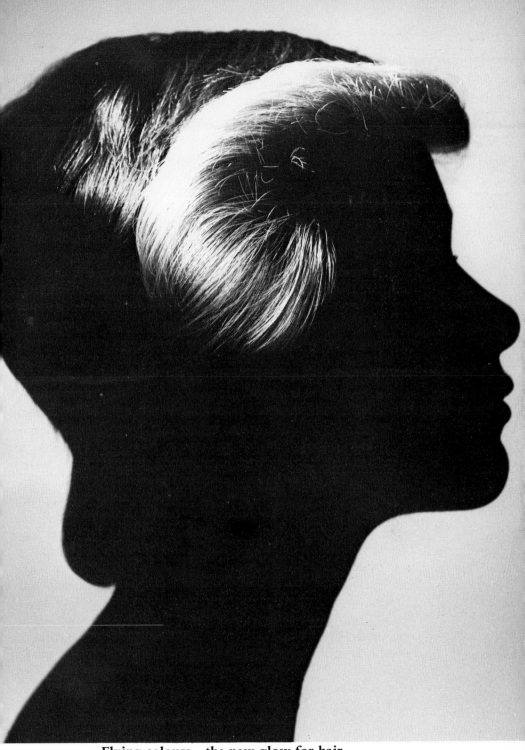

Flying colours – the new glow for hair

where the top colourists score and earn their reputations; they show their skill in determining the amount and exact shade of colour to be placed on each head. The biggest problem they face is making sure that the colour is accepted by the hair in a level way. This isn't as easy as it sounds, because hair differs naturally in its porosity. To get the same colour in the root area, for instance, as at the tip, plus achieving uniformity in a natural way (no 'solid' look of colour) colourists have to work like artists on a canvas.

They are secretive about their formulas and the way they use brand names in their own special way – and why not? Just as a chemist is known in the fragrance business for having a 'nose', the antennae for selecting the right ingredients to make a good scent (there aren't many of them – see page 345), so the top colourists are known for their inventive approach to products and people.

No wonder there's so much loyalty around in this business. There's a lot at stake when mistakes are so time-consuming and costly – in money and morale – to rectify.

Special Effects

Frosting, tipping and streaking are all special effects for the hair – effects that every woman can wear to advantage without looking in any way unnatural.

For frosting and tipping, the hair to be frosted is first pulled through the frosting cap, then lightened and toned using the double process method. A home kit will usually include a lightener, a developer, a colour rinse, a perforated cap through which individual hairs are drawn to be (double) 'processed', a hooked needle for drawing the hairs through, a mixing spoon and bowl, plastic gloves and a heat cap.

Streaking means lightening and colouring $\frac{1}{4}$-inch to $\frac{1}{2}$-inch ($\frac{1}{2}$-cm to $1\frac{1}{4}$-cm) hair sections all over the head – not recommended for hair that's already been treated or coloured.

With *hair painting*, a flat brush skims over the hair, leaving behind light ribbons with a special lightening formula (one-step process). Left on for about twenty minutes, the formula is then shampooed out, for the longer it's left on, the lighter – and so more unnatural – the 'ribbons' look. Because of the peroxide, the lights can't be washed out, and the result is shimmery and subtle. The extra beauty about hair painting is that it has only to be done every six months and it can be carried out both on hair that's already been treated by single process colouring and on virgin hair.

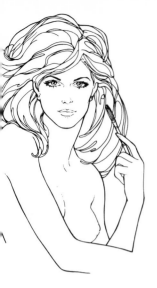

Hair painting, with a flat brush, to give 'ribbons' of lighter colour

Alas, it doesn't work as well for brunettes, as for the lighter (or mousy) haired. On dark hair, the 'ribbons' can resemble zebra stripes! In any case the lighter the hair, the more effective the result: light to medium brown being about the darkest candidate for this.

With all these effects, the object is to give a sense of light and airiness to the hair. Whenever you see 'lights' in somebody's hair, it's because light itself strikes through the translucent outer cuticle and glances off the coloured pigment deep inside the hair shaft. This 'see-through colour' is what gives hair its natural brightness, sense of life, and fascination. Modern hair colourings, whether used whole-headedly or in tipping, frosting, streaking and hair painting, help this reflection idea along. The special effects department is really for those who don't want the bother of frequent retouchings for, although the processes are permanent, as colour is not brought down to the roots where retouching has to take place with full scale colour, you get more than your money's worth.

To recap, *tipping hair* involves bleaching hair tips only. A *streaked* head is bleached in a few carefully planned sections. *Frosted hair* uses the specially designed cap described, where random strands are lightened all over the head. *Hair painting* – best on fair to mousy hair – lightens ribbons of hair with a flat brush.

Check-up at the Salon

Be sure on your first visit to a hair colourist that he or she examines your hair carefully, preferably in daylight. Artificial light can be misleading – you can end up with a shade you don't want to live with.

Make sure the colourist wraps your hair tightly around his or her finger – this way nature's own colouring mix is easily seen, the lightest to the medium to the dark. Make sure your roots are examined for the same reason.

If you don't know what colour you want, ask the colourist to make a trial run on a test cutting for security.

Don't contemplate a change of colour if you've just had a perm or straightening job. Too much chemistry in too short a time will damage hair. Leave at least two weeks between, preferably longer.

Remember that skin tone fades as you get older. Don't automatically choose the colour you remember you once were, if you're trying to hide grey. It's always safe to go a shade lighter.

If your skin is fair, stay with pale blonde shades, soft browns, even auburn. If you're under twenty-five, dark brown or even black hair can look stunning with pale skin – but only pale, *young* skin.

If your skin tends to be ruddy, it can look softer and paler with the right hair colour. Aim for beige lights. Discard anything red with a drabber, the product devised to get rid of too much red in the hair. (Every natural colouring, except pale blonde, has some red.)

Natural blondes or redheads should avoid reinforcing their natural colour when they think it's fading – it can look too harsh. Instead, they should reinstate their colouring with two-tone effects – streaking or frosting. As the kingpin Clairol advisor Leslie Blanchard puts it, 'Think of it this way, hot face (pink, rosy), cool hair (ash blonde, light brown). Cool face (pale, white), hot hair (warm mahogany, even some traces of red). Olive skin shouldn't try to be blonde, but should choose a brunette shade, and there are plenty of them.'

New York's Rose Reti, who once worked colour miracles for Mia Farrow, believes hair colouring can solve face-shape problems, too. She points out that a frame of light hair around the face 'widens' a skinny shape, but is disaster for a round one, turning it into a real moon. A round face should choose random lights throughout the hair to take the eye away from the round effect.

TOP COLOURISTS OF THE WORLD AGREE . . . Coloured hair *must* be protected from too much sun. Sun acts as an oxidizing agent, so that blonde becomes lighter but brassier, brunettes redder but harsher. Too much sun ruins the overall 'natural' effect, making hair colour patchy. It always takes away the natural oils, and so the effect of light and shine that hair colour gives.

Coloured hair needs regular scalp treatments, regular conditioning. Coloured hair is far more porous than non-coloured hair, therefore more vulnerable to every bad thing in the atmosphere.

Coloured hair must use only those shampoos and conditioners formulated for it to ensure colour is maintained correctly (no seepage, see page 185).

Do-it-yourself colouring is fine, providing directions are read as if it were a matter of life or death. It is – for the hair. Instructions are meant to be followed to the letter, and during an at-home hair-colouring session, there must be no interruptions. No 'quick phone calls'. The right timing is key!

Henna is helpful to poor hair (see page 190), providing the kind that gives colour is not used more than three times a year maximum because of the risk of colour build-up. Henna still changes colour subtly, adding lustre, and as it's a natural vegetable colour, there's no risk of irritation. Natural light blondes, however, should beware – it can turn their hair bright orange. Henna should also not be used on tinted or lightened hair.

You Can Get Addicted

If you start off with a few highlights, then move on to semi-permanent colour and finally decide on 'the works' and make a complete colour switch with a double process permanent colour job, you have to realize you've taken on a big commitment. Colour maintenance has to be part of your life, unless you intend to wear a covering hat for months, if you change your mind or are willing to shave off your hair in order to start all over again. If there's any chance you might move away from a big city, where the experts are, to an area without a pro in miles, delay any big colour switch – especially if you've never taken the step before.

Hair colouring can be a beautiful beauty treatment for hair, but for major recasting, an expert must be behind it – at least the first time.

QUICK-AT-A-GLANCE COLOUR DICTIONARY

ASH : hair colour without any red or gold tones, a natural blonde. For some extraordinary reason, many professional colourists describe it as 'drab'.

BASIC COLOUR : hair's natural shade.

BLEACH : a lightener that removes natural pigment either moderately (by a few shades) or drastically (ten to twenty shades); it always employs peroxide.

COLOUR FILLER: a product used on damaged hair or hair that's been coloured so frequently that it's too porous, and needs 'filling' in before any more colour work can be carried out or when tinting back to a one-step process.

COLOUR SHAMPOO: shampoo devised for coloured hair, to maintain the new colour for as long as possible. Lower in alkaline content than most shampoos, it's designed to keep the new hair colour from 'seeping' away.

COLOUR TEST: a test before colouring to determine formula and timing, also called a strand test.

DEVELOPER: the chemical used in 'permanent' products that mixes with the tint, and then propels colour to develop on the hair, either hydrogen peroxide or a scientifically formulated substitute.

DRABBER: used to subdue undesirable red or harsh tones.

HALO LIGHTING: the crown hair is lightened; the underneath hair remaining dark.

MARBLE-IZING: interlacing sections of light and dark shades.

OXIDATION: the development of colour on the hair through the chemical union of oxygen with the colouring materials; this term also refers to an unwanted change in colour due to exposure to strong sunlight.

PATCH TEST: a method to determine if a client is hypersensitive to a hair-colouring product. A drop of the colouring product is applied behind the ear or in the elbow crease twenty-four hours before colouring takes place.

PICTURE FRAMING: a narrow section of hair is lightened one or two shades around the face for $1\frac{1}{2}$ to 2 inches ($3\frac{1}{2}$ to 5 cms).

PLASTIC CAP: used in semi-permanent colouring treatments to help hold in heat for colour development consistency, or with holes for use in 'frosting' (see page 192).

POROSITY: hair condition enabling it to accept colour changes. Porosity is increased by constant colouring, so over-bleaching can eventually impair hair's texture. (Overperming and too much straightening can also damage hair by increasing porosity.)

RESISTANT: hair condition that repels moisture or the action of chemicals – the opposite of porous – resists hair colouring, perming or straightening. May need medical help.

SHAMPOO TINT: a tint that cleanses as it colours.

STRAND TEST: the testing of a single strand of hair with a colour product to see if the proposed colour suits hair and skin tone.

TINT: a permanent hair colour that can cover grey and lighten or darken natural pigment.

TIPPING: lightening only the ends of selected strands throughout the head, seen to best advantage on short, dark hair.

VIRGIN HAIR: hair that has never had a tint, bleach, straightener or perm – has never been in contact with chemicals of any kind.

WHITE HENNA: a magnesium carbonate, highly alkaline, added to hydrogen peroxide in order to thicken and enrich the colouring solution.

The Dieting Game

PLAYED BY MARTYRS (11 stones trying
to be size 10)
AND MISSIONARIES (the size-8 Girl Friends)

TIMES change and time changes us. Elizabeth Taylor was once
a size 8 and a decade or so ago Sophia Loren could eat her way
through three courses of pasta in one meal without a pang or a
pound showing. Now Liz has doubled in size, and Sophia keeps pasta
strictly for Sundays – once a month. They are both unwittingly – and
unwillingly – representative of people living in well-developed
countries (statisticians never see any puns), where one in three of the
adult population is officially considered overweight.

The question is no longer to slim or not to slim, but *how*. In a
single week, across the country, it's possible to pick up at least twenty
different and apparently not too arduous ways to reduce in as many
magazines and newspapers. Few bear in mind, however, that while
twenty women may be fat, they will have twenty different reasons
for it.

THE CAUSES OF OBESITY

Obesity is never due to one cause – although it has now been proved
that it can relate to the presence in the body of a greater percentage of
fat cells than found in the generally lean. The body can regulate
weight, so that whereas the normal person unconsciously maintains
his or her weight at around 10 stone (63½ kg), the abnormal and obese
will reach 13½ stone (86 kg), before starting to maintain. Further,
experiments have shown that when the very obese (20 stoners, (127 kg),
lost as much as 10 stone (63½ kg), their number of fat cells remained
the same, the weight loss deriving from each cell shrinking in size.
The conclusion? Normal weight people have less fat cells than fat

'I'm hungry . . .'

people – small comfort to those permanently on a diet. There is a genetic reason behind this, but, although in adult life extra food only distends the cells, in infancy fat cells duplicate under the stimulus of extra food. So don't bring your daughter up to be a heavyweight.

As Dr Charles Read, an American professor of paediatrics, once advised, 'I suggest to parents, throw away the scales. Tell your youngsters to look in the mirror and decide whether they like what they see. It's their 'mirror weight' which is important. A child who is self-motivated does lose weight and maintains the loss.'

Deep in the brain is the part we have in common with all vertebrate animals, the diencephalon. In man, this is the vital part from which the central nervous system controls all automatic animal functions of the body – breathing, sleeping, sex, the urinary system, digestion and, via the pituitary gland, appetite. When it comes to the control of fat, its function can be – and has been – likened to that of a bank. When the body assimilates more food than it needs to live, the surplus is deposited in what may be compared to a 'current account', easily withdrawn when needed. All normal weight people carry their fat reserves in this 'current account'. When fat deposits grow rapidly with only a small number of withdrawals (in other words, the body is taking too much in and not spending enough), a point is reached when the 'current account' becomes unmanageable. Then the control system appears to set up a 'fixed deposit' (of fat), no longer so easily withdrawn and burnt up in day-to-day activity.

This is the beginning of obesity.

Thereafter, normal fat reserves are held at a minimum, the majority of the surplus being put away in the 'fixed deposit' and taken out of normal circulation.

So the chances are, the more you put on weight, the more risk you run of not being able to take it off without a major and mighty shake-up of your whole system. 'Tomorrow, I diet' just isn't the answer when the scales start creeping up. It isn't even a calculated risk, as the banker would say.

Admittedly, luck does enter into it. If you were born with an abnormally low fat-banking capacity, it means your 'current account' of normal fat reserve will reach its limit long before most people's, so a 'fixed deposit', hard to move, soon takes over the major banking of fat. This abnormal trait will show at an early age, in spite of normal feeding, which explains why in one family, all eating the same food at the same table, one person becomes obese while the others do not.

200

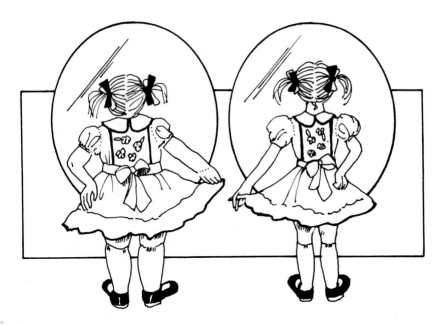

Start Thinking Thin Early

From the day we're born, eating is one of our first activities, second only to breathing in importance. By the time we're forty, we will have consumed about 50,000 meals. Add between-meals snacks, and the total is up by many thousands. We have assumed a regular pattern of eating. Because there's such an outstanding difference in dieting success between people who became obese as children and those who became obese as adults – the former finding it infinitely more difficult to lose weight – it's obviously imperative to establish the right eating habits during childhood.

In our society, it's the mother who teaches the child to over-eat, in order to earn her approval. So every mother should reflect as to whether she's inflicting the penalty of a heavyweight life on her child, and work out the right pattern of eating for every member of the family. Twiggy must have had a very sensible mother.

Some paediatricians are actually crusading for pictures of thin, trim babies on the baby food jars and tins, not chubby cherubs. These chubby cherubs may grow up to lives of misery, because fat babies invariably become fat adults.

A fat baby is likely to have inherited more fat cells than a thin baby – the fatter the parents, the more fat cells their baby is likely to have. This is not an irreversible situation, however. Fat cells continue to multiply during childhood, so, if an undisciplined pattern of eating is followed, by adolescence the chronic over-eater may have 600 billion fat cells, whereas a normal, disciplined eater of the same age will only have half that number.

Once a fat cell is 'born' it remains. However, with *constant* dieting and *regular* exercise (two words constantly, regularly and erroneously left out of many 'how-to-get-thin' edicts) it can shrink in size considerably, thus still achieving the required results.

Many fat people get discouraged when their weight doesn't tumble down accommodatingly after days or even weeks on a strict diet, even though on checking their measurements they may find – eureka – that their inches are a little less.

The reason for this is simple. When a fat cell shrinks through lack of nourishment, it first leaves a space in the body where the fat has been. That space fills up with water – and water weighs more than fat – hence no appreciable difference may be registered for quite a while on the scales, although clothes 'seem to fit better'. This is one reason why many diet doctors prefer their patients to weigh in only once a week at their surgery, when they can be on hand to explain any disappointments.

'Eat up, they're starving in India' is *not* an approach that's in keeping with the most modern way to bring up baby. 'No second helpings' is a far healthier approach.

DIETS – WHICH ONE?

At the annual dinner of that well-established, all-male club called Saints and Sinners, members – all distinguished in their various professions – choose either a white or a red carnation for their buttonhole to denote whether they consider themselves in the first or second category. It's interesting to note that most years, red carnations – the colour the club chooses for sinners – are in the majority.

When it comes to dieting, there aren't many saints around. Perhaps a better description for the ever-increasing members of the dieting club would be *martyrs* – for few people stay on a diet without indulging in long, and usually dreary, bouts of self-pity.

Whether it's a desire for a smaller size dress or a fear of coronary thrombosis, there has to be *great motivation* before even thinking of life on a lettuce leaf.

A diet plan that doesn't take into consideration the psychological reasons behind a person's over-eating habits – and remember fat means over-eating – is doomed to failure.

Motivation is the key – a size 6 dress is more appealing than a strawberry sundae

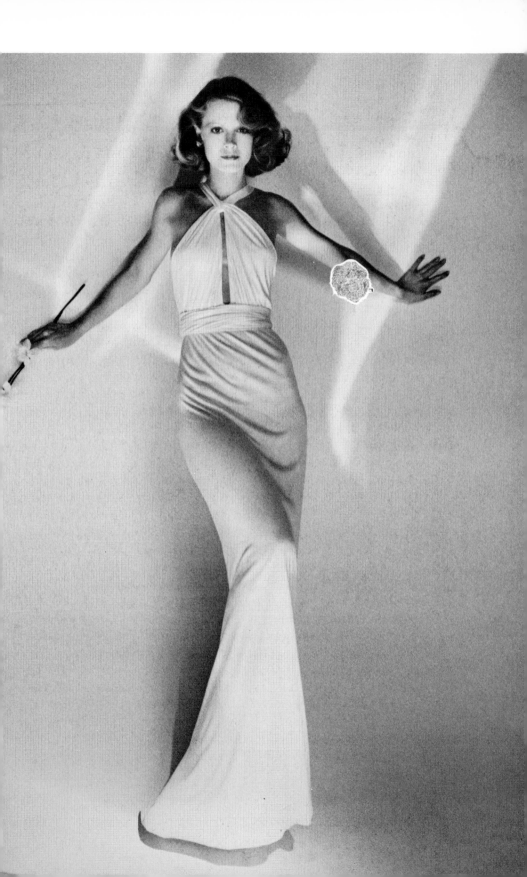

For Those Who've Almost Given up Hope ... 7 stone (44 kg) and Over Needs To Be Lost

The bigger the problem, the more drastic the remedy, which leads us to diets for the marathon martyrs, who, in my opinion, deserve everybody's (quiet) sympathy – for the first few weeks only. As results begin to show, no self-pity should be tolerated.

One diet treatment which has had considerable success with colossal heavyweights, those weighing in at around 14 stone (89 kg) and over is the one usually described as Dr Simeon's Diet, because a Dr Simeon did indeed invent it.

In 1954, while practising in Rome, Dr A. T. W. Simeon created a worldwide cyclone of human interest with his paper printed in the medical journal the *Lancet*, on 'The Action of Chorionic Gonadotrophin in the Obese.' In it he reported his findings of the past twenty years, during which time he had successfully treated over 500 overweight patients during a forty-day course with a 500-calorie (2,000-kilojoule (kJ)) a day reducing diet (a more usual, but still stringent, diet allows 1,000 calories (4,000 kJ) a day) *plus* daily injections of 125 units of human chorionic gonadotrophin, the first course followed in many cases by others of the same duration. His findings gave more than faith, hope and charity to the overweight world. They suggested a cure.

Dr Simeon stated that although gonadotrophin alone did not reduce weight, it made a drastic curtailment of calories possible; it did this by rendering fat deposits long in residence in the body (the 'fixed deposit' mentioned earlier) easily dispersable by turning them into sugar, which is easily burned up. As the blood sugar level in the body increased, the appetite became sharply depressed.

Equally, a 500-calorie (2,000-kJ) diet *alone* would not necessarily affect the 'fixed deposit', even if, by some extraordinary quirk, a person on such a low food intake had enough joie de vivre left to get out of bed in the morning!

Since that first report appeared, the obese have not been put off by their early discovery that human chorionic gonadotrophin (now known as H.C.G.) is a substance extracted from the urine of pregnant women. On the contrary, this method of treatment is eagerly sought throughout the Western world, and it's fair to say it is medically approved as being specifically helpful in the control of obesity, and applicable to a large majority of cases.

Dr Simeon explained his findings by pointing out that during pregnancy really obese women found to their surprise that they *lost* weight. Because of the enormous quantity of the hormone H.C.G. circulating naturally in their bodies, they 'weren't hungry', and so could reduce their food intake drastically. This happened without in any way affecting the child in the womb because the 'fixed deposit' of fat, generally impossible to get at, was being placed at the disposal of the growing foetus.

In the treatment of obesity alone, with no embryo to feed, a severe dietary restriction had to take the place of the embryo for the duration of the treatment – for only when the body needs extra fuel can more fat be withdrawn from the 'fixed deposit'.

DIET LET-DOWNS. Where this treatment has fallen down is where other treatments have fallen down – when an insufficient clinical, bio-chemical and personality study of the patient has been made. In other treatments, where low calorie, salt-free, low carbohydrate diets accompany injections, whether of vitamin B, appetite suppressant, liver stimulant or diuretic (always under a doctor's guidance), a patient has occasionally produced side-effects which have precluded her or him from continuing.

A person with good reflexes and general good health will obviously respond more quickly and with better long-term results than a person with a sluggish temperament, often the outward sign of a poor constitution. As a doctor who specializes in slimming says: 'There is always factor x to consider. Money or family problems, and most of all love problems.' As far as the majority of his treatments are concerned, he goes on to say, 'The purpose of the slimming injection is above all to speed up metabolism. It is the hormone balance of the body that controls its rate. Metabolism – and so digestion – is improved by getting a better blood output from the heart into the blood vessels and then into the alimentary tract where a greatly increased blood content improves the digestive powers manifold.'

Instant Cures?

Diuretic is a word often bandied about by laymen in connection with slimming treatments, but a diuretic is used solely to increase fluid output, which goes hand in glove with sodium output. Endocrinologists, nutritionists and their medical colleagues know that salt and water retention is responsible for much body bulge, and this retention is very much governed by the patient's pattern of eating over the years, the condition of various hormones in the body (the pituitary, suprarenal,

HEIGHT-WEIGHT TABLE FOR WOMEN

ft. in.	cm	Small frame, under 30 stones and pounds	kilograms	Small frame, over 30 stones and pounds	kilograms	Medium frame, under 30 stones and pounds	kilograms
4 8	142	6–8 to 6–11	41½—43	6–11 to 7–0	43—44½	6–12 to 7–3	43½—46
4 9	145	6–10 ,, 7–1	42½—45	7–1 ,, 7–3	45—46	7–0 ,, 7–6	44½—47
4 10	147	6–12 ,, 7–2	43½—45½	7–2 ,, 7–6	45½—47	7–3 ,, 7–10	46—49
4 11	150	7–1 ,, 7–5	45—46½	7–5 ,, 7–9	46½—48½	7–6 ,, 7–12	47—50
5 0	152	7–4 ,, 7–8	46½—48	7–8 ,, 7–12	48—50	7–9 ,, 8–1	48½—51
5 1	155	7–7 ,, 7–11	47½—49½	7–11 ,, 8–1	49½—51	7–12 ,, 8–4	50—52½
5 2	157	7–10 ,, 8–0	49—51	8–0 ,, 8–4	51—52½	8–1 ,, 8–7	51—54
5 3	160	7–13 ,, 8–3	50½—52	8–3 ,, 8–7	52—54	8–4 ,, 8–11	52½—56
5 4	162	8–2 ,, 8–6	51½—53½	8–6 ,, 8–11	53½—56	8–8 ,, 9–1	54½—57½
5 5	165	8–6 ,, 8–11	53½—56	8–11 ,, 9–1	56—57½	8–12 ,, 9–5	56—59½
5 6	168	8–10 ,, 9–1	55½—57½	9–1 ,, 9–5	57½—59½	9–2 ,, 9–9	55—61½
5 7	170	9–0 ,, 9–4	57—59	9–4 ,, 9–9	59—61½	9–6 ,, 10–0	60—63½
5 8	173	9–4 ,, 9–9	59—61½	9–9 ,, 10–0	61½—63½	9–10 ,, 10–4	61½—65
5 9	175	9–8 ,, 9–12	61—62½	9–12 ,, 10–4	62½—65	10–0 ,, 10–7	63½—66½
5 10	178	9–12 ,, 10–3	62½—65	10–3 ,, 10–8	65—67	10–4 ,, 10–12	65—69

ft. in.	cm	Medium frame, over 30 stones and pounds	kilograms	Large frame, under 30 stones and pounds	kilograms	Large frame, over 30 stones and pounds	kilograms
4 8	142	7–3 to 7–9	46—48½	7–6 to 7–13	47—50½	7–13 to 8–7	50½—54
4 9	145	7–6 ,, 7–12	47—50	7–8 ,, 8–2	48—51½	8–2 ,, 8–10	51½—55½
4 10	147	7–10 ,, 8–1	49—51	7–11 ,, 8–5	49½—53	8–5 ,, 8–11	53—56½
4 11	150	7–12 ,, 8–4	50—52½	8–0 ,, 8–8	51—54½	8–8 ,, 9–2	54½—58
5 0	152	8–1 ,, 8–7	51—54	8–3 ,, 8–10	52—55½	8–10 ,, 9–5	55½—59½
5 1	155	8–4 ,, 8–10	52½—55½	8–6 ,, 9–0	53½—57	9–0 ,, 9–8	57—61
5 2	157	8–7 ,, 9–0	54—57	8–9 ,, 9–3	55—58½	9–3 ,, 9–12	58½—62½
5 3	160	8–11 ,, 9–4	56—59	8–13 ,, 9–8	56½—61	9–8 ,, 10–2	61—64½
5 4	162	9–1 ,, 9–9	57½—61½	9–3 ,, 9–12	58½—62½	9–12 ,, 10–6	62½—66
5 5	165	9–5 ,, 9–13	59½—63	9–7 ,, 10–1	60—64	10–1 ,, 10–10	64—68
5 6	168	9–9 ,, 10–3	61½—65	9–11 ,, 10–6	62—66	10–6 ,, 11–0	66—70
5 7	170	10–0 ,, 10–7	63½—67	10–1 ,, 10–10	64—68	10–10 ,, 11–4	68—71½
5 8	173	10–4 ,, 10–11	65—68½	10–5 ,, 11–1	66—70½	11–1 ,, 11–9	70½—74
5 9	175	10–7 ,, 11–1	66½—70½	10–9 ,, 11–5	67½—72	11–5 ,, 12–0	72—76
5 10	178	10–12 ,, 11–5	69—72	10–13 ,, 11–9	69½—74	11–9 ,, 12–5	74—78½

HEIGHT-WEIGHT TABLE FOR MEN

ft. in.	cm	Small frame, under 30 stones and pounds	kilo-grams	Small frame, over 30 stones and pounds	kilo-grams	Medium frame, under 30 stones and pounds	kilo-grams
5 1	155	8-0 to 8-4	51—52½	8-4 to 8-8	52½—54½	8-6 to 8-11	53½—56
5 2	157	8-3 „ 8-7	52—54	8-7 „ 8-11	54—56	8-9 „ 9-1	55—57½
5 3	160	8-6 „ 8-10	53½—55½	8-10 „ 9-0	55½—57	8-12 „ 9-4	56—59
5 4	162	8-9 „ 8-13	55—56½	8-13 „ 9-3	56½—58½	9-1 „ 9-7	57½—60½
5 5	165	8-12 „ 9-3	56—58½	9-3 „ 9-7	58½—60½	9-4 „ 10-0	59—63½
5 6	168	9-2 „ 9-6	58—60	9-6 „ 9-11	60—62	9-8 „ 10-0	61—63½
5 7	170	9-6 „ 9-11	60—62	9-11 „ 10-1	62—64	9-12 „ 10-6	62½—66
5 8	173	9-10 „ 10-0	61½—63½	10-0 „ 10-5	63½—66	10-2 „ 10-9	64½—67½
5 9	175	10-0 „ 10-5	63½—66	10-5 „ 10-10	66—68	10-6 „ 10-12	66—69
5 10	178	10-4 „ 10-9	65½—67½	10-9 „ 11-0	67½—70	10-10 „ 11-3	68—71
5 11	180	10-8 „ 10-13	67—69½	10-13 „ 11-4	69½—71½	11-0 „ 11-8	70—73½
6 0	183	10-12 „ 11-3	69—71	11-3 „ 11-8	71—73½	11-4 „ 11-13	71½—75½
6 1	185	11-2 „ 11-8	71—73½	11-8 „ 11-13	73½—75½	11-8 „ 12-2	73½—77
6 2	188	11-6 „ 11-11	72½—75	11-11 „ 12-3	75—77½	11-13 „ 12-8	75½—80
6 3	190	11-10 „ 12-2	74½—77	12-2 „ 12-7	77—79½	12-4 „ 12-13	78—82

ft. in.	cm	Medium frame, over 30 stones and pounds	kilo-grams	Large frame, under 30 stones and pounds	kilo-grams	Large frame, over 30 stones and pounds	kilo-grams
5 1	155	8-11 to 9-3	56—58½	9-0 to 9-7	57—60½	9-7 to 10-1	60½—64
5 2	157	9-1 „ 9-7	57½—60½	9-3 „ 9-11	58½—62	9-11 „ 10-4	62—65½
5 3	160	9-4 „ 9-10	59—61½	9-6 „ 10-0	60—63½	10-0 „ 10-8	63½—67
5 4	162	9-7 „ 9-13	60½—63	9-9 „ 10-4	61½—65½	10-4 „ 10-12	65½—69
5 5	165	10-0 „ 10-3	63½—65	9-12 „ 10-6	62½—66	10-6 „ 11-2	66—71
5 6	168	10-0 „ 10-7	63½—66½	10-2 „ 10-12	64½—69	10-12 „ 10-7	69—73
5 7	170	10-6 „ 10-12	66—69	10-7 „ 11-3	66½—71	11-3 „ 11-12	71—75½
5 8	173	10-9 „ 11-2	67½—71	10-11 „ 11-6	68½—72½	11-6 „ 12-2	72½—77
5 9	175	10-12 „ 11-6	69—72½	11-1 „ 11-11	70½—74½	11-11 „ 12-6	74½—79
5 10	178	11-3 „ 11-11	71—74½	11-5 „ 11-11	72—74½	11-11 „ 12-11	74½—81
5 11	180	11-8 „ 12-2	73½—77	11-10 „ 12-6	74½—79	12-6 „ 13-2	79—83½
6 0	183	11-13 „ 12-7	75½—79½	12-0 „ 12-11	76—81	12-11 „ 13-7	81—85½
6 1	185	12-2 „ 12-12	77—81½	12-5 „ 13-1	78½—83	13-1 „ 13-12	83—88
6 2	188	12-8 „ 13-3	80—84	12-10 „ 13-6	80½—85½	13-6 „ 14-3	85½—90½
6 3	190	12-13 „ 13-8	82—86	13-0 „ 13-11	82½—87½	13-11 „ 14-8	87½—92½

cortical, thyroid and sex glands — affected by age), exercise (or generally lack of it) and general posture. One staggering piece of information on this subject is that there is more fluid and salt loss when *at rest* than when the patient is on the move.

Many doctors are agreed that there is little validity in injecting diuretics. I quote:

> Diuretics should only be given by injection for certain acute cardiac and other emergencies and I cannot see any reason apart from a gimmick why they should be given by injection in the treatment of obesity. They increase fluid and sodium output from the renal route, but they also increase the output of potassium. If the blood level of potassium becomes too depleted, it can cause muscular weakness, kidney and liver damage, skin rashes and bone marrow cellular depression. Such injections are also said to have sometimes aggravated diabetes and to precipitate attacks of gout where this condition already exists. They would certainly not be given for 'tired kidneys', because a definite contra-indication to their use would be renal disease.

Nevertheless, there are many kinds of chemical compounds used for the purpose of slimming and classified as diuretics, and they are widely different, not only in their effect on potassium levels but also regarding the length of time in which they act. In some cases, the action lasts for a few hours, in others for as long as twenty-four. Again, there is another type which in some people could lead to potassium retention, extremely dangerous if progress is not monitored by periodic blood biochemical analysis. Some diuretics have potassium incorporated in the pill in order to replace the potassium loss which must occur with the majority of these compounds.

The amount of fluid loss daily varies with the amount of surplus in the body. A person some 5 or 6 stone (32–38 kg) overweight could lose up to 7 lb (3 kg) a day, of which 2 lb (900 g) might be fluid, while a person only 12 lb (5½ kg) overweight shouldn't lose more than ½ lb (225 g) daily.

The overweight girl in a hurry to regain some sort of shape is the one most in danger. Taking too many pills against the doctor's orders and cutting down too drastically on calories, and particularly fluids, can result in a potassium deficiency. The girl then becomes nauseous, suffers a complete loss of appetite which precludes her from eating at all, and frequently ends up with a kidney complaint which lasts a lifetime.

Appetite suppressants are often part of a weight reducing programme. When blood sugar levels are depressed, hunger results. This can be done artificially by injecting small doses of insulin and naturally by starvation. Conversely, if blood sugar levels are raised, appetite diminishes. This is one of the effects of H.C.G., as already described. But there are other methods of doing this, employing drugs with stimulant properties; these should only be used under medical supervision, accompanied by a medically approved diet. All doctors are against amphetamines, however; while depressing appetite centres, they also cause insomnia, pulse rate rises, psychotic manifestations and anxiety attacks.

When weight 'sticks' at a certain spot, it is due to water retention, but those who make a habit of dieting are hard, if not impossible, to convince that the amount of water they retain has nothing whatsoever to do with the amount they drink. On the contrary, if fluid intake is insufficient to provide the water required, the kidneys are neglected and strained and urine becomes scanty and highly concentrated. If more water is taken than the body requires, the surplus is eliminated, so to try to prevent the body retaining water by drinking less is not only futile but also possibly harmful.

In a letter to the *Lancet* in 1962 Dr Simeon wrote,

Whenever weight is lost rapidly, two not necessarily synchronized processes are involved. One is the utilization of excess fat and the other the breakdown of adipose tissue. After a certain loss has been achieved, it seems as if the extraction of fat outruns the body's ability to break down the cellular tissue in which it was contained. It therefore replaces the fat it loses with water. As fat weighs less than water, the scales do not register any loss until the breakdown of the tissue catches up. I do not call the menstrual levelling-off a plateau [weight 'sticking'], because it occurs in almost every case and of this the patient has been forewarned. When a plateau lasts longer than five days, it is usually a sign a weight has been reached which the patient has held for several years before a further increase took place. Any plateau that is not due to careless dieting can be broken up by giving a single tablet of diuretic which relieves anxiety of those who cannot stand the strain of temporary disillusionment . . .

When it comes to the final moment of truth in a slimming programme, the vitamin or hormone injection, the diuretic pill and/or appetite suppressant all play the part of catalysts, triggering off the most vital aid to the treatment: the patient's own will to change the eating habits of years, to eat less of what she loves and more of what she doesn't – not just for a week or a month, but possibly *forever. If willpower is not sufficiently engaged, no prescribed pill or injection is worth a fig.*

Reducing with Rice

Another doctor, Walter Kempner, M.D., of Duke University, North Carolina, has spent a great part of his life combating obesity on behalf of the obese. Frank Sinatra sent his mother to Dr Kempner's clinic one year, hoping to be able to say he'd given her 'a new figure for Christmas', and Mrs Sinatra, Snr, was just one in a long line of celebrities who found themselves living primarily on rice, honest to goodness paddy field, unpolished stuff, two bowls of it a day, with or without chopsticks, accompanied by a variety of stewed, baked, tinned or fresh fruit.

During a three-week stay myself – in this instance as reporter/ companion – I can say that I saw the most astonishing weight reductions of up to 2 stone (12½ kg) in people who had been following the Rice Diet for three or four months under the all-seeing eagle eyes of Dr Kempner and his retinue of doctors – mostly female.

Dr K., a world authority on obesity, spent years studying the metabolism of living cells, healthy and diseased. He sought a diet that would not only deflate fat but also cure many of the ills associated with it: high blood pressure, diabetes, hardening of the arteries, heart diseases. He eventually came up with what is now known as the Rice Diet.

Salt is the biggest enemy of the obese, says Dr Kempner, and he maintains that we eat far more salt every day than we ever realize. Don't say immediately you never ever reach for the salt-cellar. Your salt intake is bound to be greater than you think.

To combine effective therapy with adequate nutrition in one diet,

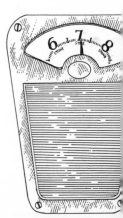

Dr K. devised a formula in which salt, protein and fat are kept as low as possible, while the body still receives the amino-acids and fatty acids essential for life and growth. The combination of rice, fruit and fruit juices completely fulfils those requirements.

The diet is unique in that while it is low in protein, it is comparatively high in carbohydrate – usually a dirty word as far as diets are concerned. In fact, the Rice Diet contains almost twice as much carbohydrate as all other diets, only a quarter as much protein and less than one twentieth as much fat. As the carbohydrate intake is tailor-made to provide the body's heat, light and power, not one calorie left over to stay on the hips, the unusually low protein intake has been proved to be sufficient.

Why rice? Diets usually stress the importance of protein but few go to the trouble of explaining that proteins, made up of various amino-acids, differ from each other in type and in the proportion of amino-acids they contain.

Some are more useful to the body than others, and rice protein comes top of the list. It 'approximates', as Dr Kempner has said for years, 'closely in biological value for man to beef, is easily assimilated by the body, and the amino-acids compare exceptionally favourably with those contained in other proteins'. He goes further. 'So far as the metabolism of the kidney cells is concerned, rice protein cannot be replaced at will by any other.' In other words, rice is good for you and better still for your figure.

Breakfast at one of the Rice Houses consists of a piece of citrus fruit, prune juice, and a cup of tea (no milk, but sugar if you like) or decaffeinated coffee. Lunch is a big bowl of rice, cooked any way you like, providing there's no salt or fat involved, together with two types of fruit – say, half a tin of peaches with a large piece of melon or stewed apples with a large bunch of grapes – and tea or coffee. At dinner there is again a big bowl of rice with other fruits plus tea or coffee.

Apples and pears are always peeled – there's salt in the skin – and fluid intake is restricted to between 24 and 32 fl oz (710 and 950 ml) in each twenty-four-hour period, the fluid varying from milkless tea or coffee to water or fresh lemonade.

Unless you have a doctor totally familiar and in agreement with Dr Kempner's methods, it cannot be advised you try the Rice Diet at home, for thorough daily medical checks are necessary and are made every morning at the Rice Houses, where patients take their meals.

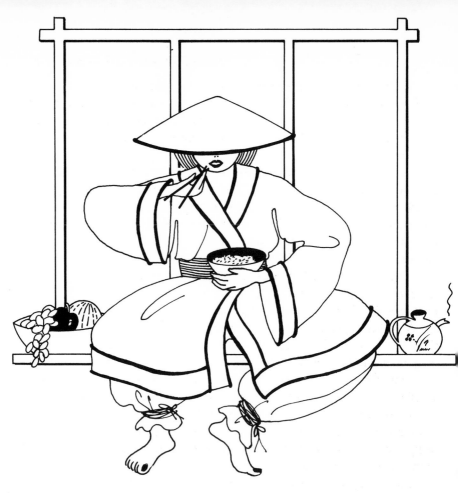

No pills, no injections, just rice, fruit and fruit juices, make up the menu, while rest after every meal is obligatory, as is exercise for half an hour six times a day. Most people walk, cycle or play table tennis. If anyone cheats, they're out of the clinic at once – the waiting list's too long to bother with anyone who only wants to pretend they're slimming.

Low Carbohydrate Diets

The great law of life is replenishment. If we don't eat, we die. So our bodies depend on us for a fair deal. Often we eat and forget what the menu was, but our bodies have to remember *and* cope with whatever we put into them. Most fat people put a lot of carbohydrate into their bodies, mainly on the assumption that they're not going to lose weight, anyway, even if they do go without their buttered toast at breakfast and their bouef-en-croûte at dinner, so why should they suffer one unnecessary hunger pang.

On the other hand, once a fatty sees the light, however far away at the end of the tunnel, it's ten to one he or she will go for a low carbohydrate diet, because *everyone* knows that although we need *some*, we don't need that *much* carbohydrate. Excess just turns the body into a great big warehouse.

Another growing body of opinion re the villain of the piece, carbohydrate, is that it is generally less hunger satisfying than protein, which means one is able to consume more (and usually does) at any one sitting. There also seems to be evidence that carbohydrate helps the system retain natural moisture, thus filling out any curves the body happens to have.

The low carbohydrate diet has had many aliases, and new ones are always cropping up. Staying the course are the Drinking Man's Diet, the Air Force Diet (nothing to do with the boys in blue, says the Air Ministry), and the Mayo Clinic Diet (from which the Mayo Clinic in Rochester, Minnesota, completely disassociates itself), not forgetting the Grapefruit Diet, about which a top nutritionist says: '. . . grapefruit . . . supposed to chew up and dissolve body fat is an asinine proposition. No food has such properties.'

Chewing up fat or not, lurking beneath all that grapefruit at every meal is the oldie: no more than 50–60 g of carbohydrate a day, this being put to work by the body, so that it never gets stored as fat (look at the carbohydrate counter on page 232).

For some people, there's no doubt that this type of diet has worked miracles, because they have genuinely set out to find a new pattern of eating, eschewing the old and the bad, guided by nutritional values, which is what good dieting is all about.

Gimmicky titles take away from the fundamental purpose of the low carbohydrate theme – which is to enjoy an eating pattern that is (a) sociable, (b) nutritious and (c) as palatable as possible. This is found in a low carbohydrate diet, providing it isn't decked out with red herrings (no calories) to beautify the citrus industry's profits or the martini makers' balance sheets.

If such a diet is properly organized, it's sociable, because you can eat most of the same food as the rest of the guests at a dinner party, only avoiding the bread, the potatoes and, if possible without making a T.V. production out of it, the dessert. It's nutritious, containing meat, fish, eggs, some vegetables and at least half a pint (250 ml) of milk – foods rich in amino-acids, vitamins and essential minerals. Most important, it's palatable. Once we've quelled our addiction to sugary and starchy foods, it's obvious there's more subtle taste in meat, fish, egg and cheese dishes, often swamped with extraneous flavours.

Calorie Counting

When one finally gets down to the nitty-gritty of losing pounds and inches, every doctor agrees that **calories have to be counted.** Crash diets of bananas and brazil nuts every four hours or alfalfa sprouts on wholewheat every three may take away a few pounds, but they'll take a lot of the joy out of life, too – if you have any left after a while.

Worst of all, crash diets don't work. After the first thrilling plummet of the scales, the pointer inexorably creeps back up again.

For the majority of us, those who need to lose about 10–12 lb (4½–5½ kg) sensible dieting vis-à-vis the daily calorie count *does* work, and I know that from my own experience, as an active participant, *not* as a reporter and/or companion.

Whether you received A's or D's for arithmetic, everyone can work out this sum: 1 lb (450 g) of fatty tissue equals in energy 3,500 calories (14,000 kJ). Every time you eat 3,500 calories (14,000 kJ) less than you expend, you use up 1 lb (450 g) of fatty tissue (out of that 'current account', remember?). A deficit of 500 calories (2,000 kJ) a day (eating 2,000 (8,000) and using up 2,500 (10,000) for instance) can lead to a loss of 1 lb (450 g) a week – 52 lb (23½ kg) a year. Get to a deficit of 1,000 calories (4,000 kJ) (the best number for a not too awesome eating programme) and you can lose 104 lb (47 kg) a year. Will you be able to see yourself in the glass?

The reason calorie counting sometimes goes awry is the number of misconceptions connected with it. Too many believe there's a whole area of non-fattening food, where they can indulge their hunger pangs to their pituitary's delight. They piously dive into steaks the size of Gulliver's shoe and gulp down king-size glasses of fresh orange juice, averting their eyes and their mouths scrupulously from all that 'dreadful fattening food – bread, potatoes, pasta'. They don't lose weight. They throw their calorie counter into a coconut fudge sundae and bewail the injustice of it all.

The serious student of calories – and therefore the serious dieter, too – has to study facts and learn that a 3 oz (75 g) slice of roast beef, enough to cover a slice of bread, contains 260 calories (1,040 kJ), and that a tall glass of fresh orange juice, straight out of the peel, is 110 calories (440 kJ) concentrated out of a tin, it's 300 (1,200). As for that

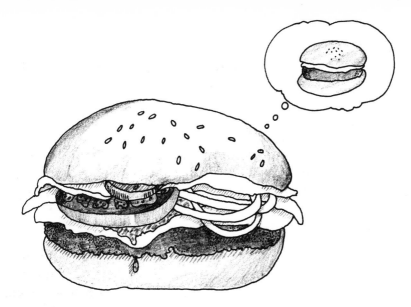

coconut fudge sundae, it's 500 calories (2,000 kJ) – is that spelt out enough?

Steak is a problem in itself, whatever its size. It is widely believed to be pure protein and so able to be consumed *ad infinitum*, allowing the consumer to emerge as skinny as Twiggy. It is conveniently for-gotten that *all meat contains fat*. Three ounces (75 g) of sirloin, for instance, or a deboned Sunday joint, is likely to contain 20 g protein (80 calories (320 kJ)) and 20 g fat (180 calories (720 kJ)). A 3 oz (75 g) hamburger contains on average 20 g protein (80 calories (320 kJ)) and 26 g fat (230 calories (920 kJ)). Ham contains even more fat in relation to protein content.

Size is just as important a factor as selection, when it comes to choosing from a menu or cooking at home. Eating a large hamburger, but counting it as a small one, will make the difference of 2 lb (900 g) of fat staying in place. Self-deception only leads to a hidden surtax which destroys the calorie budget just as effectively as the coconut fudge sundae. Peanuts, you say? Sorry, 850 calories (3,400 kJ) for a couple of handfuls – however much President Carter may beg to differ.

Millions of people are deluded by the word protein, thinking it is some magical panacea to diet and that if they stick to it alone, pounds will fall off. Instead, with a carbohydrate and fat deficiency the health will suffer and the pounds may not fall off either.

Protein contains about 120 calories (480 kJ) per 28 g, the same as carbohydrate (fats are more costly at about 280 (1,120) per 28 g), but when too much protein is eaten, and it's in the presence of carbohydrate,

215

the protein is converted and stored in the body as fatty tissue, too. When there is no carbohydrate present (which is rare), excess can be absorbed and stored as muscle tissue. Depending on the type of protein – and so amino-acids – present and the type of person you are, the fatty tissue may or may not be reconverted into protein for the body's requirements. Where there is a tendency to obesity, the fat stays as fat.

It isn't easy to work out how many calories you personally burn up each day. As mentioned previously, factor x is at work, governing the way you cope with life, apart from how you happen to spend it.

As a simple guide, you can work out an approximate figure from the following:

1 Sitting, relaxing, the body burns up from 13 to 16 calories (52 to 64 kJ) per pound (450 g) of body weight.

2 Doing sedentary work – secretarial or light housework – the body burns up from 18 to 20 calories (72 to 80 kJ) per pound (450 g) of body weight.

3 During hard work – exercise, making love – the body burns up from 28 to 35 calories (112 to 140 kJ) per pound (450 g) of body weight.

Let's say your ideal body weight for your age (over thirty), height (5 ft 5 in (165 cm) and body structure (medium, see chart on page 206-7) is 136 lb (9 stone 10 lb) (62 kg) and that you're an executive secretary, a fairly high-powered job, which means you probably burn up on average the top rate of 20 calories (80 kJ) per pound (450 g) of body weight during most of the day. You multiply 136 by 20, which means to stay the same weight you need to consume 2,720 calories (10,880 kJ) each day. *To lose weight, you must eat less.*

The sad fact remains, as you get older, you'll need to eat still less to remain that curvy 136 lb (62 kg). Ask Liz and Sophia. Body functions slow down, exercise isn't so attractive, while food, for some unaccountable reason, gets more and more irresistible.

When you're on a conveyor belt of luncheons, cocktail parties and dinners; when, if you're not going out, you take second helpings at home to encourage guests to appreciate the cook, then you can be in trouble – particularly as this usually happens a little later on in life when your husband, and/or you yourself, have become successful.

When you're in the social boat, it takes extra motivation, more than diuretic pills, to break through the food barrier and win back measurements. It takes cunning not to be boring (and so fall easy victim to an over-eager hostess anxious to break your diet rules – why do women want to do that?) and not to be bored yourself with an ever-lasting eating syndrome of grapefruit, steak and/or fish.

To keep your bounce and social nounce, certain foods, low in calories, ought always to be on the menu to equip the body naturally in its diet endeavour. Lettuce, onions, celery and spinach all contain natural silicone, which is a natural body brightener, helping prevent nervous exhaustion and mental fatigue. Oysters, clams, raisins and leeks are natural but low sources of sodium, helping endurance, clearing sinuses and reducing moodiness, while seafood is always good for you (if you're not allergic to it in some way), containing as it does complete protein, which supplies the essential amino-acids the body can't manufacture and must get from food. Milk is important, because, together with other dairy products, it can provide nearly two-thirds of the body's calcium demands. If there's a lack of calcium, it shows up most in nervous tension. Whether taken straight or used in a low-calorie soup, sauce or shake recipe, one ½-pint (225 ml) glass of skimmed milk or buttermilk should be taken every day. Eggs, a good source of protein, are tricky because of their cholesterol value. However, four or five a week is a safe margin, providing you don't lose count when using one in a recipe.

Best Food for Dieters

One of the most underrated – and in some cases wrongly accused – foods is the avocado – underrated because it is in fact a beauty armoury containing eleven vitamins and seventeen minerals (just to start with) and wrongly accused of being fattening because it isn't when you compare it to a multitude of other far less deserving chow. One average size half contains 132 calories (528 kJ), less than a cup of plain gelatin or 2 oz (56 g) of the dieter's perpetual lunch, grilled hamburger. It's head and stalk above so many other fruits because of its numerous nutritional qualities: the protein content is of equal status to many kinds of meat. It contains little starch and practically no sugar (both devils to diets as we know); it offers generous quantities of calcium, magnesium, potassium, sodium, copper, phosphates, manganese and iron, and is even more valuable because of its high percentage of polyunsaturated fatty acid, which gives the fruit its mellow texture and nutlike flavour. The Mexicans call it 'butter growing on trees', and they use it like that, too, spreading the pulp on their tortillas. It's an amazingly complete meal in itself, and if you lunched on one half every day you'd find it a great incentive to losing the last few obstinate pounds that refuse to budge.

VITAMINS ARE VITAL, YET EASY TO FORGET ...

Vitamin A, marvellous for helping to produce a flawless skin (known as the 'Beautiful Skin' vitamin) and promoting good eyesight, it is found in all green (especially leafy) and yellow vegetables, yellow fruits, chicken, liver, butter, egg yolks and cheese.

Vitamin B complex includes all members of the vitamin B family, which must be present before any living organism can burn glucose, the fuel that keeps us on the move. It helps supply oxygen to the vital areas of the body – especially the brain. Eat it in liver, kidney, oysters and all grains. Wholemeal toast is a marvellous way to start the day.

Vitamin B12 is an energizer, fighting disease, age and nervousness. Eat it in broccoli, crab, mushrooms and skimmed milk.

Vitamin C (ascorbic acid) is the body's way of making the cement that holds the cells together. A poor vitamin C intake leads to tooth decay and bruises that last. Bean sprouts, oranges and peppers are all rich sources.

Vitamin D is a body builder, and a slimmer in that it helps the body burn up sugar more efficiently. Sunshine is a beautiful source (watch that ultra-violet, though, see page 53), so is milk, and wine when it's made from grapes.

Vitamin E is thought to increase hormone production and so retard age and do wonders for your sex life – but so far it doesn't have the official stamp of approval. Fish, apples, liver, some cheeses and eggs provide E – which can't do any harm at all!

Vitamin P fights illness through acting on the capillaries. Spinach, parsley, lettuce and all citrus fruits are good sources of P.

MINERALS ARE A MUST, TOO. Check you're mobilizing the right ones for health, strength, and shape:

Calcium is necessary for strong bones and teeth, relaxed nerves and muscles. Drink milk, and eat yogurt, clams, kale and cheese.

Phosphorus is calcium's running mate; the brain tissues are rich with it. Nearly all vegetables and fruit provide some phosphorus.

Potassium is a directing force, 'posting' the right nourishment from the blood stream to the cells. If there's a deficiency, constipation is one result, skin rashes another. Leafy green vegetables and fruit for you.

Sulphur suits your blood, prompting the liver to absorb what's good for it. Brussel sprouts are sweet with sulphur.

Iron helps oxygen reach muscle and blood cells, an essential task. When there's a short supply, anaemia (and a poor skin colour) is one result. Parsley, kidneys, shellfish and fresh fruit for iron.

Iodine is a gland fuel, helping produce the hormones that control many of life's processes – the metabolism and other timings for the body. Garlic may be anti-social, but it's high in iodine, so is seafood. Langouste Catalan anyone?

Psychological Aids

Don't knock them. They're as important as weights and measures in reminding you about your great shape crusade.

1 Sit near a mirror at mealtimes, so you can see how you've bloated the shape nature gave you.

2 Wear something tight about the house, but not when you're going out. Then, something 'tight' can 'show on your face' and ruin your looks (and your evening), like tight shoes.

3 Before a special night out weigh yourself and write your weight down to glance at when you powder your nose in the ladies room.

4 Eat slowly. Chew well, and eat from a smaller plate.

5 Take the edge off your hunger before a meal with snacks of bouillon, a heart of lettuce, a handful of raisins, a spoonful of yoghurt.

6 Season food with spices or herbs or tart fruit juices. Sprinkle sunflower seeds on salads, or soups, coconut meal on vegetables – all to add variety to your willpower.

7 Cut down dramatically on alcohol by asking for something you don't like. If you've been on martinis for years, ask for scotch-on-the-rocks. Hate vodka? Ask for a long one. You may grow to like it eventually, but you'll have consumed a lot less in the indoctrination period.

8 Pamper yourself in other ways. If breakfast in bed is your idea of heaven, indulge yourself. Make a good start to your diet with an ideal breakfast of orange slices, one poached egg on whole-wheat bread, coffee with skimmed milk. Then put a make-up mirror on your breakfast-tray and take your mind off your weight by looking at your face. Experiment for fifteen to twenty minutes with make-up or face packs or anything you fancy.

9 Rest more anyway.

10 Exercise more, too, not enough to frighten the neighbours, but in a relaxed, pleasant way. Try not to bend your knees when you retrieve the glove you dropped or put the lead on Fido (buying a dog is one way to exercise more). Stretch up to reach for something – even if it's out of reach, stretch up anyway. Climb up and down a couple of flights for a couple of days instead of taking the lift. See how the pavement feels under your heels. Walk if you can for at least fifteen minutes each day, Fido or no Fido.

There's no doubt about it. If the only muscles you ever move are the chewing muscles, it makes the whole slimming down process far more difficult.

New Diet Tricks

One of the latest things nutritionists and diet doctors advise the overweight to do is to exercise the intestinal tract. Apparently after years of eating overcooked food, most of us have softened the muscles of our intestinal tract. In other words, our mechanism for breaking down and utilizing our food the right way is, to say the least, rusty and out of condition. Eating mostly overcooked food is bad for another reason. A great deal of nutritional value is lost in cooking any-way, so when food is *over*cooked, the situation is clearly a losing one. For example, to obtain as much vitamin C from cooked cabbage as you receive in 2 oz (56 g) of the raw stuff you have to go on a cabbage eating marathon and try to plough your way through $2\frac{1}{2}$ lb (just over 1 kg). Cabbage soup, anyone?

A certain female professor of nutrition I know uses unorthodox methods to get her point across. Sharing a stage with her on a beauty tour, I was as surprised as the audience when she opened a pad of fine writing paper and instead of writing a letter proceeded to chew the pages. After this promising start, she explained she was attempting to get across the following information: that some of the better quality 'slices' of paper around are more nutritious or certainly *as* nutritious as some of the food we choose to put in our mouths. She then proceeded to analyse the paper and a favourite hamburger. Certainly their chemical formulations were astonishingly similar. However, there was another underlining point to the professor's paper eating performance: the importance of exercising the intestinal tract by consuming a fair amount of roughage every day – not paper, but food that as the word suggests needs more effort to eat. It generally means raw food, for the more food gets cooked the less 'rough' it becomes. She maintains, along with many of her colleagues, that if you aim to include roughage in the form of fruit, leaf and root of the plant at least once a day, you're on the way not only to improving your digestive system but – something you may be more aware of – improving your skin, hair and psyche.

Assuming that everyone likes their body mechanism to run smoothly, eat the fruit of the plant in tomatoes, cucumbers and even pumpkin; the leaf in lettuce (natural silicone content is a body brightener), chicory and parsley; the root in the form of onions, radishes, carrots and potatoes, which can be parboiled.

Spend a minute more in the kitchen and squeeze fresh oranges and grapefruits for juices – you don't get the cellulose content in tinned or cartoned juice, and cellulose is helpful in retoning that intestinal tract again. Get used to whole grain cereals for breakfast every morning. Grated nuts add a plus because of their vitamin B content, which also helps calm the nervous system. Grains and nuts need extra energy to be expended on the part of the internal machinery to do their best for our bodies. Rough and Raw are two new r's that you should learn to assimilate for the sake of your looks.

R.S.V.P. (*répondez s'il vous plaît*, as if you didn't know) has another meaning in the world of bariatrics (the field of medicine devoted to the control of obesity). Many bariatric doctors have found that by using snappy lingo ('girth control as well as birth control') their patients remember more easily a new pattern of eating, a pattern which incidentally they may have to follow for life and not just for a couple of months of martyrdom.

Where does R.S.V.P. come in? Roughage, salads, vegetables and protein – that's where. All four add up to what many medics consider the ideal reducing diet, low in fat, equally spread between high quality carbohydrate and protein intake. Eating more roughage, as just mentioned, produces a more efficient digestive system, which in turn can lead to a natural bloom on your cheek and shape in your body.

High quality carbohydrate comes from salads, fruit and vegetables, but you must be aware that some contain more natural sugar than others. You can obtain enough fat from your protein allowance when it's devoted to meat. That trim looking steak contains fat whether you can see it or not.

Water is part of the diet, too, to help you stick to the rules, filling you up or giving you the *feeling* of being full, which is just as important. It will also help the metabolism, your body's motor, to tick over at top rate. All nutritionists agree that drinking eight glasses of water a day helps the skin to look its best and the body to shape up faster – but, of course, only if the other dietary rules just mentioned are observed.

The No-Nonsense Low Carbo Diet

RULE ONE: before embarking on any diet, have a check up and talk it over with your doctor.

RULE TWO: no more than 50–60 g of carbohydrate every day.

RULE THREE: no large or second helpings (probably ever again).

RULE FOUR: no more than one alcoholic drink per meal (before, during or after – and never, ever in between).

All numbers in brackets refer to grams of carbohydrate, not calorie content.

Breakfast, choose from: poached egg (0) or a medium-size piece of haddock (4) or 2 pieces of lean grilled bacon (0) with grilled tomato (6) plus 2 slices of diet bread (8) or 1 piece of rye or white (12) or wholewheat (11), 1 pat butter (0), coffee or tea, dash of milk if required (4), sugar substitute (0)

Lunch, choose from: grilled trout or plaice or sole, sliced tomato salad with French dressing, 1 oz (28 g) cheese, 2 water biscuits, coffee (13 in all) *or* ½ teacup tinned crab (8) with ½ teacup asparagus (3) plus butter sauce (0), coffee *or* 1 serving baked, boiled or devilled ham (0) with 1 oz (28 g) courgettes (1) plus half a medium-size cantaloupe melon (9), coffee.

Dinner, choose from: onion soup (4) plus filet mignon (0), ½ teacup brussel sprouts (6), 1 fresh plum (7), coffee *or* 1 medium artichoke (5) with butter sauce (0) plus baked or tinned salmon (0) with cucumber salad (2) and French dressing (2), ½ teacup jelly (18) *or* oyster cocktail (8), spareribs (0), barbecue sauce (2), 1 oz (28 g) Camembert (½), 1 cracker (5), coffee. If you add a Manhattan before dinner, add 7 g to

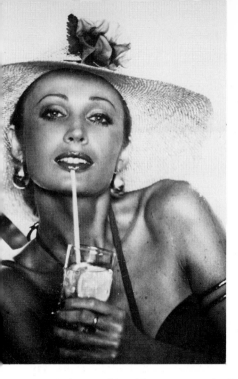

Alcohol is no help on a diet. Ask for something you don't like, to learn to do without it

your daily total. Add a martini before lunch, and it's another 1. If you're a wine drinker, the tax is heavier: 12 g carbohydrate for most medium dry to sweet white wines, 14 for red – but you can celebrate occasionally with a glass of champagne, for 3 fl oz (85 g) of the bubbly stuff totals only 2 g of carbohydrate.

Count up to 1,000 Calories (4,000 kJ) a Day to Lose the Weight You Need to Lose
(and not a Single One More!)

RULE ONE: before embarking, have a check-up and talk it over with your doctor.

RULE TWO: count every calorie you consume – see calorie counter on page 232.

Breakfast every day (and don't skip it – breakfast whips the metabolism into shape to keep you on your toes throughout the day): orange juice (1 small glass), 1 poached egg, wholewheat toast (1 slice), coffee with skimmed milk.

Lunch, choose from: frankfurter (1), asparagus (6 spears), 1 yogurt, coffee with skimmed milk or tea with lemon *or* 3 oz (85 g) crabmeat with lettuce and tomato, 1 teacup tinned cherries, coffee or tea *or* tomato juice, turkey or chicken, lettuce and tomato sandwich (brown bread only, please), coffee or tea *or* clear soup, salmon salad with a little mayonnaise, lettuce and 1 tomato, coffee or tea.

Dinner, choose from: grilled lean lamb chop, peas and carrots, 1 slice brown bread, coffee or tea *or* 1 medium slice of roast beef, ½ teacup rice, tossed salad with lemon juice, 1 slice plain cake, coffee or tea *or* grilled cod with cabbage, 1 raw tomato, 1 flavoured yogurt, coffee or tea *or* grilled shrimps, 1 baked potato, 1 teacup beetroot, half a grapefruit with a spoonful of honey, coffee or tea.

Happy Counting.

GROUP THERAPY

Most people have heard of Weight Watchers today, and the founder, Jean Nidetch, is always anxious to point out that W.W., as it's familiarly called, is a programme, *not* a diet.

Once a fat lady herself, Jean created W.W. out of her personal experience, realizing she had become thin through a sense of competition entering into her slimming campaign – once she started to exchange progress reports with her friends.

Based on the old theory that it always helps resolve when you know others are suffering the same pangs, W.W. grew into a worldwide business through a re-education programme for eating habits.

At the weekly class and lecture, everyone is weighed and publicly congratulated or otherwise. Everyone receives their weekly menu, which may include a potato or even spaghetti, but all compensated for in the overall scheme of things.

Of course, the meals are planned around a calorie count – they have to be – but the calorie content is not discussed because W.W. believes that counting calories can lead to a person 'saving' them and eating a piece of chocolate layer cake in the happy assumption they are well within their limits.

The overall philosophy is that anyone can go on a diet and lose weight – momentarily – but it means nothing if *food habits have not been basically changed* to a lifetime of well-balanced, healthy, nutritional meals.

To W.W. – and anyone who has any sense – *nutrition* is the most important aspect of dieting – and eating.

SWEET 'N' LOW

When you feel depressed for no reason, snappy when somebody smiles, anxious though you know you've got nothing to be anxious about, stop and think about your diet. Today we're all bombarded with suggestions that one set of symptoms refers to another set of circumstances, and as nutritionists, chemists and physicists turn out more evidence our diet is often held responsible for much of our behaviour. One of the most overworked words in medical journalism is hypoglycaemia, which means a low blood sugar condition – the reverse of diabetes, when blood sugar is too high, because the body is not manufacturing enough insulin.

A friend of mine who had brought on her own crisis through excessive irritability and lack of *joie de vivre* (she lost her job and her beau) finally wound up at the doctor's surgery wondering if by any chance something by the name of hypoglycaemia could possibly be responsible for her woes.

Her doctor found that indeed her level of insulin was far too high, causing the blood sugar level to fall too low. The reason? A contemporary one of skipped meals, and hasty, poor quality carbohydrate snacks instead of balanced protein and high quality carbohydrate meals. Smoking was to blame, too, plus the use of a glass of white wine as a placebo to replace food. All these things produced a sick pancreas, which in panic suddenly stimulated the output of insulin, lifting the blood sugar level momentarily, only to be followed by a disastrous downward curve.

The emphasis on dieting has caused millions of us over the past two decades to yo-yo up and down in weight, placing a burden on the usually well organized digestive system, particularly where the pancreas is concerned. When calorie intake is severely restricted, as in the case of many 'crash' programmes, this immediately creates a low blood sugar level, producing in many cases an irresistible craving for something sweet plus intense fatigue, depression and the crankiness described. Frequently a sufferer will revert to cup after cup of black coffee, which unfortunately only makes matters worse, because caffeine alerts the adrenal gland to produce more adrenalin which in turn causes the pancreas to release *more* and *more* insulin. Help!

The only permanent way to get relief from hypoglycaemia (caused by an irregular eating and drinking pattern) is to start eating sensibly *immediately*. Cut down on all white sugar and starch. No more white bread in any form whatsoever. And cut out alcohol and cigarettes.

Doctors also advise their patients to eat as many as six small protein meals a day, maybe a hard boiled egg, a slice of cheese, a bowl of bran with sliced bananas and milk, four or five nuts, a small lamb chop – the choice is endless and delicious.

Coffee should be restricted to two cups a day, and to help the digestive processes get back to normal, at least eight glasses of water should be a daily habit, too.

If after a month to six weeks there's no personality change and the patient is sweating for no apparent reason and suffering from tremors and headaches, the doctor usually advises a sugar tolerance test in case the pancreas is malfunctioning for other reasons.

No one should embark on a new pattern of eating without a doctor's advice in any case.

With hypoglycaemia the right diet can probably have you on your way back to your own sweet temper – which ought to be the only sweet thing about you.

HOW TO GET FATTER

When You've Been Too Thin All Your Life

Maria Beatrice de Savoia, daughter of ex-King Umberto of Italy, is a member of the most envied minority group in the Western World – the skinny people, around 7 stone (44 kg) in total, size three to four variety. Other members of the group are Gloria Vanderbilt Cooper, Audrey Hepburn, Twiggy and Mia Farrow – even when she's pregnant she only looks as if she's swallowed an olive.

Medically speaking, the lightweights are way ahead of the heavyweights in the lifespan race, but the line between lightweight and underweight is, understandably, a thin one.

Underweight can also mean under-nourished, which calls for a diet just as urgently as any case of obesity – a diet which would seem delightful to most people, obviously being based on a high calorie intake.

It's practically impossible to get thin people to admit to liking their shape. They always say they want to gain but can't; just like fat people, they say, 'But I eat like everybody else.' The fact is they don't. They only think they do. Just see your thinnest friend eat – it can resemble a sparrow at work.

Why They Stay Thin

Unless there's a medical dysfunction – a chronic infection, a hormonal imbalance, an underactive adrenal gland or an overactive thyroid, all of which obviously need medical attention – the forever slim and willowy or underfed and skinny (depending on how you look at it and whether they know how to dress) stay that way because there's rarely any feeling of acute hunger in the body. A low calorie intake maintains the status quo.

Experiments prove that habit factors greatly affect our shape.

For instance, when a fat and a thin person were put into a room furnished only with a table, a chair, and a clock, the fat person asked for something to eat when the clock told him it was lunchtime, while the thin person showed no reaction. In fact the clock was rigged to go twice as fast as normal, but one look at the time was enough to activate hunger signals fast from the hypothalamic appetite-regulating portion of the fat person's brain, affecting saliva and even stomach ache from hunger.

A lack of appetite is frequently behind a lack of measurements and this in turn can be caused by anorexia, a nervous condition which dissipates any interest in food. Some doctors with a number of too skinny patients observe that a minuscule appetite can be stimulated artificially with medical help, but as they are likely to have some sort of blood disturbance – diabetes or the reverse, low blood sugar – a glucose tolerance test is a wise course of action before embarking on any gain programme. Even if there is no medical explanation behind an obstinate inability to gain pounds and inches, doctors maintain that excessive sugar intake is a mistake. With a correct blood sugar level, appetite *can* be regained more easily and maintained. To that end, ironically, *diet* drinks, weak tea and sugar substitutes, are sometimes recommended even when you are trying to gain.

The Easiest Mistake to Make

The most common pitfall is to think a gain-weight diet is the opposite of a reducing one. Gulping down rich ice cream, cakes, extra portions of spaghetti, sugar and sweets won't help the picture, for these foods deliver the 'empty' kind of calories, which *fill us up* without *building up* nutrition.

The best gain-weight plan increases calorie intake with the building kind of foods. As 3,500 calories (14,000 kJ) is roughly equivalent to 1 lb (450 g) of body weight, it really means consuming about 1,000 calories (4,000 kJ) a day more than your body uses up for fuel. To add to average eating habits, it's best to choose portions of unrefined carbo-hydrate – potatoes (from 95 to 230 calories (380–920 kJ), depending on

The Dieting Game

cooking method), peas (105/420), corn (165/660), wild rice (395/1,580), olives (40/160), avocados (320/1,280), bananas (175/700), lima (150/600) and red kidney beans (320/1,280). In fact, most types of Mexican and Chinese food help achieve extra curves. Carbohydrates are less satisfying than proteins, so one can consume more. There's also evidence that carbohydrates help the system retain natural moisture, 'plumping' out the figure in the bleak spots. Nevertheless it's still wise to choose more of the unrefined type than the refined (foods which are heavy with sugar, flour or cornflour). If you smoke and/or drink more than moderately, cutting down or, best of all, completely *giving* up cigarettes and alcohol can only help spur the appetite.

Vitamins are Vital

Whatever vitamins you're taking now, there should be an increase in vitamin E and vitamin B complex intake, as well as more concentration on foods already packed with them naturally, like liver (85/340), whole grain (50/200) and enriched cereals (95–310/380–1,240), bread (30–190/120–760) and nuts (95/380).

It's been proved that the fastest way of gaining weight is eating snacks, which is why nibbling is taboo to the other, more commonplace kind of dieter. Three or four snacks taken throughout the day can add an amazing number of extra calories. For instance, by adding a cup of skimmed milk powder to a cup of soup, custard, or a hot drink, you immediately gain an extra 435 calories (1,740 kJ). By adding an instant food mix to an 8 fl oz (225 ml) glass of milk (160/640), you add 290 calories (1,160 kJ); add 3 tablespoons of malted milk powder and increase the whole total by 405 calories (1,620 kJ). These tricks make it easy to add 1,000 extra calories (4,000 kJ) a day – which will eventually show on the scales – and curves.

HYPNOSIS – CAN IT HELP AND HOW

She is hypnotized, not like Trilby by Svengali, or Walter Scott's Lady of the Lake, not asleep, not awake, not unconscious, but, to quote Dr Herbert Spiegel, Associate Professor of the Department of Psychiatry at Columbia University, 'she is in a form of *intense, aroused, attentive concentration*. Responsive concentration.'

Dr Spiegel is describing the hypnotic state as it really is, not mystical or frightening, or hocus-pocus either, but a condition induced by many doctors today to help in the treatment of a number of

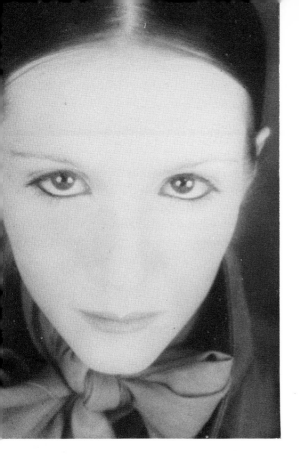

She is not asleep, not awake; she is hypnotized for her health's sake

self-inflicted sicknesses – brought about by over-eating, drinking or smoking.

Hypnosis is also a valuable ancillary towards overcoming a number of phobias (fear of flying, heights, crowds, cats or dogs), it also helps to assuage grief and shock, and to relieve pain in childbirth – in fact pain generally.

Today hypnosis is accepted as *aiding treatment*, providing it takes place under the auspices of skilled doctors.

Obviously, the august medical bodies would only recognize qualified treatment, but actually most laymen can be taught to hypnotize others.

What distinguishes the skilled practitioner from the layman is *knowing what to do once hypnosis is induced and having the ability to recognize who is hypnotizable and who is not.*

According to Dr Spiegel, about 70 per cent of the population can be hypnotized, which means 70 per cent have the ability *to concentrate well.* 'It's a complete fallacy,' he says 'that only the weak-minded can be hypnotized, for it is the weak-minded who are unable to concentrate for any length of time and so discipline their thoughts. The lower the intelligence, the poorer the subject for hypnotherapy.'

What Does It Feel like to be Hypnotized

Patients have described it as a totally relaxed, languid feeling of tranquillity, pleasant, peaceful, giving a sensation of floating. People who sleep deeply may even doze momentarily, while light sleepers feel completely awake.

Physicians describe it as a state that occurs *normally* somewhere between the diurnal rhythm of being asleep and being awake. This midway state is deliberately extended by the doctor, so that treatment can be carried out within its bounds.

Once hypnotizability is established, the entire emphasis in treatment is on replacing or superseding negative ways of thinking, feeling and acting (perhaps engrained over the years as habits) with totally new, *positive* ways; it is rather like using a projector on the mind, focusing on a new slide, giving the patient a different aspect of the situation.

The human mind, one-ninth conscious, eight-ninths sub-conscious, is extremely suggestible and becomes more so under hypnosis – 'the state of receptive attention', as practitioners often call it. Their object is to put forward a view that the patient is *for* rather than against.

For example, the unsuccessful dieter caught in a permanent on-and-off diet syndrome is helped to be positive and so more successful in her weight loss campaign by the doctor putting deep into her mind three basic but forceful facts:

1 Over-eating and over-drinking are damaging to your body.

2 You need your body to live. It is the precious physical plant through which you experience life.

3 You owe your body respect and protection.

These facts are put there to distract her attention completely away from her constant urge to eat the foods she knows defeat her objective. *Like all urges, if repeatedly not satisfied by being ignored, it eventually withers away.*

In trying to cut down or stop anything one knows is detrimental to health and spirit, the most frequent mistake is to put all the emphasis on *not doing so*. I must not eat ice cream. I should not eat ice cream. I will not eat ice cream.

As Dr Spiegel reiterates: 'This kind of thinking is dead wrong. It makes about as much sense as if you concentrate on not having an itching sensation on your nose. What happens if you concentrate on *not* having that itch? You have it all the more.'

The same thing happens when you concentrate merely on avoiding fattening foods. You end up more preoccupied with them than ever. The person accustomed to freedom is not helped with permanent sanctions against the urge that is uppermost in her mind, but she can affiliate with and arouse her compassion for a worthwhile and obviously self-preserving goal: *respecting the body, protecting it.*

Critics of hypnotism bring up the fact that it takes up so much time. The fact is, it doesn't. Today the most significant progress relates to the success of self-hypnosis, taught by the physician after only the first session. The patient using twenty seconds ten times a day is taught to float into her own island of awareness, and there to *reimprint* the new positive aspect for living already shown to her under hypnosis.

Hypnotism can't be forced on anyone who doesn't want it and neither can hypnotism induce anybody to act totally out of character. In other words, a basically moral person cannot be made to behave immorally, or vice versa. On the contrary, hypnotism frees people of inhibitions and their surface 'personality', allowing them to behave as they really are.

There are many programmes in existence that had their basis in hypnotism, such as the rerouting of consciousness used in Dr Grantley Dick-Read's method of natural childbirth, where the mind is distracted, led away from pain and directed with programmed breathing towards a specific job in helping give birth to the child. Programmed motivation, using tape systems to help one become more receptive to new thoughts – 'diet without drugs', 'listen and stop smoking' – work in the same way that one learns a language through repeated sessions with cassettes or recordings.

Research carried out in universities and medical schools has revealed that the shifting of awareness into another health-based, self-preservative category in response to a signal from another permits more intensive concentration upon a designated goal and, in this way, is of enormous benefit to medicine.

This means only one thing: *hypnosis.* You can't underrate it.

CALORIES COUNTER

Note: for convenience all metric measures of quantities of food have been rounded off into units of 25 gm or ml.

	CALORIES	KILO-JOULES	CARBO-HYDRATES
Beverages			
Beer (½ pint/275 ml)	170	680	18
Brandy (1 tot, 1½ fl. oz/38 ml)	120	480	0
Carbonated beverages – Cola (½ pint/			
275 ml)	107	428	20
Champagne (1 glass, 3 fl. oz/75 ml)	80	320	2
Chocolate beverages with milk			
(⅜ pint/225 ml)	205	820	18
Cider, sweet (½ pint/275 ml)	124	496	26
Coffee, black, sugarless (1 cup)	0	0	0
Cordials (1 small glass)	121	484	6
Gin, dry (1 tot, 1½ fl. oz/38 ml)	120	480	0
Rum (1 tot, 1½ fl. oz/38 ml)	105	420	0
Sherry (1 glass, 3 fl. oz/75 ml)	85	340	10–12
Tea, without milk (1 cup)	0	0	½
Whisky (1 tot, 1½ fl. oz/38 ml)	110	440	0
Wine, dry (1 glass, 3 fl. oz/75 ml)	85	340	10
Wine, sweet (1 glass, 3 fl. oz/75 ml)	160	640	12
Bread and Cereals			
Biscuits, salted (1)	15	60	3
Biscuits, soda (1)	30	120	4
Bran flakes (½ cup)	145	580	21
Bread, brown (1 slice)	90	360	11
Bread, raisin (1 slice)	65	260	13
Bread, rye, dark (1 slice)	57	228	12
Bread, wheat, cracked (1 slice)	60	240	12
Bread, white enriched (1 slice)	64	256	12
Bread, whole-wheat (1 slice)	55	220	11
Cereal foods – Infant, Dry-precooked			
(½ cup)	103	412	18
Cornflakes (½ cup)	96	384	18
Cracker, whole-wheat (1)	30	120	5
Doughnut (1)	125	500	17

	CALORIES	KILO-JOULES	CARBO-HYDRATES
Macaroni, cooked (½ cup)	209	836	80
Macaroni with cheese (½ cup)	215	860	84
Matzo (1)	80	320	5
Noodles, egg, cooked (½ cup)	200	800	49
Pancake (1)	90–105	360–420	18
Popped corn (1 cup)	54	216	10
Potato crisps (10)	108	432	10
Pretzel (5 small sticks)	18	72	11
Rice, cooked, white (½ cup)	160	640	30
Rice flakes (½ cup)	118	472	27
Rice, puffed (1 cup)	55	220	13
Roll, plain (1)	118	472	20
Roll, sweet (1)	178	712	20
Shredded wheat (1 bar)	85	340	18
Spaghetti, plain, cooked (3 oz/75 g)	165	660	35
Waffle with syrup (1)	216	864	30
Wheatgerm (2 tbsp.)	35	140	10
Wheat flakes (1 oz/25g)	125	500	23

Dairy Products

	CALORIES	KILO-JOULES	CARBO-HYDRATES
Butter (½ oz/15 g)	50	200	0
Cheese, blue (1 oz/25 g)	104	416	½
Cheese, Camembert (1 oz/25 g)	85	340	½
Cheese, Cheddar (1 oz/25 g)	113	452	½
Cheese, Cheddar, processed (1 oz/25 g)	105	420	½
Cheese, cottage (1 scoop)	225	900	3
Cheese, cream (1 scoop)	106	424	½
Cheese, Swiss, natural (1 oz/25 g)	105	420	1
Cheese, Swiss, processed (1 oz/25 g)	101	404	1
Cream, single (1 tbsp.)	30	120	1
Cream, double (1 tbsp.)	49	396	1½
Ice cream (1 scoop)	120–260	480–1,040	15
Milk, chocolate flavoured (½ pint/ 275 ml)	205	820	18
Milk, condensed, sweetened (1 tbsp.)	60	240	15
Milk, evaporated, unsweetened (1 tbsp.)	22	88	
Milk, malted, beverage (½ pint/275 m)	281	1,124	18

	CALORIES	KILO-JOULES	CARBO-HYDRATES
Milk, skimmed (½ pint/275 ml)	80	320	5
Milk, skimmed, dry (1 tbsp.)	28	112	2
Milk, whole (½ pint/275 ml)	166	664	11
Water ice (1 scoop)	236	944	28
Yogurt, plain (1 cup)	120	480	5
Yogurt, fruit (1 cup)	260	1,040	27

Desserts and Sweets

Apple strudel (1 small slice)	344	1,376	48
Cake, angel (1 small slice)	120	480	30
Cake, cup, iced (1 small slice)	161	644	31
Cake, fruit, dark (1 small slice)	140	560	45
Cake, plain (1 small slice)	180	720	31
Cake, pound (1 small slice)	130	520	15
Cake, sponge (1 small slice)	75	300	22
Chocolate, bitter (1 small bar)	142	568	12
Chocolate, sweetened (1 small bar)	133	532	24
Chocolate, syrup (1 tbsp.)	42	168	11
Cocoa (1 tbsp.)	21	84	12
Custard, baked (½ cup)	283	1,132	14
Fig biscuits, commercial (1)	55	220	12
Gelatin, dessert (½ cup)	80	320	18
Gelatin with fruit (½ cup)	140	560	21
Honey (1 tbsp.)	62	248	17
Jams, marmalades, preserves (1 tbsp.)	55	220	14
Pie, apple (1 wedge)	410	1,640	50
Pie, cherry (1 wedge)	420	1,680	45
Pie, custard (1 wedge)	365	1,460	35
Pie, lemon meringue (1 wedge)	355	1,420	35
Sugar, brown (1 tbsp.)	45	180	12
Sugar, granulated (1 tbsp.)	45	180	12
Syrup, golden (1 tbsp.)	57	228	15
Syrup, maple (1 tbsp.)	104	416	25

Fruit

Apple, fresh (1)	90	360	18
Apple sauce, no sugar (1 tbsp.)	100	400	20
Apple sauce, sweetened (1 tbsp.)	184	736	25
Apricot, raw (1)	18	72	13½

	CALORIES	KILO-JOULES	CARBO-HYDRATES
Avocado, raw ($\frac{1}{2}$)	160	640	6
Banana (1)	175	700	23
Blackberries, raw ($\frac{1}{2}$ cup)	41	164	10
Blackberries, syrup pack ($\frac{1}{2}$ cup)	85	340	12
Cantaloupe ($\frac{1}{2}$)	60	240	9
Cherries, fresh (1 cup)	65	260	8
Cherries, tinned (1 cup)	122	488	16
Cranberries, fresh (1 cup)	45	180	12
Cranberry sauce, sweetened, tinned (1 cup)	549	2,196	100
Dates, dried, pitted (1 cup)	490	1,960	7
Figs, dried (1)	40	160	15
Figs, tinned in syrup (3)	85	340	36
Fruit cocktail (1 cup)	110	440	50
Grapefruit, fresh ($\frac{1}{2}$)	40	160	14
Grapefruit, tinned (1 cup)	140	560	42
Grapefruit juice, sweetened ($\frac{1}{2}$ pint/ 275 ml)	175	700	18
Grapefruit juice, unsweetened ($\frac{1}{2}$ pint 275 ml)	75	300	9
Grape juice (1 cup)	145	580	21
Grapes (1 cup)	105	420	16
Honeydew melon ($\frac{1}{4}$)	49	196	10
Lemon, fresh (1)	25	100	6
Lemon juice (1 tbsp.)	4	16	1
Lime juice (1 tbsp.)	5	20	1
Olives (10)	220	880	2
Orange (1)	75	300	16
Orange juice, fresh (1 glass, $\frac{1}{2}$ pint/ 275 ml)	110	440	18
Peach, fresh (1)	35	140	10
Peaches tinned (2 halves)	79	316	24
Pear, fresh (1)	40	160	25
Pears, tinned (2 halves)	79	316	43
Pineapple, fresh (1 cup)	65	260	20
Pineapple, tinned, crushed (1 cup)	204	816	54
Pineapple juice (1 cup)	140	560	15
Plums, raw (1)	29	116	7

	CALORIES	KILO-JOULES	CARBO-HYDRATES
Plums, tinned (1)	186	744	25
Prunes, cooked, unsweetened (5)	120	480	22
Prunes, dry (4 uncooked)	73	292	20
Prune juice (1 cup)	190	760	22
Raisins, dry (1 tbsp.)	30	120	30
Raspberries, fresh (1 cup)	75	300	20
Redcurrants, raw (1 cup)	60	240	20
Rhubarb, stewed, sweetened (1 cup)	375	1,500	96
Strawberries, fresh (1 cup)	54	216	13
Strawberries, frozen (3 oz/75 g)	90	360	25
Tangerine (1)	45	180	10
Watermelon (1 wedge)	235	940	29

Meat, Fish, Poultry, Eggs

(3½ oz/100 g cooked weight wherever quantities are not specifically given)

	CALORIES	KILO-JOULES	CARBO-HYDRATES
Bacon, 2 rashers	97	388	1
Beef, hamburger chuck	316	1,264	0
Beef, rib roast, boneless	266	1,064	0
Beef, steak	257	1,028	0
Brains	106	424	6
Caviar (1 tbsp.)	24	96	0
Chicken	332	1,328	0
Chicken, fryer, breast	210	840	5
Cod	106	424	½
Crab	89	356	0–5
Egg (1)	77	308	0
Yolk	57	228	0
White	14	56	0
Flounder, baked (8–10 oz/225–250 g)	200	800	0
Frankfurter (1 large)	124	496	1
Haddock, fried (8–10 oz/225–250 g)	165	660	4
Halibut, grilled (8–10 oz/225–250 g)	215	860	0
Ham, fresh or smoked, cooked	338	1,352	0
Herring, smoked, kippered	210	840	0
Lamb chop	356	1,424	0
Lamb, leg, roasted (2 slices)	230	920	0
Liver (2 slices)	75–85	300–340	8

	CALORIES	KILO-JOULES	CARBO-HYDRATES
Liver sausage (2 slices)	80	320	1
Lobster (2 oz/50 g)	78	312	0
Mackerel (8–10 oz/225–250 g)	190–305	760–1,220	0
Oysters (6)	200	800	8
Pork, loin	240	960	0
Salmon	180	720	0
Sardines, drained (8–10 oz/225–250 g)	171	684	1
Sardines in tomato sauce (8–10 oz/225–250 g)	195	780	6
Sausage, pork	150	600	0
Scallops, raw (4 medium-size)	89	356	11
Shrimps	115	460	0
Swordfish, grilled	175	700	0
Tongue, beef	160	640	1
Tuna, tinned, drained (2 oz/50 g)	135	540	0

Nuts

Almonds (18)	130	520	7
Peanut butter (1 tbsp.)	92	368	3
Peanuts (1 cup)	840	3,360	28
Pecans (1 cup)	700	2,800	16
Walnuts (1 cup)	654	2,616	20

Sandwiches

Chicken salad	245	980	19
Cream cheese and nut	267	1,068	30
Egg salad	280	1,120	18
Ham	280	1,120	18
Ham and cheese	413	1,652	20
Hamburger	400	1,600	20

Sauces, Fats and Oils

Chilli sauce (1 tbsp.)	17	68	4
French dressing (1 tbsp.)	59	236	2
Margarine (1 tbsp.)	50	200	0
Mayonnaise (1 tbsp.)	110	440	0
Oils (1 tbsp.)	124	496	0
Tomato ketchup (1 tbsp.)	20	80	4
Tomato purée (1 cup)	100	400	15

	CALORIES	KILO-JOULES	CARBO-HYDRATES
Soups			
(all 8 fl. oz/225 ml portions)			
Bean	191	764	19
Bouillon, cube	2	8	0
Bouillon, ready to serve	9	36	0
Chicken	75	300	7
Clam chowder	86	344	10
Creamed soups	201	804	10
Noodle soups	117	468	6
Oyster stew	209	836	10
Pea	120	480	23
Tomato	75	300	16
Vegetable	65	260	13
Vegetables			
Asparagus (6 spears)	22	88	3
Beans, kidney (1 cup)	230	920	42
Beans, lima (1 cup)	152	608	30
Beans, navy (1 cup)	642	2,568	30
Beans, green (1 cup)	27	108	10
Beans, tinned, baked (1 cup)	310	1,240	48
Beetroot (1 cup)	68	272	16
Broccoli (1 cup)	44	176	8
Brussels sprouts (1 cup)	60	240	12
Cabbage (1 cup)	40	160	10
Carrots, raw (1 cup)	21	84	10
Carrots, tinned (1 cup)	44	176	12
Cauliflower, cooked (2 oz/50 g)	30	120	6
Cauliflower, raw (2 oz/50 g)	25	100	6
Celery (1 stalk)	18	72	1
Coleslaw (2 oz/50 g)	102	408	12
Corn, sweet, fresh (1 ear)	100	400	16
Corn, sweet, tinned (2 oz/50 g)	165	660	40
Cucumber (2 oz/50 g)	15	60	2
Endive (1 lb/450 g)	90	360	10
Kale, fresh (1 cup)	45	180	10
Lettuce (2 leaves)	7	28	1
Mushrooms (1 cup)	35	140	10

	CALORIES	KILO-JOULES	CARBO-HYDRATES
Onions, raw (1)	40	160	11
Parsley	5	20	1
Peas, fresh (1 cup)	100	400	28
Peas, tinned (1 cup)	105	420	32
Peppers, green (1)	16	64	3
Pickles, dill (1)	15	60	2
Pickles, sweet (1)	150	600	5
Potatoes, baked (large)	140	560	21
Potatoes, chipped (10)	140	560	16
Potatoes, mashed (½ cup)	95	380	30
Radishes, raw (5)	10	40	2
Sauerkaut (1 cup)	25	100	6
Spinach, boiled (1 cup)	40	160	6
Sweet potatoes, baked (1)	140	560	36
Sweet potatoes, candied (1)	115	460	60
Tomato, raw (1)	35	140	6
Tomato, tinned or cooked (1 cup)	46	184	10
Tomato juice (1 cup)	50	200	5
Turnip (1 cup)	30	120	10

11

For Women at Work - 3

HOW TO INCREASE YOUR PRODUCTIVITY WITHOUT LOSING YOUR BREATH

HAVE you ever related early morning apathy at the type-writer to the absence of a boiled egg in your life, or linked the loss of your usual good telephone manner to the doughnut you decided to have, throwing your usual caution to the winds? If the two experiences seem familiar and yet totally unconnected to your food intake, think again. Your energy level depends very much on what you happen to put in your mouth, and your state of mind is intimately associated with your energy level.

As the great nutritionist Adele Davis once said, 'For the sake of your health and stamina, eat breakfast like a king, lunch like a prince and dinner like a pauper.' For most of us that's difficult to swallow (literally!), and yet all those I know who strive to live by it are healthy and have great stamina to prove it.

Energy

The biggest obstacle to building energy and so productivity at work is unfortunately often canteen food, with the tea wagon going round the office or factory at 10 a.m. and/or 3 p.m. to ensure just the right quota of sluggishness is served up for the day. If you want to prove me wrong go along with an easy test period. Set your alarm clock for half an hour earlier than usual (and, hopefully, go to bed earlier the night before) in order to serve yourself a breakfast of body brightening foods, guaranteed to set your metabolism going at the right rate and to exercise your intestinal tract – probably sleepy and sluggish after years of eating too much overcooked soft stuff.

Ideally serve an alphabet of vitamins: A, essential for producing a

240

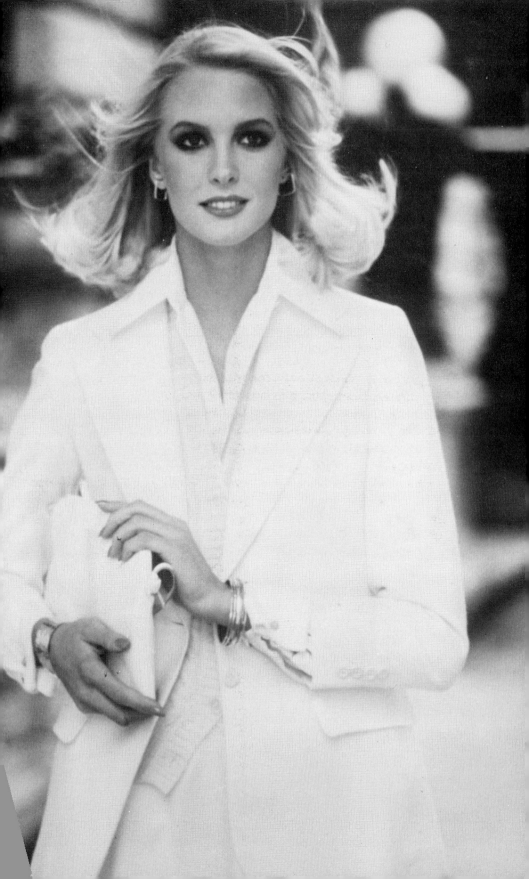

firm clear skin, found in yellow fruits, vegetables and eggs; B complex, essential for 'burning' our food, turning carbohydrate into glucose, the fuel we literally need to keep going, directing nutrients in food to blood cells, 'rejuvenating' all our vital organs – found in all grains and nuts; C, essential to fight infection, found in all citrus fruits, straw-berries, watercress, and celery; and D, essential for strengthening bones and teeth, found in milk, grapes, tomatoes and sunshine.

An early morning energy menu that's easily followed and quickly prepared is this: a banana (vitamin A plus the all important potassium), wholemeal toast (B complex) and honey (D), a large glass of orange juice (C), and, if you must have coffee or tea, at least make it with milk (more D). Add an egg twice a week, and let me know if your energy level doesn't improve and along with it your early morning sense of humour.

'Roughage'

Without stressing the point, your work will suffer if you don't give your body some time in the morning to eliminate what it has to. One way to ensure 'regularity' is to make 'roughage' part of your daily menu. Start by not straining fruit juices; the cellulose is valuable in stimulating the intestinal tract to perform beautifully. If the food you have available in your lunch hour is only the junk kind, don't weaken, thinking it can't do you any harm. It can and probably has already, if only to make you feel more tired than you really are.

Take along with you a 'roughage' lunch or snack to speed up your own body machinery. Take it in plant form – in fruit (apples, full of acids your body needs, tomatoes or cucumbers), in leaf (lettuce, cresses, chicory or parsley) and in root (carrots, radishes, cold cooked leeks or shallots). Add a piece of chicken or cold fish and you have the perfect working woman's lunch, geared to building stamina (and so speed) and improving skin *and* shape at the same time (the kind of self-productivity we can all be proud of).

How to Fall in Love with Exercise

AND EVERYTHING YOU EVER WANTED TO KNOW ABOUT THE SUBJECT

NOBODY owns up about exercise, owns up to the fact that it bores the leotards off most of us, unless it's attached to a favourite sport. Tennis anybody?

While exercise teachers, gymnasts, calisthenic tutors and yoga gurus seem to grow in number every year, pupils mostly come and go – admittedly always to be replaced by more pupils, who also come, but, alas, then go. Staying the course is really the exception rather than the rule, which is another reason, statistically speaking, why we are so out of shape as a nation (see Chapter 10, page 198).

Psychoanalysts point out that the relationship between posture and mental attitude is illustrated for all to see in paintings and sculpture dating back hundreds of years. The man who is depressed is crouching up there on the canvas. The man or woman who is confident and happy *stretches* out with exuberance – which, as every exercise-happy psychoanalyst will tell you, is the first and most fundamental exercise, one that starts every worthwhile exercise class.

The fact is we know that stretching and much more are good for us. We know we should do our exercises every day as diligently as we brush our teeth and, as I've written myself at least 2,000 times, 'only a few minutes every day will help'.

We also know that for some reason exercise is like daily medicine, something that we tend to pretend we forget to take. We're too busy. We work too hard, so we're too exhausted. It's too cold in the morning. Too tiring at night.

The truth for most of us is that WE DON'T LIKE IT – except as far as I'm concerned I *used* not to like it, but I've learned to. How? Through being brainwashed by contact with so many experts, and also through seeing with my own eyes *the end results*.

THAT FEW MINUTES EACH DAY

What isn't boring about exercise is undoubtedly the beautiful end result, as many can testify, like, for instance, the Man Who-Wanted-To-Be President of the U.S.A., Ronald Reagan, Frank's daughter, Tina Sinatra, Barbra Streisand and Vidal's now sleek and svelte American wife Beverly Sassoon.

All of these neat people 'had no time' for exercise once, until they came under the influence of an expert body shaper – in the first three instances, a well known Hollywood one called Marvin Hart, in the case of Beverly Sassoon, a guru named Bikram Choudhury.

They all quickly discovered that *supervision* from someone you respect is the easiest way to beat man's ancient enemy, laziness.

Marvin Hart, whose 'outwit-your-body exercises' I'll tell you about later (see page 271), has transformed more sluggish shapes than Daryl Zanuck ever transformed starlets into stars. Because of *results*, people like Ronnie, Tina and Barbra keep at it day after day, because, as Marvin says (in common with all exercise experts), *'to be effective exercise has to become as much part of your lifestyle as eating and sleeping'*.

This brings us right back to those 'few minutes every day'. It's a fact that has to be faced: those few minutes have to be devoted to daily practice for RESULTS. Curiously enough, the right set of movements carried out every day *does* eventually lead to a feeling of well-being and, best of all, better looks. Unfortunately, nothing is achieved if exercise is a once-a-month, or even once-a-week, act of martyrdom. The right mental attitude is as important as the exercise itself. The trim, must-be-slim-at-all-costs, from Jackie Onassis to Farah Diba, the Shah's wife, work at it with tenacious concentration wherever they happen to be. As far as Jackie and Farah Diba are concerned, they happen to believe in jogging, rain or shine.

How to Get the Most out of Exercise

Whatever kind of shape you're in, it's a good idea to begin any approach to exercise in front of a full-length mirror, working out as a dancer does, whether you're copying movements from a magazine or

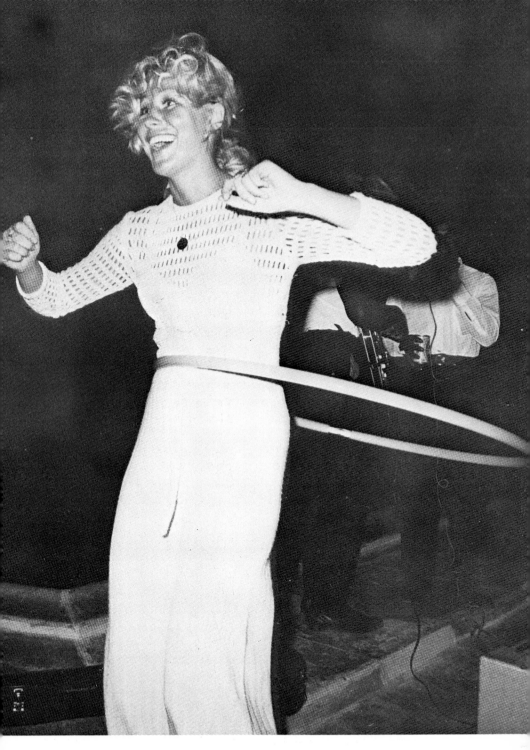

A few minutes each day – a little exercise never hurt anybody

book or listening to a T.V. or radio tutor. As any expert worth his wall bars will tell you, 'exercise must be taken at a comfortable pace'. Any continuing pain or strain attached to movement is a no-no. If you find touching your toes an insurmountable task, don't fret. Start by touching your calves or ankles instead. Do what you can and you'll end up doing more – and more. If music helps, use it. Try to exercise without stopping for the duration of one side of a disc – about fifteen minutes of listening time. Don't stop for a tea break or even to say 'yes' on the telephone. You'll find your momentum gone and the magic wasted. It may seem hard to believe, but when you're at your most fatigued, from a day at the office or the backgammon board, exercise can give your body more of a lift than a gin and tonic or a glass of champagne. You don't have to swing from the chandeliers or climb the nearest mountain to find out I'm right. Simple stretching exercises, arms up, then down to the floor, while breathing the right way, will restore energy, moving fresh blood up to the brain to get you in good shape for whatever life holds in store.

LEARN HOW TO BREATHE

No instructor will start anyone moving a muscle without first teaching and preaching correct breathing. Yes, *breathing*. It's a curious fact that, generally without realizing it, beginners tend to *hold* their breath when attempting their first exercises, hoping that way they'll achieve more, because they're used to tensing up that way whenever they have to *achieve*!

Double breathing is the way to break the holding habit. This means a combination of inhaling and exhaling at given times during the exercise.

1 At the beginning you should concentrate on *inhaling* through the nose. This guarantees that more oxygen will flood the lungs to move on to your bloodstream to give extra life and energy to your body.

2 Towards the middle of the movement *exhale explosively*. This rids the body of carbon dioxide and waste matters filtered from the bloodstream.

3 *Inhale* deeply once more (more oxygen).

4 Finally *exhale* just as noisily as before.

If you learn to *be conscious* of your breathing when you start to exercise, inhaling and exhaling as described, this will develop the diaphragm, enlarge the rib cage, and strengthen all muscles connected with the breathing apparatus – very useful in just keeping up with life's hustle and bustle without getting breathless.

Watch a sleeping baby to learn about correct breathing. See how the stomach expands and relaxes rhythmically as the baby breathes. Nothing else moves. Unfortunately, as the baby grows older that natural breathing pattern changes. You will see for yourself in a mirror that you are now breathing differently than from when you were a baby. Probably your bosom will be rising and falling while your stomach doesn't move a muscle. This is shallow breathing, taking in very little air and using only the uppermost part of the lungs, something forced upon us by the rush-rush-rush of modern civilization. Today we have to relearn correct breathing to cope with day-to-day life, to improve both the colour and strength of our skin and to build our stamina.

When our lungs process air (about 21 per cent oxygen, 79 per cent nitrogen) we naturally extract the oxygen our body needs and exhale the rest. The more oxygen we take in, the healthier we can become. Oxygen helps burn the food we eat to turn it into the fuel that literally produces our energy. Oxygen builds up our blood supply which in turn delivers nutrition to every part of our being – the condition of our teeth, nails, scalp, every inch of us, depends upon the condition of our bloodstream.

Because the brain requires at least three times more oxygen than the rest of our body, take time for some deep breathing exercises before solving a knotty problem or facing a room full of people. A well conditioned body is often connected to an alert, bright brain, because anyone in good shape inhales more air (more oxygen) for longer periods and exhales more waste, as the muscles around the lungs are in shape to do more work. All exercise improves oxygen intake, which is why a morning constitutional came into being for many of those engaged in affairs of state.

'A man can think better after a run around the park,' one was heard to say, and that goes for a woman, too.

To pep up your body and brain, practise deep breathing by an open window (not in a polluted area). Crosslegged on a comfortable rug or blanket and keeping your spine straight, inhale smoothly through your nose, silently counting to five. Inhale from your diaphragm, if you can, feeling the muscle between your bosom and your stomach. As your lungs fully inflate, feel your diaphragm contract. Hold for ten, then exhale just as smoothly and slowly through your mouth, relaxing your diaphragm, rib cage and abdomen. Do this as many times as you like, for there's more power behind this simple breathing exercise than people realize. On inhaling, nature uses our built-in filters to strain out impurities in the air, allowing only the pure oxygen through, changing it to body temperature before it reaches the lungs. On exhaling, the smoker, for example, gets rid of cigarette smoke as well as carbon dioxide and other waste matters from the body. If you carry out that simple exercise throughout the week you should feel renewed energy and interest in life. Also, if you are experiencing pain or tension, concentrate on deep breathing to get you through until you can get positive help. Deep rhythmic breathing is used to control pain in natural childbirth because the extra oxygen helps the brain to help you think positively.

Whenever you're feeling frazzled, carry out the inhale-and-exhale 'exercise'. You'll be surprised how refreshed you'll feel.

WHICH EXERCISE METHOD IS FOR YOU?

Men and women have turned mental somersaults searching for exercise methods that would not only bring results, but might be fun, too. In cities like Stockholm, Hamburg, San Francisco and Copenhagen, sex is suggested as part of the exercise manual, with positions, gyrations and gymnastics based on the supposition that as muscles begin to shrink from about twenty onwards, stretching them back can be accomplished with a member of the opposite sex. Nobody has suggested, however, that sex helps achieve a well articulated pelvis – yet.

The dance method of exercise, however, can do this – if carried out correctly – so can calisthenics (exercises using only the body, no real 'equipment'), gym (with equipment) or yoga (with or without guru). But where to start and what to choose?

Contrast is the key thing to look for in any exercise plan – look for one that's in direct *contrast* to your usual life.

If you're a desk-bound, typewriter-trapped, sedentary secretary, join a gym where you can work off buttock boredom on a vast array of equipment, or join a club with a swimming pool, so that water can help deliver results.

If you're a house-bound, child-tied, husband-happy housewife, get introduced to yoga – to grab some contemplative moments along with shape-making movements.

If you're a happy, horsy, hippy, jolly hockey sticks sort of lady, try a svelter form of exercise, and join a dance class with mirrored walls and evocative music to help you move more sinuously.

Three things to remember:

1 If you laugh at yourself or others while exercising, you'll accomplish nothing. Laughter means you're too relaxed. Your movements can't have the necessary thrust.

2 Pain means the exercise isn't working properly – and exhaustion isn't the object of the exercise either. Move, but don't over-exert yourself.

3 Panty girdles can inhibit exercise, particularly restricting the flow of blood to and from the area being exercised. Panty girdles are a deceptive crutch anyway, for, apart from restricting the blood flow to the lower part of the body (the part most put upon by flab), they don't give lazy muscles any chance to work. Imagine every time you wanted to lift your arm, someone lifted it for you. It wouldn't be long before the arm muscles became so flabby and weak you wouldn't be able to lift it yourself. So the panty girdle encourages muscles to be lazy in just the area where flab likes to sit and do nothing. They should be for 'sometimes', never *always*, and buttocks should practise contracting several times a day to act as nature's own girdle. Try it now as you read the next section. Contract, relax, contract, relax and on . . .

Who Wants to Dance Their Way to Shape?

Not since Fred Astaire made every girl want to Ginger up has the dance method of exercise (dance classes for non-dancers) been so in demand. Ballet, modern jazz, Afro, West Indian limbo – it's been proved that all these dance movements correctly taught and practised bring as much tone to the body as the hula hoop.

Plenty of *plié* (kneebends) in the morning and some *relevé* (stretching) at night appeal to some far more than jogging or, as the disenchanted call it, 'dreary exercise'.

Since few people have even a smidgen of Margot Fonteyn, the beginners' dance-exercise class can seem downright ordinary, because the most conscientious teachers set out to prove in slow motion how each dance movement can tone various parts of the body, rather like swimming on dry land. (Swimming and exercising in wet water is another story, see page 258. Even the most basic breast stroke exercises every part of you, providing your feet are off the bottom.)

Most dance-exercise classes start with a standing or sitting warm-up – swinging arms vigorously back and forth, head down, head up, to eliminate tension. Then there's a lot of lateral movement involved because, as is usually pointed out, 'We don't move from side to side in daily life – so this movement wakes up muscles that rarely get used.' *Contrast is all.*

When lying down, students may be asked to flex their muscles in time to music or the teacher's finger-snapping tempo. Each area is moved separately – head, neck, shoulders, rib cage, pelvis, ankles, stomach, buttocks and thighs – hopefully in time to get tuned up.

If the dance class is classically orientated, this means *barre* work – ballet's way of describing movements carried out at a bar attached to a (usually) mirrored wall. The bar is great to anchor those unused to deep kneebends and sideways leg stretching, with shoulders kept *back*, the head *up* in as lofty a manner as possible. Ballet movements help people with problem legs, whereas jazz exercises – stretching and shaking – affect the body all over *if* carried out *consistently*.

There are teachers who believe that in the early stages of the game pupils should work with their eyes closed, so they're not conscious of what they look like (!) but, hopefully, start reflecting on what's happening *inside* as movements get more and more away from the movements used in daily life.

In the modern dance-exercise classes, initial work-outs can be tough, students being expected to bend and flex in time to rock music with beachballs wedged between their knees.

Later, trained by the beachball technique, they move on to waist trimming with music, undulating on bended knee to tone the pelvic area.

GETTING INTO THE HAREM. Belly dancing has reared its solar plexus aggressively in the last few years – offered not as a titillating Turkish treat, but as a direct method of decreasing flab without increasing the size of the belly. It's claimed there are over 450 different steps and combinations (dance steps combined) to belly dancing. When carried out to Middle Eastern music, under the stern eyes of a lady who perhaps gives no indication of ever having been near a harem, poise, grace, stamina and shape *can* still improve. As a way of bringing young mothers back to pre-pregnancy shape, belly dancing has been given the once-over by hospital physiotherapists and pronounced okay for toning stomach muscles.

Yoga for Constant Youth

The relationship between dancing and yoga is distant, yet definite, says the guru. 'Dance movements loosen the muscles, strengthen the body, *and relax the mind and spirit.*'

This is key, because yoga, one of the most popular yet not altogether understood forms of exercise in the Western World, relates as much to the mind as to the body.

In California, Vidal Sassoon's wife, Beverly has improved her shape with yoga, as she says, 'out of all recognition'. She also says she sleeps better, her skin is clearer, and most important of all, she is more able to cope with a hectic life, involving three young children, a college course, a full social programme, plus travelling the world with Vidal to help him publicize his hairdressing empire.

Beverly says she owes even a new equilibrium to yoga, taught to her whenever she's home six days a week by guru Bikram Choudhury, a graduate of the Yoga College of India in Calcutta.

As he explains his 'science', 'Yoga psychology recognizes mind and body as interdependent. Just as the mind cannot function perfectly when the body is suffering, so the body is in trouble when there are mental disturbances.'

At his yoga class or at any given by a *true yogi* (there is a big difference between the real McCoy and the sham), you start by learning how to achieve control over your body to further self-discipline.

The majority of students who turn to yoga as a means of maintaining, attaining or retrieving a beautiful shape learn about forty exercise movements fundamental to yoga, along with the vital breathing techniques that enable them, if necessary, to be able to go through life practising satisfactorily alone.

The main accomplishment of hatha (physical) yoga is toning and firming the body by releasing muscle tension and learning to utilize breathing, literally, in the most refreshing way. *Ha breathing* is a positive exercise devised to help cope with the negative aspects of life. Providing there's privacy to ensure concentration, it can be practised anywhere at any time. The extra beauty about yoga is that it is a time-honoured system of physical culture that allows anyone of any age or condition to exercise according to his or her capacity and at his or her own pace.

To breathe the ha way, stand with feet well apart, arms at sides, and breathe *out*, *out*, *out*, as if to lose every breath in your body. Slowly raise arms up over your head, and inhale through the nose. As you lower your arms s-l-o-w-l-y to the sides, exhale once more.

Ha breathing is part of hatha yoga, the discipline or science concerned with perfect health that's most generally taught in the West. Because there are *sixteen* systems of yoga, not surprisingly there's often confusion, even fear, in the Western mind about this complex but fascinating Indian philosophy.

The sixteen systems were first recorded by Patanjali, who lived three centuries after Buddha and greatly admired his teachings. The yoga wheel developed by Patanjali was largely inspired by the Buddhist wheel of life, and comprises of sixteen spokes, eight outer ones concerned with the *physical* world, eight inner ones concerned with the *spiritual* world. Significantly, the wheel collapses without one of its spokes.

There are practitioners among the Eastern mystics who have complete grasp and control over all sixteen 'spokes' – the final step is called *raja yogi* – who can feel heat or cold at will, sleep on a bed of nails, go without sleep or any apparent food and, it's said, practise the act of self-levitation.

There are no Western raja yogis – sufficient comment on the serenity to be gained in this part of the world – but *hatha yoga* has many disciples here, all gaining a sense of peace and mastery over their problems – through exercises that rely on mind and body working together in perfect harmony, exercise carried out with special thoughts.

AN ELEMENTARY YOGA CLASS. This is the sort of thing that might happen at your first yoga class.

You will be asked to kneel to listen to slow rhythmic music, your head folded on to your crossed arms.

As you listen you will be asked to show you love the music by hugging your arms to your body, all the time inhaling deeply, and to relate the music to nature and the nature of things by enacting a scene, following the yogi, but thinking your own thoughts. You stretch back still on your knees, moving your arms as far back as you possibly can. Then, like the yogi, you fall forward into the 'earth' and are told to imagine rain pouring down to make things grow, stretching forward with your arms, following your arms with your body, pressing your head down 'becoming a seed'. Outstretched you keep down, exhaling, holding that position until you start to inhale again. Again you will be asked to think only of nature as you listen to the music. This time, stretching back up, you inhale fresh oxygen from life's power – air – using stretching as a tranquillizer, one used by man and animal alike. You will shake and sway, imagining the wind blowing, flowers quivering, then you will be asked to fold down gently, slowly, as seeds do, relaxing completely, back to your first position on your knees, head folded into your arms, as if to sleep till next spring.

Elementary, but surprisingly effective, and, of course, that's just the beginning.

SHOW BUSINESS YOGA. Two favourite yoga exercises for actors and actresses are called the Lion and the Gargoyle, both aimed at developing a supple spine *and* spirit.

In the Lion position, you kneel, hands on knees, with buttocks resting on heels. The Lion springs into action as you lean torso forward, tensing all muscles, making even your hands tense as your fingers spread apart to touch thumbs while your fingertips brush the floor. Stick out your tongue as far as you can and feel your face and neck muscles tense. Slowly roll the tongue back until the under side of its tip presses against the roof of the mouth. Relax, return to your kneeling position and repeat ten times. Singers say this exercise relieves tired, even sore, throats.

From the Lion position, more advanced students move on to the Gargoyle, retracting the tongue but with the head still down. Then the mouth should be opened as wide as possible, bending the head back as far on the neck as it will go. The last movement is to clench the teeth (not lips) three times. I'm told this is a sure-fire preventative for grinding teeth in one's sleep (see page 328), while both Lion and Gargoyle are exercises that are anti-double chin, anti-crêpy neck, and anti-jowls.

Still quoting show business sources, opera singers tell me they love a triple breathing exercise from yoga, which as it strengthens the neck also strengthens the voice, giving it new quality. They say when they carry out this breathing exercise before a performance, it gives the face a special radiance.

Inhale and exhale so deeply through the nose that it creates a 'bellows effect', even making the neck veins stand out. When inhaling, try to blow out the stomach as if it were a balloon filling with air; it isn't easy because it feels as if you're working at cross purposes, but that's the object.

When exhaling, try to draw in the stomach. Yogis say it's necessary to do it at least twenty-five times in the beginning before you're able to get the rhythm, then it comes easily after only seven or eight times.

Deep breathing helps your skin, too. By taking in more oxygen, you take in more water molecules, which form moisture in the body, the vital ally to skin texture (see page 32).

Surprising as it may seem, even if you've never seen the world the other way up, you will probably be encouraged to try a headstand at your first yoga class. Yogis and gurus believe in it – so do all exercise experts – because the headstand (or even a near miss) sends fresh blood to nourish the brain structure, *benefiting every other part of the body* and also increasing coordination. The brain and heart receive stimulation from the change of gravity and the increase in oxygen and blood. Every muscle and organ benefits. The aorta, carotids and arteries receive the bonus blood, which finally reaches the entire body, spinal cord and central nervous system, so sharpening intellect and memory and relieving asthmatic discomfort, headaches and dizziness. High wire workers often do a headstand before getting on the trapeze. They find they have less accidents that way.

UPSIDE DOWN DO-IT-YOURSELF. To get that way up, first practise kneeling with weight firmly resting on your forearms and elbows, hands on mat, fingers interlocked, cupping head to keep it steady. Rise on your toes and with bent knees move slowly forward until you feel the weight of your body balanced on your arms. Practise until you feel in control and comfortable, then slowly raise legs, remembering your weight is being held by your arms resting on the floor, while your hands hold your head steady, stomach muscles and spine assisting.

Everything about yoga requires *thinking*, so that a tedious job becomes an exercise for improving your muscles – and so your shape. Yoga is a continuous process – for, as thousands have discovered, the more body and mind become one in endeavour, the fitter, shapelier and happier they become.

Physiotherapy – You May Not Know You Need It

The physiotherapist's job is to help you mobilize your muscles – although you may not always know your muscles need mobilizing. Here the expert helps you educate or re-educate the muscles that con-

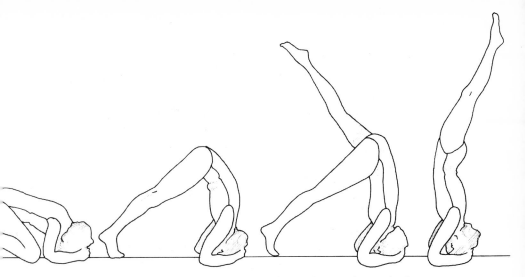

trol posture and movement, so that they perform their tasks with the ease and symmetry nature intended.

In the medical and surgical world, physiotherapy is a vital ancillary science aiding recovery from illness or accident. In the world of beauty, it offers a scientific route to elegance and shape.

EXERCISING THE NECK. Whether you go through life burying your head in the sand or are known for your remarkable stiff upper lip, the wear and tear on your lily-white neck is tremendous. This is where much back trouble can stem from and the pun is deliberate.

Take five seconds off to think about *how much* depends upon the neck's state of health, its ability to move freely – the larynx, the thyroid and lymphatic glands, and the various nerve roots need a healthy neck to perform well, as do the large blood vessels which supply the brain.

The neck muscles not only fight a constant battle against the downward pull of gravity, but are easily dispirited by emotional upset, tension, worry, fret and fuss – and whoever knew anybody who was never subject to any of that?

Yet the neck is neglected, frequently left out when it comes to daily and/or nightly beauty rituals, when skin care so often stops short at the chin – and it's rarely if ever *exercised*.

It's a pity, physiotherapists tell me often enough, because the right set of neck exercises can help relieve *all* feelings of congestion and pressure inside the head and generally contribute a feeling of well-being to the whole body. *Practised regularly* like the pianoforte, neck exercises can even improve one's appearance, cutting down to the right proportion the ancient problem of how-to-win-friends-and/or-influence-the-right-people.

How to Fall in Love with Exercise

The following do-it-yourself exercises were originally devised by physiotherapist Norman Sandieson, D.O., M.R.O., for those *not* under medical care for any spinal complaints. Used as part of an overall exercise programme at the Sussex spa, Forest Mere, they may appear to affect only the neck, but they do affect the back muscles, too, which they are meant to do, hence the medical warning.

Basically there are four movements to concentrate on for homework. *Side bending:* keeping the face to the front throughout, bend the head first to one side, then to the other, trying to bring the ear as close to the shoulder as possible. *Forward and backward bending:* bring the head slowly forward until the chin is pressing on the chest, then up and back as far as possible, keeping the mouth open slightly, so that the lower jaw is relaxed and doesn't retard movement. *Head rolling:* start with the side bending movement, then continue trying to 'roll' the head as far as it will go around to the back, then move slowly forward again to the opposite side, before reversing the entire movement. *Another 'rolling' exercise* involves turning the head s-l-o-w-l-y, trying to peep over your own shoulder, stretching so that by glancing down you can almost see your heels, first one side, then the other.

Carried out tortoise slow ten times in front of a mirror twice a day, the best results come with practice, gradually pressing a little harder each time so that the muscles really get stretched. Creaking and cracking may go on, especially in neck rolling, but not to worry – it merely shows how much the exercises are needed. The physiotherapist always employs massage, along with special exercises, during treatment, bending legs back, 'cracking' arm muscles, alternating muscle workouts with soothing, stroking movements.

Everyone should make a point of checking over their muscles with an expert physiotherapist once a year – whether they 'hurt' or not.

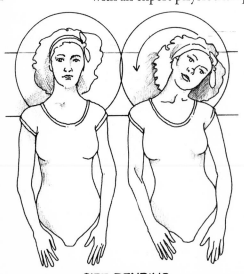

SIDE BENDING

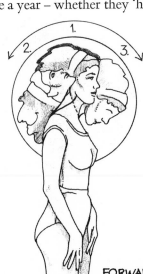

FORWARD AND
BACKWARD BENDING

THINKING 'UP' CAN PREVENT BACKACHE. Posture isn't just a pretty word. It's a pretty look. Without it you can look and feel years older. On the other foot, with good posture you can be noticed and admired even if you happen to have a big nose, a receding chin or other irritating facts of life.

To get down to basics, poor posture simply means there's poor coordination between one set of muscles and another, one set of limbs and another part of the body. It can create problems, related not only to the attractiveness of a look, but to something as real and as painful as backache, possibly the most talked about ailment in life today.

Muscle is the raw material of movement; without it we would be floppy and immobile. Over 650 muscles provide body movement and the necessary support for us to stand upright. There are other muscles in the body, but these 650 skeletal or voluntary muscles are the ones we depend on. As the word 'voluntary' suggests, it's up to our brain to tell these voluntary muscles just how we wish to stand or slump, smile or frown. Acting in the same way as cables, muscles pull on our bones to produce the movements we 'voluntarily' signal we want to produce, involving the contraction and shortening of muscle fibres. Even when we're relaxed, our muscles contract partially but don't shorten.

The gluteus maximus, which gives shape, or should give shape, to our buttocks, is a large muscle and so easy to use; yet it is often neglected and so unused. Flexed in and out and contracted *voluntarily* throughout the day, the buttocks can easily become attractive, shapely, firm and well toned. Just sat on all day and unused, and the largeness of the gluteous maximus is a complete waste of space in the body.

When we stand still, much coordinated muscular activity is actually being carried out though we can't see or feel it. We are forever

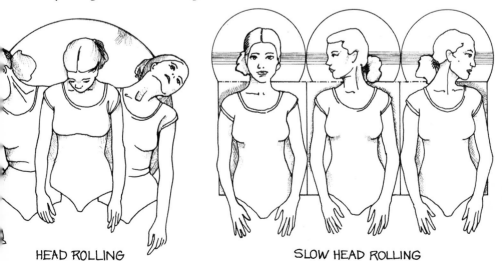

HEAD ROLLING   SLOW HEAD ROLLING

fighting the pull of gravity downwards. In order for us to stand upright, our muscles are at work, requiring a great amount of energy on
the body's part, from the feet on up to the legs, the pelvis, the abdomen
and the shoulders, constantly adjusting and readjusting the alignment
of bones, transmitting our weight to the ground. That's why a cocktail
party, however entertaining, can also be tiring, even more tiring to
some than jogging for half an hour, although all we may do is stand
more or less in one spot, holding nothing weightier than a martini
glass. Think about this because the most important thing to do is to
use your skeletal '*voluntary*' muscles correctly. Once you start thinking
about how you're standing, sitting and moving, you will voluntarily
alter your position (using your muscles) into one you know suits the
way you want your body to look.

As you read this, lower your shoulders, straighten your back, hold
your head a little higher and contract your abdominal muscles. You'll
end up looking graceful. When you get up to go about your daily
business, continue to hold your head high and 'think' your shoulders
low, your head held in a plumb line straight down to your heels.

It makes a world of difference to your looks and your feelings when
you try to both look and think 'up' – and thinking 'up' is definitely
one way to help prevent aches and pains.

POOL WORK. To give muscles the perfect chance to play exhibitionist
the physiotherapist likes to put you in a swimming pool – or at least
enough deep water to swim in.

Swimming exercises *all* the muscles, providing you don't rely on
doggy paddle once out of your depth, for, as any expert will say,
underwater exercises are the telling kind. You're not cheating if you
keep your head above the surface, though.

For the benefit of neck, stomach, arms and legs, try this: holding
head erect, start to breast stroke, then move into reverse, first pushing
water *back* with your arms, *then* pushing it *forward*. At the same time,
move one leg straight up and down underwater with a slow scissor
movement. After thirty kicks, move the other leg. It isn't easy, but
(just like riding a bike) once you've mastered it you will wonder what
all the fuss was about.

Keeping one foot flat against the side of the pool, stand on the
other foot. Bend forward from the waist, arms out, thumbs locked
together. Inhale. Hold breath as you push away from wall. Glide

relaxed for as long as you can. Exhale slowly before you regain footing. Repeat twenty times.

Another good exercise for the whole body is to kick from the hips with relaxed legs, holding on to the wall bar if you can't swim. Better still, if you can, do it without a prop. Slap down on the surface of the water with the instep of the foot. Short, quick strokes are faster and less tiring.

If you haven't enough water around to get out of your depth, make do with a plunge bath, and loofah your legs, thighs and buttocks underwater moving *upwards* all the time, keeping first one side of your body taut, then the other.

Out of the bath, massage with a loofah sprinkled with surgical spirit – it can ignite the circulation faster than a four-minute mile, and it's a great way to banish goosepimples.

SCARED OF WATER? Swimming movements can be helpful for the non-swimmer, too.

Take the backstroke, moving anybody who cares fast through the water, with legs kicking away. Out of the water, the arm movements of the backstroke can shape up the upper arms (one of the most difficult parts of the anatomy to slim), and you can carry them out sitting at the kitchen table. If you want to help your gluteus maximus (the buttocks' muscle) it's better to stand up and contract your buttocks as you swing. Make sure nothing is in your way, then start one arm at a time, moving it up and back making a wide circle as you go. As one arm reaches the top of the circle, start up and back with the other arm. You can go on like this indefinitely. It's more fun in the water, but backstroking on land can still be an effective exercise.

Don't overlook the landlocked breaststroke either. It does a nifty job of strengthening the pectoral muscles which support the breasts.

Lying on the edge of the bed, so your torso is on it while your legs are mostly off, is one way to get some of the leg shaping benefits derived from the kick of the American crawl. That is, if you kick your legs rhythmically up and down, up and down. It isn't as easy as 'crawling' in the water and you may even stub your toe, but it can firm and trim thigh and calf muscles and has even been known to slim a few waists, too.

As we all know, water helps exercise to be more effective. Because the water pressure adds resistance to movement, you have to push and kick and work harder to move.

The best answer for non-swimmers who want to trim themselves up is to summon up their courage and work out in the shallow end. However, if water is definitely not for you, don't forget that swimming exercises on land *can* help shape.

Calisthenics – Instant Exercises that Work

If you're irritable without cause, if you toss and turn and feel you aren't sleeping properly, if you ache although you haven't been exerting your body, these are messages you can't ignore. Your brain is telling you clearly you will have to change your ways.

To quote an eminent doctor friend, 'An over-taxed body is more vulnerable to injury. You have to learn to listen to what your body is telling you and then do something about it.'

That 'something' for many people could be a slow turn to calisthenics, a clumsy word for the simplest exercises in the world, those we can all do, anywhere, at any time, at our own pace.

To get some relief from a tense, taut back, for instance, simply lie on your back with a pillow tucked beneath your knees, under each arm and under the back of your neck. Shake your neck, shoulders, arms, thighs, legs and feet until they wobble. Raise your arms slowly and then let them drop like stones. Raise your legs and feet, then let them drop. Finally, drop your head to the left, to the right and on to your chest, inhaling and exhaling deeply and slowly (see breathing section on page 246). Start thinking about feeling heavy – as if you were carrying each one of your own pounds. Close your eyes, let your jaw sag, exhaling as you go. Continue on this cycle of shaking, wobbling, lifting and relaxing until you feel less tense and maybe even start to doze. This is a regular calisthenic routine adopted by top athletes after a race or competition to help them 'wind down' and to prevent the build-up of lactic acid in the muscles.

If you've been on edge because of a speech you had to make or a personal appearance of any kind, wind down this way to prevent a painful lactic acid build-up in neck and shoulder muscles. Ouch!

Eileen Ford is the name behind the largest model agency in the world. She uses calisthenics as a way of life, starting her day by *literally* rolling out of bed on to the floor where she immediately carries out her kneebends and toe touching routines. While brushing her teeth she puts her foot on top of the basin and flexes her knee, first the right, then the left – good for the inner thighs. 'I do my chin exercises driving to work. People think I'm sticking my tongue out, but it's all part of my shape-up programme. My office is my world so I sometimes do

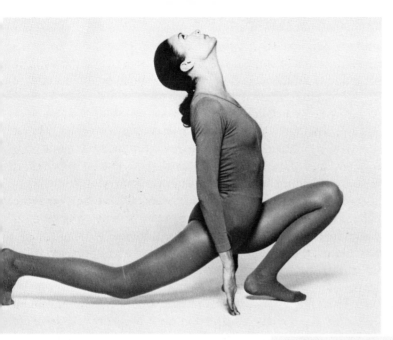

'You don't need to do anything strenuous', says actress and singer Julie Wilson, who admits to her fifty-one years of age. 'Simple limbering-up exercises are fine if you do them every day.'

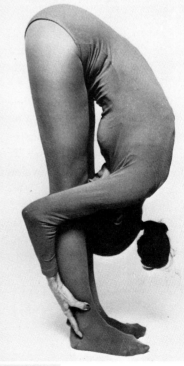

leg lifts while talking on the phone or dictating to my secretary.'
Instant exercise, in other words.

Everyone, but especially extra tall girls like Vanessa Redgrave and
Germaine Greer, should sometimes follow an exercise that's based on
thinking of the body as a building of several storeys with each storey
being placed properly on top of the other so that the building (the
body) is in correct alignment. The feet are obviously the foundation –
and it's important to be aware of that 'foundation' and stand with feet
a few inches apart and parallel, the weight of the body placed on the
balls of the feet. Keeping legs straight, knee joints should be relaxed,
buttock muscles tightened and abdominal muscles pulled in. The torso
should be stretched so that one is immediately aware of the waist.
If the torso is 'pulled up', almost as if it were being drawn to the crown
of the head, the result will be a perfectly aligned body – the head
aligned to neck and spine, the spine to legs, the legs to feet – (the thigh
bone's connected to the hip bone, remember that old song?)

This 'exercise' is especially vital for the extra tall woman because
without good posture she can easily look 'bent' (and so 'crouched' and
older). The very tall Mrs Henry Kissinger, for instance, should learn
from this. She's round-shouldered through years of thinking 'short'
not 'tall'. When the rib cage is up, better posture results automatically,
and when shoulders are lowered the neck feels longer. Try it, you'll
like it.

There are a variety of short snappy exercises that can also be part
of your everyday life which can help shape, such as:

Turning the knob of the next door you open with your left hand
(if you're left-handed do it with your right).

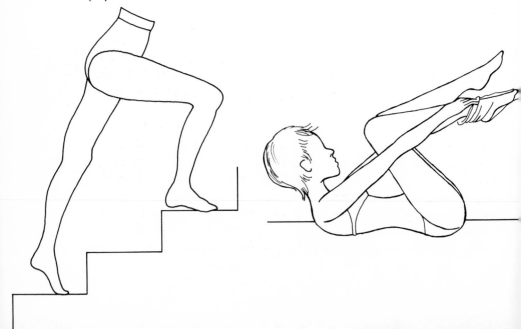

Picking up something from the floor without bending your knees, then using your left hand to do it.

Going upstairs and downstairs two at a time – this is very good for the thigh muscles.

Lying down to put on tights, extending legs up in the air, pointing toes while pulling stockings up.

Walking downstairs toes first, then lowering the heel, good for foot and leg.

Reaching up for something on a top shelf, standing on your toes to do it – stretching first with the left, then with the right hand.

Jogging whenever you want to get from one room to another – for at least part of the day.

REDUCING EACH SPOT. For some people, general exercise may not give them what they really want, that is *spot reducing on the one spot that defies trimming*. In the Western World, it's the thigh area that's the number one trouble zone, hard to tackle, mainly because we're all too *sedentary* by habit and so inclination.

Calisthenics can be broken down to direct the action to one problem area – but, as with every other exercise, at least fifteen minutes should be spent carrying out the movement, mornings and evening. But not too near bedtime, for too much exertion can bring on insomnia.

But remember, experts all over the world will advise: 'Always begin any exercise session with a special breathing session. Stand very tall. Close eyes. Inhale deeply and hold for a count of six. Exhale deeply. During breathing exercises think about and visualize air entering and leaving body. Repeat ten times.'

FOR HIPS, WAIST AND ABDOMEN. Marjorie Craig of Elizabeth Arden is a name (and a gorgeous shape) that will bring several illustrious ladies out of their chaises longues to rush to the wall bars. Her influence over exercise has been felt for many years because of the most logical reason: results.

For waist, abdomen and upper hips, Miss Craig's favourite exercise is the following: lie on the floor on your back, arms out at shoulder level with palms up. Bend knees to chest, then drop both knees to the floor directly out from hips to one side. Keeping knees close to the floor, pull them up towards elbows. Hold, then roll knees back over chest. Hold. Repeat exercise on the other side. Do this ten times (page 264).

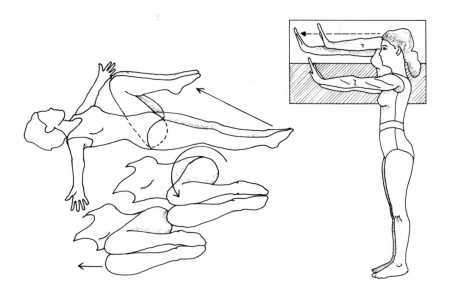

Here are some other exercises for hips and waist:

1 Stand upright with good posture, lift arms overhead and bend torso eight times to the right, eight times to the left. Next, bend knees eight times, keeping buttocks tight, abdomen pulled in. Then bend upper body from the waist, arms and knees relaxed, eight times. Repeat all these movements in the same order eight times.

2 Place hands on hips, then swing torso to the right, forward, to the left, and then reverse. Sixteen times.

3 Stand tall, tucking stomach in well. Raise arms perpendicular to torso and hold palms up as if stopping the traffic. Push out with right hand as far as possible in a horizontal and steady direction. Repeat eight to ten times with alternate hands.

4 With legs wide apart, stand tall, head up. Raise elbows to horizontal position with palms down, pelvis forward. Twist body to left side; pause, face forward; twist to right side. Repeat eight to ten times each side.

5 When a waist really becomes *tiresome*, with emphasis on the spare *tyre*, stand, raise arms above head, and in a sweeping motion

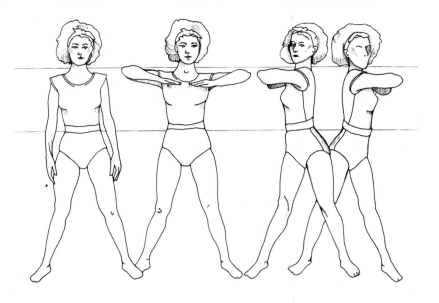

twist body from the waist to the right, then sweep down to the toes, around to the left and back up to the original position – always keeping arms outstretched. This is really acting out a windmill. Repeat twice to the right, then reverse. Move from the waist only. The lower part of the body should face *forward* all the time.

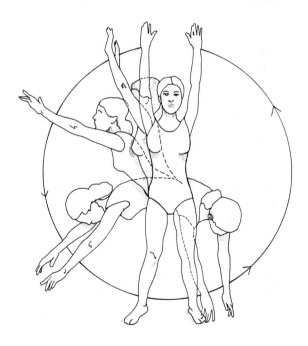

6 One exercise that works well if carried out with that old military discipline: lie flat on back with arms extended wide at shoulder level. Bend knees and roll from side to side, keeping shoulders flat as you roll. The more you bend your knees the higher you will roll. If thighs and lower hips need the most work, bend knees only slightly. If higher hips and waist are in trouble, bring knees to chest. Roll five times to each side, working up to twenty.

Another person to influence exercise for the better is Lotte Berk, encouraging the likes of Lee Radziwill, Lady Whitmore and novelist Edna O'Brien to *follow* instead of trying to *lead* their own brand of shape making. Lotte has a school across the Atlantic, too, which is already a great success. Lotte's age is difficult to assess, because she has the shape and vigour of an eighteen-year-old, yet the experience and knowledge of someone three times older.

Her exercise for the stomach and waist region is easy to follow:

Lie flat, tucking feet under sofa or bed. Press small of back into floor. Slowly pull yourself up from waist into half sitting position. Keep small of back straight, while reaching forward with hands, bounce backwards and forwards from waist, then slowly return to lie flat on floor. Relax, repeat. Take it slowly. It's difficult, but it gets a little easier each time.

Or, sit on floor with legs wide apart. Rest palms on floor between legs. Keep back straight. Lift legs an inch or two off floor and stretch them straight. Keep weight on hands. Bend legs and continue rhythmically to bend and stretch, not letting legs touch floor. Relax, repeat two or three times. Increase with practice.

FOR THE THIGHS. Also from Marjorie Craig, this exercise is a good attack on thighs and helps a fatty back too. Stand with legs apart. Bend knees slightly and pull hips under you. Raise both arms over head, hands clasped, palms turned up. Keeping hands joined, bend to touch floor in front of right toes. Bend knees as you bend down. Come up, bringing arms up over head, again pulling stomach in and up. Repeat movement, this time touching floor between feet; come up, arms back over head. Bend again, knees bent, to touch floor in front of left toes ... and so it goes on, ten times (see page 268).

Arlene Dahl, not just a lovely face, but a worker for better looks, sought out several exercise experts before releasing her *Slim-Down for Thighs Movement:*

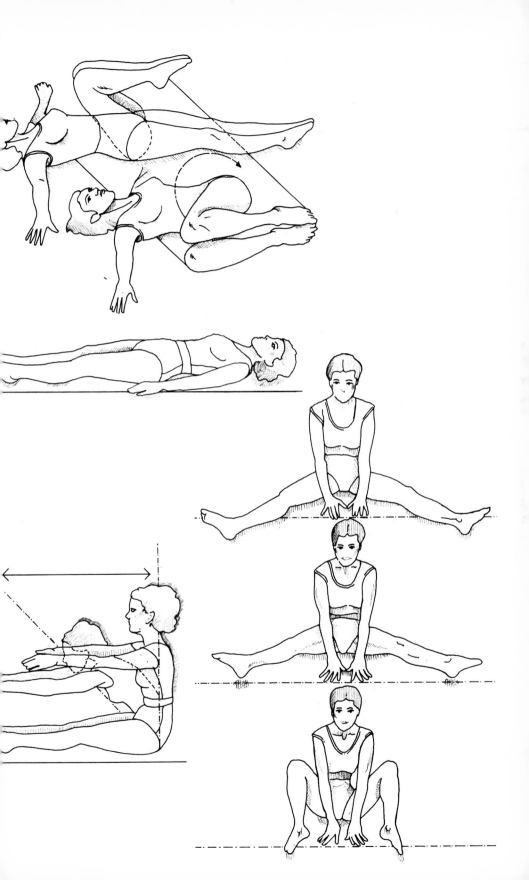

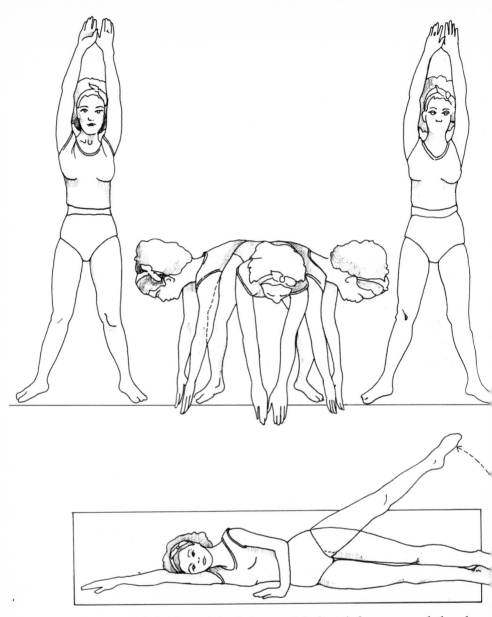

Lie on left side with body in a straight line, left arm extended under head, right hand placed in front for balance. Raise the right leg to make a 45 degree angle with the floor, if possible, contract buttocks, hold, then lower slowly to the floor. Repeat six times before rolling over to do the same for the left leg.

At the Greenhouse Spa in Dallas, Texas, where comfort and luxury go hand in hand with rigid streamlining (see spas, page 83), the thigh

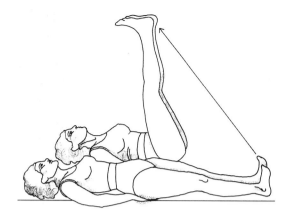

exercise that brings most results is the one where you lie on your back with hands beneath buttocks, head relaxed, feet flexed, and lift legs straight towards the ceiling, inhaling as you open and close legs, exhaling on the next split – this carried out twenty times.

Also from the Greenhouse: lie on back with hands under buttocks. Keeping spine flat on floor, raise legs and cycle in large circles, inhaling as you lift right leg, exhaling on the left. Forty times medium fast.

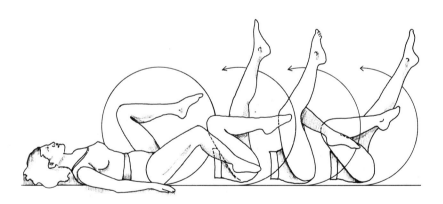

FOR THE UPPER ARMS

1 Towel exercises are helpful because seeing a towel can jog your memory to get going in the early morning. Stand upright with legs apart and hold a towel behind your left knee in both hands, with thumbs facing upwards. Attempt to push backward with leg but *resist* with the towel held taut, using arms only. Switch

269

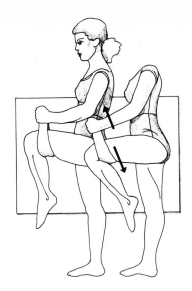
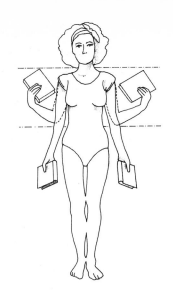

towel to behind your right knee and again attempt to thwart leg movement. Alternate legs.

2 Standing upright, grasp a book in each hand (or use a pair of dumb-bells), keeping thumbs down, arms at sides. Curl arms up to shoulder level, without moving upper arms. Lower to sides, then repeat. Always stand erect.

3 Grasp a book or weight in each hand and lean out and forward from the waist, keeping upper body in parallel position to floor.

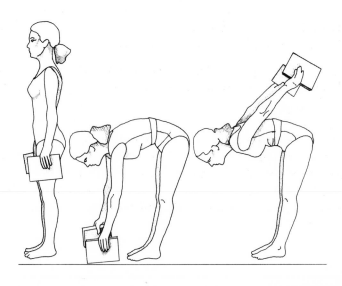

To work upper arm muscles, extend arms back and as high as possible without moving body. Return arms to sides, bending elbows, attempting to point books towards ceiling. Continue exercise as many times as possible. *Don't* get exhausted.

FOR BACK MUSCLES (AND ABDOMINAL ONES, TOO)

1 Lie flat on back, arms at sides, and try to bend knees to chest as far as possible.

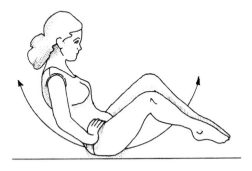

2 Sit on floor and slowly lean back as if sitting in a rocking chair. With hands on hips and knees slightly bent, feet just touching floor, try to rock backwards and forwards.

(*For the following three exercises see page 272*).

3 Lying flat on floor with arms at sides, raise first one leg as far as it will go, then the other, then both together, returning to floor one at a time and starting again.

4 Lying on your stomach, reach back to hold ankles with hands. Rock backwards and forwards twenty times, then relax, breathing in and out deeply. Repeat another twenty times.

5 Standing upright, feet together, raise arms over head and hold hands. Bend from side to side, attempting to get as near the waist as possible.

WHAT NEEDS EXERCISE MOST. To discover just where your muscles are letting you down – mostly through lack of use, covered up with flab, encouraging more flab – Marvin Hart, shapemaker to the stars (see page 244), devised six simple tests you can try for yourself to assess if and where you need the most help.

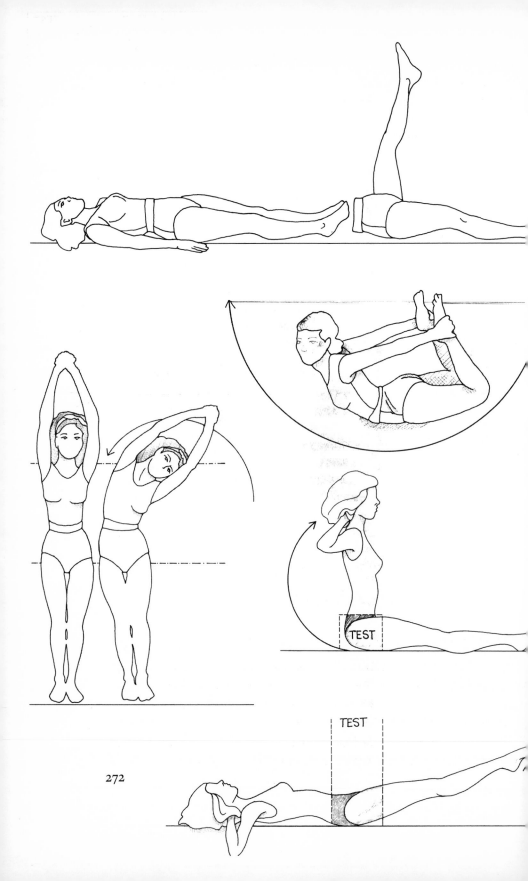

TEST

TEST

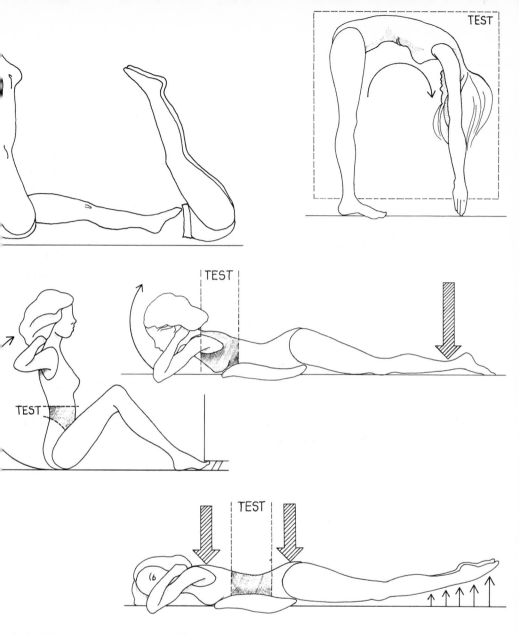

(*The following six exercises are illustrated opposite and on this page.*)

1 To test *hip muscles:* lie on your back, hands behind neck, legs straight. Raise both feet at least ten inches from the floor, holding them still for ten seconds. If you can't do it, you need to concentrate on exercises for your hips.

2 To test *hip and abdominal muscles:* lie on your back, hands clasped behind your neck, legs straight, with your feet under a heavy object, desk or dressing table. Try to get into a sitting position without moving your hands. If you can't your stomach and hip muscles need work.

3 To test *stomach and waist muscles:* lie on your back with hands behind your neck, this time with knees bent, tuck feet under a heavy piece of furniture. Again try to sit up – without the use of your hands. No luck? Get to work on stomach and waist exercises.

4 To test *upper back muscles* (often where tension ties a knot of pain during a busy working day), lie on your stomach with pillow under your abdomen, hands behind your neck. With someone holding feet and hips down, try to raise the top half of your body and hold for ten seconds. You should feel your back muscles really working here. (Marvin Hart frequently acts as the *resistance* against which his pupil has to exert his or her muscles.)

5 Again in the position for the above exercise, this time have someone hold your shoulders and hips down, and try to raise your legs, keeping them straight and holding for ten seconds. This is a test for *muscles of the lower back*, where fat loves to accumulate.

6 For *overall muscle flexibility*, test yourself by standing erect with shoes off, feet together, knees stiff, hands at sides. Try to touch floor with fingertips. If you can't do it, try again. Relax, drop head forward and attempt to let your torso 'hang' from your hips, keeping knees straight. Chances are you'll do better the second time. If this eludes you, you must think about an exercise programme that gives you an overhaul overall.

EXERCISES TO START THE DAY. One easy exercise you hardly need to think about is a great start to the day as it firms not only the waist but *the sides of the waist*, shoulders, hips, back and front of legs and thighs, as well as helping the spine become more flexible. Stand upright, with legs apart, holding a fair-sized book in each hand. Swing forward,

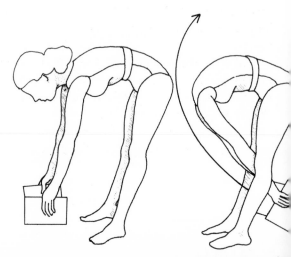

bending loosely at the waist, then swing your hands through your legs as far as you can go – still holding the books, of course. Swing hands up again over your head and as far back as possible. The most important point: KEEP BREATHING, inhaling through the nose, exhaling loudly through the mouth. Repeat the exercise at least three times at first, working up to ten by the next day, twenty by the end of the week.

On waking, blink your eyes, stretch like a cat from head to toe, throw back the covers over your ankles, bend your knees and sit up. Lie down again, sit up again. Do this several times to get your 'motor' on the move.

If you oversleep and have to run for the train, be conscious of your running, and breathe the *right* way as you run, inhaling and exhaling. Once on board, stretch every muscle as you put your bag on the seat or coat on the rack. *Think* shape all the way to the bank and don't forget the word if you're sitting in front of a typewriter all day. Occasionally, contract your abdominal muscles, tighten your seat, straighten your shoulders and hold that position as you work for a few minutes. Walk that way to lunch, and if you sit that way at lunch you'll find you won't eat so much.

HOW TO START EXERCISING. The easiest way to start exercising by yourself, following the exercises mentioned here, is to *start slowly* – telling yourself you will carry out five exercises every day the first week, increasing the number until it becomes second nature.

The most important thing to remember is that once you *start*, you must *continue* for any results to show.

Don't find excuses. If the thought bores you, tires you, exhausts you, exercise first thing in the morning before you brush your teeth, as soon as you wake up so that it's out of the way. *Don't* leap out of bed to start work. If you need an alarm clock, set it a few minutes early and before you start thinking what a drag and fall back to sleep, look at an unflattering photograph of yourself you've placed by the clock to remind you what you need to do.

Marvin Hart thinks repetition is the main drag about exercise. For this reason, he has many variations of each shape-making movement to give the body a change and, he thinks, to give his obviously delighted clients the interest to keep at it.

The key words are *consistency, breathing and stretching* for *your own exercise programme* to do *you* all the good in the world.

275

If You're a Jane at Heart, Tarzan or No Tarzan at Home

Apparatus is not the crutch the kneebend girls think. All over the world apparatus work is one way that certain of the species get their bodies in trim and keep them that way.

A regular date at a gym, run by well qualified people, is far more exhilarating, this type of positive thinker thinks, than half-hearted attempts at body stretches all alone at home.

The important point about gym work-outs is that they offer an endless variety of movements and *lots of challenge*. You may start on the floor, but end up literally flying through the air.

Some of the basic routines for physical fitness that play a part in the Olympic gymnasts' regime are fitted into these classes – which, with numbers kept to a minimum, say six at a time, are always full.

In case you think I'm referring to the natural athlete or super-Amazon type, I'm not. Gym can be for tired, old bodies, too – sufferers learn how to lose fatigue and stand up straight, and emotional tension is relieved physically because it is recognized that tension causes incorrect breathing and cramps. Most leading gymnasts recommend that to begin with 'students' should study for two hours a week at a good gym with a daily routine of ten minutes' exercise at home, mostly breathing and bending – not forgetting a good helping of sport, the best introduction to gym work.

A coordination test is one of the first things many gyms insist upon before work-outs begin, to discover how soon – if ever – you will be performing. Work-outs are devised with light dumb-bells to help posture, stretches on specially devised bars, handstands and tumbling with instructors at the ready to hold you up until you hold yourself up.

Mat work trims waists, strengthens backs.

Routine exercises on wall bars firm hips.

Work on incline boards and balance beams is good for hips and knees.

Back bends, headstands and weight lifting are for all-over toning.

Rings are for balance and to increase co-ordination.

Many gyms have ingeniously devised apparatus that use springs, pulleys and sliding blocks to provide extra resistance against which students work.

The incentive is obvious – better shape for out-of-shape areas – but some gym groups are so anxious for their students to succeed that they offer a prize, say a magnum of champagne to anyone who can kick a horizontal bar way above their heads ten times. Needless to say, you don't get to the horizontal bar class until you've worked your way through many dumb-bells routines. Not even a glass of beer for that – *especially* not a glass of beer.

Whatever apparatus work appeals to you, by the end of the first lesson you may find you are exhausted – so say pupils who've been through it. But when they have the willpower to return for the next class and the next, until it becomes a regular part of their lives, they also say they experience an extraordinary new sensation – relaxation with exhilaration. Physical tuning *does* affect the psyche.

THE PREGNANT POSITION

Why do dancers, skiers, mountain climbers and crack tennis players so often have easy pregnancies and deliveries, while backgammon players, pianists, palmists and P.R. girls don't? The answer in a barbell is great muscle tone, overall fitness and stamina. Even if you don't play ball or read palms, in common with those that do you may have back pain during the latter months of pregnancy. The degree of pain usually depends on the extra weight involved, but back pain of any degree can be nasty. Again, the right set of movements can help.

To strengthen the back and cut down strain: lie on your back with knees bent, feet flat on the floor some inches apart, then literally try to press your spine into the floor, contracting your abdominal muscles as you do, holding for a count of ten. If you carry out this movement about ten times a day, it will definitely strengthen your back and hopefully preclude that old backache.

Getting Back into Shape

If you were in top shape before the baby, it won't be much trouble getting back there again. If you were in less-than-top shape, it isn't so easy, particularly if you've cheated and put on too much weight. Once your doctor has given you the okay to start working your way back to normal weight and shape, limber up on waking up by stretching every part of your anatomy, one area at a time. Still lying in bed, on a hard mattress if possible, bend your right knee up to your chin, holding it there with your hands. Slowly lift head, neck and shoulders up as you pull your knee closer and closer, hold for a count of five, and then release as you lower your head back down. Repeat with the left leg and so on.

Another helpful movement to get back in shape is to sit on the floor with legs stretched out in front, arms stretched high overhead. Keeping your back straight, bend your head and aim to catch hold of your toes. Bounce back with arms stretched above, then lean forward once more. Repeat at least five times. *Warning:* Don't do any exercise too near bedtime – over-exertion can lead to insomnia and you must have the remedial quota of sleep.

LAZY WAY TO NEW SHAPE – SOMETIMES

Classes, salons, spas and studios offering *equipment* are not necessarily offering apparatus. The two are far apart and qualified gymnasts are anxious to have them differentiated. *Apparatus* needs *your* muscles, *your* participation, *your* work for anything to happen. *Equipment* generally means you lean your body against *it* in a certain way and *it* attempts to do something to you while you could – if you were so inclined – read your horoscope, manicure your nails and, we hope, breathe consciously and correctly as you do during any other body endeavour programme.

Today, you can find mechanical wonderlands, with spine correctors, reformers, towers, 'wundachairs', tensors, pedi-puls and trapeze tables, but whatever the piece of equipment is called it usually has to be plugged in to the electricity so that with one click of the switch parts of the machine wallop away at your posterior or abdomen or stretch your arms and legs. It doesn't do you any *harm* – but unless you're watching your calorie intake and moving your own muscles yourself, as well, it doesn't do much good either!

Faradic machines are popular, too, perhaps more so – faradic meaning moving muscles involuntarily with a low frequency current. You lie there counting sheep and except for a slight tingling sensation don't feel anything at all – no aches and pains, no strains – although your muscles alternately contract and relax.

Then, again, you can turn to a machine using jets of hot air to get at your flab. This often looks like a hair drier with fat tubes, which direct the jets of hot air under considerable pressure on to your bulges. The hot air produces a ripple effect on the skin, as you might expect. It does stimulate circulation, and to a certain extent may be considered as soothing and relaxing, but, frankly, again it cannot have any dramatic results without you putting in a great deal of work, too.

HOW MANY CALORIES/KILOJOULES YOU BURN UP IN ONE HOUR'S ACTIVITY

	CALORIES	KILOJOULES
Jogging on the spot at home	300	1,200
Jogging out of doors	500	2,000
Throwing a ball	200	800
Flying a kite	30	120
Ice skating (depending on the vigour of your figure eights)	200–600	800–2,400
Cycling (uphill)	200–600	800–2,400
Walking slowly	115	460
Walking fairly fast	215	860
Walking as fast as you can	550	2,200
Window shopping (for one day)	900	3,600
Museum viewing – the National Gallery	1,250	5,000
– the Tate Gallery	750	3,000
Dancing (depending on the music)	200–400	800–1,600
Rowing (depending on how many in the boat)	500–900	2,000–3,600
Tennis (doubles–singles)	500–700	2,000–2,800
Skipping with a rope	300	1,200
Riding a horse	150	600
Galloping	600	2,400
Judo	800	3,200
Exercise class (depending on the class)	250–1,000	1,000–4,000
Skiing	350–600	1,400–2,400
Cross-country skiing	650–1,000	2,600–4,000
Cross-country running	500–700	2,000–2,800
Cleaning the house (scrubbing, etc.)	165	660
Ironing	50	200
Washing up	50	200
Painting	150–200	600–800
Wallpapering	150–200	600–800
Mowing	300	900
Golf with no cart	145	580
Card playing – with money involved	100	400
– no money – no emotion	50	200
Billiards	250	1,000
Table tennis	180	720
Standing at cocktail parties 30 minutes	20	80
60 minutes	50	200

CELLULITE – THE TRUTH

Hot air, heated water and low current machines are at work right now somewhere in the world trying to affect the controversial affliction known as *cellulite*.

Does it exist or doesn't it? The French are convinced it does. The Americans – some of them at least – maintain cellulite is just plain ordinary fat that shows up more on some women than others, depending on the thickness of the skin. As for us, I'd say we're non-committal.

How do most French doctors describe cellulite? As an association of fat, water and waste created by too much toxin in the body. Because of this, they say, the tissues lack normal elasticity, so you can literally *see* 'bubbles' or 'lumps' of fat imprisoned in the flesh, particularly in the thigh and upper arm areas, creating a look that has been described variously as chicken skin and orange peel, and in other similarly attractive word pictures.

Whatever it's called, and whatever it really is, ordinary or extraordinary fat, cellulite doesn't look pretty; it can ruin the line of a dress and makes some people paranoid about going to the beach.

Cellulite appears more in the thigh area than anywhere else, and it often goes, lump by lump, with poor circulation (which can lead to varicose veins) and weak pelvic muscles.

Apart from this favourite resting place (the front, inside and back of thighs) cellulite also likes the inside of the knees, hips and buttocks, upper arms, ankles and sometimes but not often the abdomen. And what are the main offenders in creating this condition? Tension (extra fluid can be retained under emotional stress), air pollution, poor breathing and poor diet are the main ones, *with lack of exercise backing them all up.*

How to Lose Cellulite

The objective of any cellulite treatment is to rid the body of this trapped mixture of fluid and fat, draining it through the usual elimination points of the body. In Paris, machines loosen the lumps electrically. Sponges impregnated with thyroid base and silicone medicaments are applied to the cellulite areas, with metal plaques placed on top; these are then plugged into an instrument, which shoots through the current, causing mild muscle spasm. At least ten treatments are advised, but often many more are needed before any difference can be seen.

As cellulite is often found around muscles, hot air jet machines are also used (often by French operators) to get between skin and muscle and so attack the hated lumps. The hot air can be helpful because it zips up the circulation, too.

If you use these machine treatments regularly and back up their use with an anti-cellulite diet, you may well cure or at least improve the condition.

A regular diet of food containing anti-cellulite minerals – particularly iodine – can be helpful: this means liberal helpings of seafood (no hardship for most), asparagus, cabbage (a valuable and underestimated food) and bananas, plus at least 2 pints (1 litre) of water a day to flush the system and decrease salt retention.

One piece of equipment you can use to help your own shape along, away from the salon, and/or gym, is the simple garden hose. In the summer aim it at your thighs for a few seconds to create your own 'machine' – not using hot air but pleasantly warm water, which can also attack the 'lumps', but don't forget, you also need to *move* more.

AVOIDING A PAINFUL P.S. TO EXERCISE

In case you didn't know it, our beauty flow (better known as blood flow) has an enormous amount of work to do in the body. When we're in a sedentary position, sitting, lounging or sleeping, our muscles only receive about 12 per cent of our blood supply. When we jump up in the morning to do our physical jerks or rush to the tennis courts or jog to the office, the supply goes up to about 80 per cent.

When a sedentary person suddenly decides to join a 'keep fit' movement after years of inactivity, it's often not realized that the body needs time to adjust. As we grow older our blood vessels become less elastic, our ligaments are more brittle. If, after years of passing on only about 12 per cent of our blood supply to the muscles, the blood vessels are suddenly called upon to deliver 80 per cent, you can visualize why they're likely to suffer and, alas, even snap under the extra stress.

As a number of leading orthopaedic surgeons and physiotherapists will be quick to tell you, for every year of a sedentary, non-active life, it takes a month of regular exercise to get into shape.

If, after months of sitting at your desk, you suddenly decide to water-ski, swim and go on long uphill walks one weekend, don't be surprised on Monday morning if you can hardly crawl out of bed. It isn't that you've aged overnight. Your normally passive leg muscles, joints, tendons and ligaments have suddenly been subjected to an enormous load of extra stress. Your circulation isn't used to providing your muscles with all the extra blood needed to deliver the nutrients for all the extra activity. The consequence? Lactic acid, a waste product of the blood, builds up in the limbs and that often results in horrendous aches and pains.

The remedy is that after any bout of unaccustomed sport, you *must* take time to wind your body down *slowly* with stretching exercises. You mustn't just plop in a chair after throwing off your waterskis to stretch out a languid hand in the direction of a gin and tonic. Far better to jog and then walk slowly along the beach for fifteen minutes.

Better still, don't participate in strenuous sport only at weekends. That way you're giving your body bouts of stress, which can be harmful. Instead, build a bridge between Monday and Friday. Stretch every morning and evening in bed. Skip with a rope every day or walk briskly with long strides.

In other words, don't slump all week and stomp all weekend. It's bad for your body and can lead to problems you'd rather be without.

13

Stepping Up Foot Care

POOR relations to our legs, our feet get stepped on in life, just as much figuratively as physically. When our feet hurt, it literally wipes the smile off our faces, and yet, despite the fact that most of us will walk at least 100,000 miles in our lifetime, we neglect our feet, rarely giving them more than a cursory splash in bath or shower, only really noticing them when a toe is stubbed, a nail is broken or they just hurt.

The majority of us don't know why our feet hurt. There are a variety of reasons that converge to help develop corns, callouses and all sorts of bony abnormalities. Many of us are suffering from a condition we don't even know we've got. Our metatarsal bone (the 'arch' of the foot) has dropped through consistently choosing and wearing the wrong kind of shoes.

THE SHOES WE WEAR

In case anyone is contemplating a return to the stiletto heel, take heed now: that tiny heel base was responsible for more varicose veins than anything else in the history of chiropody. *It forced* the ankle to take on extra work to provide *some* balance for the foot/leg/body, inevitably leading to swollen ankles and eventually to varicose veins.

Tights that fit too snugly also add to the woeful picture. As we generally wear our tights longer during the day than we wear our shoes (which we can always kick off for a blissful few minutes of respite), too small tights lead to all sorts of unpleasant and maddening things like blisters and callouses, quite apart from causing the feet to perspire profusely, trapped as they are in oppressive plastic. One size fits all – phooey!

The astonishing thing is that few people really even know the exact size of their feet. Most of us just make a wild guess at what we think our feet measure, even though foot measuring apparatus is easily available. Even if you're certain you know your size, you should check it every time you go shoe shopping, preferably at the end of the day when foot size is at its largest.

If you wear the same heel height all day and all night, too, you must get resigned to a lifetime of limping. If, instead, you vary your heel height throughout the day, you'll have found a quick way to give feet and legs a good rest.

As a general rule, remember the longer the leg, the higher the heel can be, *providing* the heel has a decent-sized base. A 3-inch (7½-cm) heel will cause the calf muscle to flex and usually make ankles look trimmer. But the merest fraction over and wrinkles can appear at the sides and back of the lower calf, actually making the ankles look thicker. Perish the thought.

If you have short legs, too high a heel can throw your whole posture out of gear and make you look totally out of proportion.

In some states in the U.S.A. they feel so strongly about the dangers inherent in high heels that they have a law stating that no woman can wear heels higher than 1½ inches (3¾ cm) or less than 1 inch (2½ cm) in diameter. When a woman wants to tower above her 'sisters', she has to apply for a special permit at the town hall, and to agree to bear any liability for damage to herself and/or to others 'caused by falling down on public streets while wearing such shoes'. Hard to credit, but those Americans do believe in taking precautions.

The problem with continually wearing high heels is that they throw an enormous, *unnatural* strain upon the feet, because a greater proportion of weight than normal rests on the arch, already the weakest part of the foot. If we didn't wear shoes at all, our feet would be in better shape. Although different heel heights do exercise different leg muscles, generally the lower the heel, the better the legs are naturally exercised.

The main problem with shoes is that whereas feet are like finger-prints – one person's will differ from another's – shoes don't differ (un-less they're custom-made). Made on standard lasts, with identical right and left feet, is it any wonder that feet hurt when they're cooped up in such inflexible objects for such long periods?

As any good chiropodist will tell you, the best shoes for feet are the open-toed kind, which is why to please him you should aim to wear open sandals as much as possible in summer, enabling your feet to encounter as much fresh air as they can before colder weather means months of being trapped again. If you can't stand open-toed sandals, the chiropodist will also tell you to choose shoes with a *square-shaped toe* and a *good solid heel* – that is if you care about foot health and your gastrocnemius (calf muscle to you and me). If you have a pair of shoes that doesn't fit perfectly, the same wise chiropodist will also tell you to give them away or even throw them away, but '*don't wear them*'. It sounds extravagant, but it could be the best advice your feet will ever have.

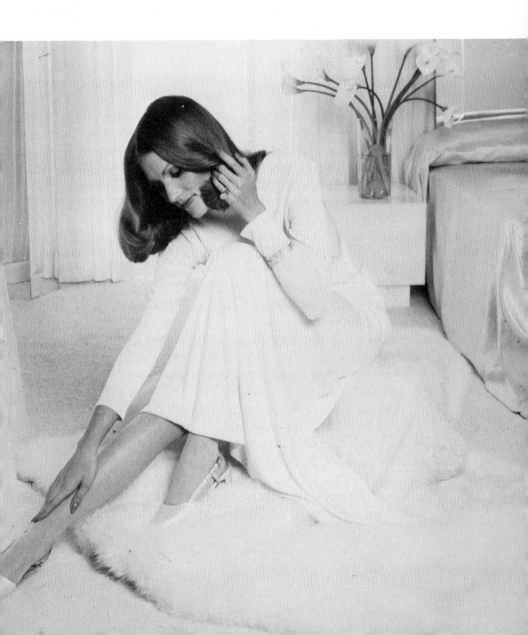

WHAT HAVE YOU DONE FOR
YOUR FEET LATELY?

We rarely sit – or stand – with our weight firmly resting on the balls of our feet, the very foundations of our body, yet ignoring nature's own little 'cushions' often puts so much out of alignment. Once we concentrate on sitting and standing the right way, with our feet planted firmly on the ground, it's possible to have a totally new viewpoint on life. We're just not used to standing or sitting that way. Once we do, every step we take can be an exercise. Try it.

Never stand around too long in one position – even if you are correctly balanced on the balls of your feet, it's still putting intolerable pressure on them. Remember that at your next cocktail party. It's a marvellous excuse for escaping the party bore.

In winter, feet are particularly abused, cramped up in boots all day (and sometimes in the evening, too) plus overheated tights. Feet crawl into bed often without the courtesy of a real wash – and I'm not saying that their owners don't take a shower. It's just that in the shower the water goes right past them down the drain. They only *stand* in the water, they don't actually get *washed* in it. Does that ring a bell in anyone's life? Once you take off shoes or boots that 'have been killing you all day' (pinched nerve endings sending piercing signals all over the body) it's up to you to make it up to your feet with some good remedial treatment.

Every other night, at least give your feet a good long soak in warm fragrant water. If your soles feel irritated, add cucumber slices to the water, cooling and soothing. Use the old-fashioned pumice stone to rub away all rough spots, particularly on your soles. Smooth a body or hand lotion all over the feet, in between every toe, massaging it around every nook and cranny.

People I know whose jobs keep them on their feet all day long recover after hours by giving their feet icepacks a couple of times a week. Alcohol rubs are stimulating and refreshing, too. Then everyone in this sort of job goes barefoot around the house (or even better on grass or sand) as often as possible.

Walking barefoot strengthens not only the feet but also the calf and thigh muscles. As Aristotle and Leonardo da Vinci observed before me, the mechanics of walking show that the heels make the first contact with the ground, followed by the outer border of the foot, then the ball of the foot and finally the toes.

Today, shoes abound that are higher at the front than at the back, encouraging us to walk the most natural way – a help to those who have no opportunity to go barefoot, but who want the same advantages on city pavements. These kind of shoes need practice to stand in, let alone walk in, but once you get used to them you quickly realize they *do* place the feet in the ideal position for walking, forcing the body to stand correctly, strengthening ankles, fallen arches and leg muscles and even improving circulation.

Exercises for the Foot

Unless it's done barefoot, walking isn't the kind of exercise that best helps feet to carry out their life's work. The key to healthy feet is: switch heel heights during the day and exercise as often as you think of it: simply rise on tiptoe ten or twenty times, to strengthen the arch and increase the flexibility of the toes; pick up coins from the floor with the toes; jog on tiptoe from room to room (or as far as you can manage).

Don't wear tights every day and every evening, particularly in the summer – your feet need air. Use talc in the bottom of your shoes to absorb excess perspiration (particularly if you're going dancing), and to avoid that hot burning feeling; this also precludes infection from any bacterial build-up.

At the office, morning and afternoon, stretch your feet up and down. Draw circles in the air under the desk with your shoes off and when you get home massage in and out of your toes, pulling each one out. Try to move each one independently – difficult, but it can be done.

After a long, or even short, day, put your feet up, with your head at least 12 inches (30 cm) lower if you can, so fresh blood can whirl around that area, refreshing and relaxing all of you.

Once you're in bed, try to rub the soles of your feet together. This stimulates the circulation, which is good for the feet.

Pretty Up

Have a heart for your feet, silent champions that bear the weight of *all* of you. Realize that from the purely visual point of view, anything short of totally groomed means ugly feet because nature wasn't particularly generous in the looks department here. Nothing looks worse than broken toe-nails with enamel half on and half off.

Give yourself regular pedicures, being sure to clip toe nails straight across. If clipping nails is a painful experience, see a professional chiropodist right away. Don't ignore the problem. It can only get worse.

Just as in manicuring, use a cuticle remover with an orange stick to loosen cuticles. After bathing, push them back softly with a corner of the towel. Apply a base coat, enamel and then a protective top coat, too. Think twice about using bright colours in the summer. They chip easily, if you have a lot of beach life in store. Naturals and pale frosteds look prettier on tanned skin anyway.

In the morning before your lemon tea, rub half a lemon all over heels and soles to soften and whiten them. Incidentally, use lemon on your elbows, too, and anywhere else you'd like to feel softer and look whiter.

YOUR FEET BELONG TO ALL OF YOU

In many parts of the world, feet are regarded with so much respect that there are special schools and clinics devoted to their care and foot therapy, known as Zone Therapy, is an important part of the curriculum.

Practitioners learn, for example, how for centuries Asian physicians have treated problems affecting other parts of the body by treating the feet (see acupuncture, page 302). Even major ailments are diagnosed and then treated with a special foot massage. Why? Because for every important muscle in the trunk and head, there's a tiny area that relates to it on one or both feet.

One of the best massages I ever had in my life was directed totally to my feet. It was done by a Zone Therapist from Germany, who told me the feet are a repository of a number of junction points and nerve endings, which expertly manipulated can help alleviate many other problems present in the body.

I only know that when I left this remarkable lady, my digestion definitely improved and I didn't have hiccups for months. If you don't know of a Zone Therapist, a little do-it-yourself foot massage can certainly do no harm and, who knows, may even do a great deal of good.

GIVING YOU A LEG UP

One make-up rule you apply to your face – emphasize good points with light shades (light attracts light), de-emphasize poor points with dark shades (dark absorbs light) – you can also apply to your body, and in particular your legs. If you're blessed with a shapely pair of legs like some lucky ladies I know, you should play them up by wearing pale, café-au-lait-coloured stockings with a darker, contrasting coloured skirt above.

If, on the other leg, you're in the majority with legs that refuse to shape up, however scrupulously you follow an exercise regime, stick to dark stockings, repeating the same colour in your shoes and echoing it with your skirt, so you create the effect of a long line from waist to toe-tip.

If you're a patient kind of girl, leg shaping *can* be done with exercise. Stand with toes on a telephone book, the bigger the better, with heels on the floor. Lift up on to tiptoes, then come back down. Repeat ten times night and morning. Easier to do, but more time consuming, try to tear up one of the Sunday newspapers with your toes. This also helps ankle shape. Make sure the family have read it first, though.

Try some lateral sliding across the room, also known as dancing the mashed potato. Don't know the steps? Simply move across the room sideways, bringing toes together first, then heels, toes, heels, toes, heels. Music helps. Another ankle shaper is to use lateral movement by walking sideways on the outsides of your feet. If it gets too painful, stop promptly.

Roll an empty bottle across the floor with your bare feet, even trying to get it out of corners with your toes like a cat playing with a mouse. The total objective of all this is to get you to use your toes and feet more in order to shape up what is immediately above them.

Every time you find yourself sitting with your legs crossed, particularly high up, one thigh resting on the other, uncross them immediately, for you're impeding your blood flow, actually helping to increase the size of your thighs. You probably won't remember every time, but at least try to cross your legs at ankle level gracefully. I'm not trying to fool you into thinking that graceful movements alone will transform chunky legs into the streamlined kind, but they do at least relay a shapelier impression.

Bare-legged Truth

When legs are bare, good shape or not, skin texture is important. Nothing looks worse than legs covered in fuzz, whatever the shape.

As far as I'm concerned, if you happen to be lucky enough to know an expert in waxing, that's the easiest way to a velvety, thoroughly smooth surface – the only kind to have.

If there's no way you can book a wax session, don't turn your nose up at using a razor, ladies' version or otherwise. It's quick and efficient, but it does mean – like constantly weeding a garden – you have to keep after hair growth more assiduously than if you literally nipped growth in the bud with wax or electrolysis.

Apart from nature's contribution of fuzz, there's the environment's contribution of wind and cold to fight, making the skin rough and scaly, so that it catches on tights – and yet you still wonder where that sudden snag came from. In winter, it's essential to use a body lotion on your legs or even the moisturizer you use on your face. There are no oil ducts in the legs to keep the skin there naturally well lubricated, so unless you want to look as if you have 'patterned' skin, keep rough patches away with outside help.

14

For Women at Work - 4

HOW TO IMPROVE YOUR BODY LANGUAGE WITHOUT BEING MISINTERPRETED

IF YOU want to do well at your job, but you also know you don't always *look* alert for the simple reason that you don't *feel* it, start stretching the minute you wake up and keep yawning, too. Again and again. A yawn is simply the body's way of asking for more oxygen. Yawn stretch, yawn stretch – keep on with that regime even in the bath or shower, and if you happen to take the underground to work don't sit down even if the train is empty. Strap-hang, because that way you'll be stretching, too. If you happen to yawn on the way, it will not attract attention. It's that time of day, isn't it?

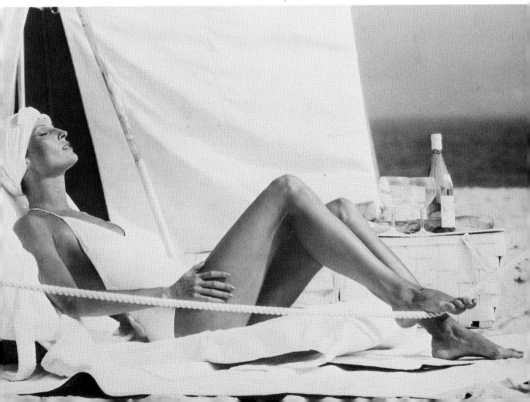

Lunch-time Lessons

If you work in an area where there's little or no evidence of the day outside, be sure to go out at lunch to grab as much oxygen as you can. It's vital for your legs to stretch, too. A day spent sitting in more or less two or three positions is asking for fat thighs and swollen ankles. Walk a little at lunch time, even if only to window-shop. If you can stretch somewhere as high in the air as possible, you will be improving your work performance for the afternoon, make no mistake about it.

To look as if you care about the job in hand, get into the habit of sitting fairly near the edge of your chair, with your weight resting on the 'balls' of your feet (which should be kept fairly far apart). Every time you realize you've crossed your legs, uncross them. Keep your shoulders 'down' and you'll find, because of your position on the chair, it will be difficult for you to slouch, which invariably looks slack, even if at heart you're conscientious and caring.

Save time by responding to commands quickly. Don't think you can 'just finish that sentence or read that line or fill that container'. If your boss buzzes or calls for your attention and you're able to give it to him or her, act at once. Alacrity on the job is prized in the big world of commerce, where minutes literally cost money.

'Conscious Breathing'

To feel alert, pay more attention to the way you breathe. If for no other reason than a late, late night you feel horribly sleepy at work, go to the ladies' room for some 'conscious breathing'. Stand upright and concentrate on inhaling deeply through your nose. This will flood your lungs with more oxygen, which will then move on into your bloodstream to give your whole body extra vitality and life. When you can't inhale any more, exhale explosively, literally making a sound of getting rid of something – in this instance carbon dioxide and waste matters from your body, filtered from the bloodstream. Inhale again (more oxygen), exhale again (more elimination). In the couple of minutes you spend on this breathing exercise you will banish any thoughts of sleep and regain your sense of purpose.

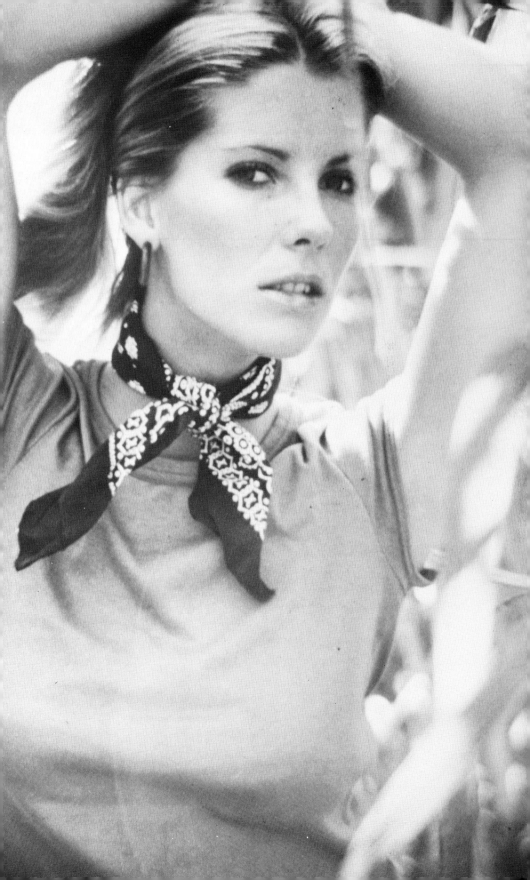

The Contemporary Curse

ACHES AND PAINS AS A WAY OF LIFE

ONE of my own Shirley Lord polls, conducted by somewhat unorthodox methods, has revealed that at seven out of ten dinner parties 30 per cent of the guests will admit with varying degrees of authenticity to aches and pains of some sort; that on four or sometimes five days out of seven, I will run across friends, acquaintances and/or business colleagues who will stretch and creak and complain of vague backaches and/or various kinds of headaches.

What does it all mean and what can we, as a nation of stiff upper backs and lips, do about it?

HAS ANYONE HAD A GOOD BACKACHE LATELY?

'Our lives are too comfortable. We eat too much and exercise too little. We forget about posture immediately we leave school. We ride instead of walk. We deliberately look for and buy furniture that's soft to sink into rather than to support us. We've become a nation of slumpers and the vertebrae weren't built for slumping ...' It's a leading orthopaedist speaking to me and I know that every word he says is true.

What were the vertebrae built for? To hold us *up*, of course, *up* being the operative word. This is what our twenty-four detached vertebrae starting at the base of the skull and the nine vertebrae of the lower back were created for.

The detached vertebrae, connected by a jelly-like substance, are somewhat misleadingly called 'discs', and 'slipped disc' has been all the rage for years as a neat explanation of a variety of back ailments (frequently as unrelated to a disc having 'slipped' as to an ankle having twisted).

When a disc really 'slips', causing an immediate stabbing back pain,

294

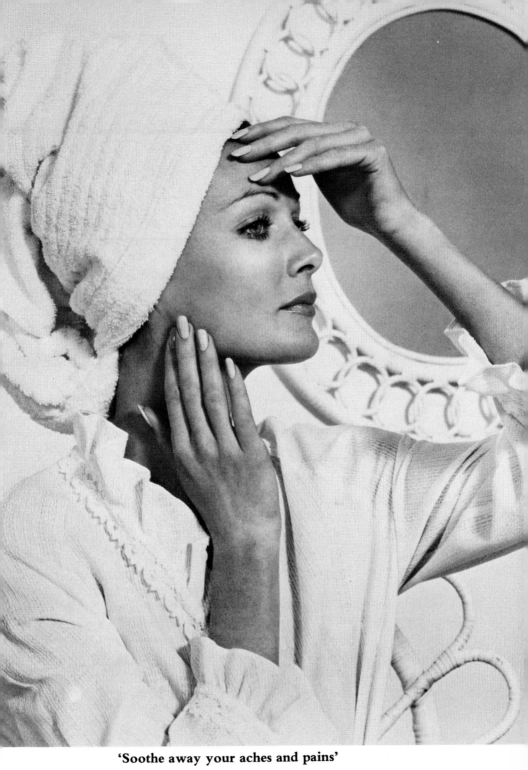

'Soothe away your aches and pains'

it means some of the jelly has slipped out of place and is pressing on the nerve ending, causing inflammation and so pain.

It's natural when this happens for the sufferer to want to cease moving altogether, but unfortunately no movement can be the worst policy, often aggravating the problem rather than lessening it. Spending weeks in one position, or as near to one as is possible, weakens the muscles that support the lower back, denying support to the upper vertebrae and so pulling muscles, ligaments and spinal vertebrae further out of their true place. For this reason many doctors today believe in getting their patients moving as soon as is practical, even after major surgery.

Statistics have proved that chronic and constant backache can often be traced to an emotional rather than a physical reason. Tension, a common part of living these days, seems to attack the back, particularly the muscular structure, which tightens up as if to ready the body for action.

As life rarely presents an opportunity to let fly, and so release tension, this tightening and readying up of the spine often leads instead to excruciating backache. The best antidote for this tension-linked pain is exercise, followed by massage and a warm steady shower on the area crying out for attention.

Preventative anti-backache action means starting new habits: maintaining the right weight, sleeping on a hard mattress, exercising regularly, whether in a game, at a gym or doing a daily ten-minute work-out at home. If you do all these things and your back *still* hurts, obviously you must get a check-up with your doctor for another set of remedies and don't delay.

HEADING OFF THE HEADACHE

When your head aches, it isn't, as you may think, that your brain or even skull is aching. There are three kinds of headaches, but the painful area for all these usually lies outside the brain in the surrounding muscles, veins and arteries.

If you've got a vascular – migraine – headache, the pain comes from *vasodilation*, when blood vessels inside and outside the skull dilate because of certain chemicals present in the bloodstream. Because the blood vessels enlarge, they can press on nerves and . . . ouch, ouch! Alas, a migraine isn't necessarily triggered off by anything you do; more likely it's because you come from a family of migraine sufferers.

But, though inheritance plays a big part, research has now revealed that the vascular kind of headache can be the result of an allergy, for some foods definitely produce the chemical in the bloodstream that triggers off the ache in those already predisposed towards it.

What are the foods on the 'headache' list for the unfortunate few? Cheese (except cottage cheese), Chinese food, vinegar, chicken livers, frankfurters, pickled herring and chocolates, while it's believed beer, bourbon, gin and red wine can start the action going, too.

Some doctors believe the classic hangover headache is caused by vasodilation and can be alleviated by speeding up the metabolism of the alcohol with spoonfuls of honey. Try it!

A diet high in roughage is recommended to the migraine sufferer, too, with plenty of raw vegetables, vegetable juices, fruit and fish, and as little meat as possible to avoid having acid-forming substances in the bloodstream. Whether the right diet can actually cure migraine is debatable, but medical opinion agrees that the right diet can certainly help alleviate the problem, which, as anyone who's ever had a 'good headache' knows, is better than nothing.

The most common place for migraine to strike is along one half of the forehead, at one temple or around and behind one eye. Frequently the pain is accompanied by nausea, depression or even what appears to be the start of a cold. Doctors believe it can be the body's way of telling you to slow down, sending you a warning that something is amiss with the way you're living your life.

Both acupuncture and hypnosis (see pages 302 and 229) are being used to help the chronic migraine sufferer, but rest and silence are immediate musts when it comes to coping with an attack.

There are multitudes of migraine drugs on the market aimed at preventing the dilation of the blood vessels and encouraging relaxation. So far the drugs are short-term relievers and in no way a cure, but if the attacks come on a regular basis medication can be prescribed early to help prevent the chemical changes which force the blood vessels to go into spasm, thus causing the intense pain.

The organically caused *headache*, attacking from outer space without any apparent cause, is often related to a hidden infection, perhaps in the eyes, ears, nose or teeth. Any pain in the head that recurs regularly, for however short a duration, should be checked out with your doctor. If it's organically based, it can usually be cured by finding and then tackling the infection at its source.

The headache the world spends most on is the tension-related one, often starting around 2.30 in the afternoon after a steady day of meetings and not letting up till sleep takes over. Conversely, it also often starts just when the pressure's off, at the beginning of a holiday, for example, when something biochemical seems to happen in the body to upset the system.

Over-the-counter medication can help, but if you feel you get *more* headaches than you used to and they're growing in intensity, a thorough check-up is the only solution to learn what they're all about.

Apparently most people don't like to trouble their doctor with a headache. It seems too insignificant to mention, but, 'better safe than sorry' is the only answer to this point of view.

Tension headaches are prevalent because the muscles of neck and scalp pull on and irritate nerve endings all too easily when one is sitting at a desk for long periods of time, coping with a seemingly endless series of problems, telephone calls, visitors.

One of the best cures is sleep, going to bed as soon as possible after getting home from the office. Warmth helps, but too much warmth can cause headaches. Many office managements go by the date rather than the temperature in switching central heating off and on. Whatever your thermostat states, it is important to keep the neck and shoulders comfortably warm during a working day, for this can preclude a lot of the tensing up we all subconsciously do – tensing up that leads to irritated nerve endings and finally to the tension headache.

LEARN ABOUT MASSAGE – IT'S GOOD FOR YOU

'I know when a body is out of tune,' said the lady with the magical hands. 'I can retune it as well as my cousin retunes a Stradivarius.'

Many top masseurs are large people, which must have something to do with their muscle power, although they never show it, their touch, often as light as a feather, working wonders on tired out, tense bodies.

Massage is a panacea to many pace-setters and people who feel they must try to keep up that pace.

But massage is not a medicine, as many think, and the masseur who offers it as a cure for arthritis or to banish wrinkles or to help you lose weight *is the masseur to avoid*.

In the hands of a trained physiotherapist, however, massage makes you feel better psychologically and physiologically. It can help the body in many different ways, affecting nerve endings, muscles and blood circulation.

The best time to have a massage is when you feel worn out – an improvement on rest alone, as from the right hands it unknots bunched muscles and stimulates the blood flow to cleanse the body faster of waste matters, toxins.

The psychological benefits depend largely on the response from the nerve endings – important in that the sense of touch conveys a great deal of information to the person being massaged. Indifference or sympathy is relayed via touch – one reason why one pair of hands will relax you to the point when you are lulled to sleep, while another pair will make you wish you'd never come in the first place. When it is as it should be, *tranquillizing*, massage works faster than alcohol or drugs – and is obviously much better for you.

There's an analogy to be drawn between tight shoes and massage. When you wear tight shoes or ones that aren't comfortable, the 'touch' receptors in the feet which record pain (1,300 of them to each square inch of skin (200 to each square centimetre)) signal 'it hurts' and go on recording the message until somebody does something about it – hopefully yourself.

In the Orient, the wearing of tight, painful shoes is considered a sin, as it is considered this affects the meridian lines of the body (see page 302), and so the entire health and balance.

With massage the object is to activate the touch receptors that record pressure (there are about 160 to each square inch of skin (twenty-five to each square centimetre)) in such a way that the signals sent to the brain are pleasurable, relaxed and tension-free.

The better the massage, the better the delivery service to the brain through these built-in skin receptors, ensuring speedy relaxation and release from nagging problems, if only momentarily. This is the most important and obvious result of a good massage.

The effect on muscles is actually minimal, although a good physiotherapist will be able to reduce muscle spasm caused, for example, by the whiplash produced in minor collisions. The difference between a masseur and a physiotherapist is that the latter has to know a great deal about anatomy, pathology, physiology, the muscular and skeletal structure, and the nervous and circulatory systems of the body.

Circulation isn't significantly changed by a full body massage; a brisk walk will deliver the same results. However, when a physiotherapist works on a particular area for any length of time, blood circulation will increase and so bring the necessary benefits. With this kind of expert massage, constricted blood vessels can be opened to enable the flow of blood to move through normal routes, besides removing the waste matters that help cause the blockage in the first place.

The techniques used by a physiotherapist differ from those used by the masseur, in that the former nearly always concentrates on the afflicted area, not on giving a full body massage. Each stroke the physiotherapist makes moves towards the heart, the better to move the blood in the veins in that direction. Often the movements are connected with other treatments such as heatpacks or infra-red sessions.

For special aches and pains all this can be helpful. If aches and pains aren't the problem you can certainly find rest and relaxation with massage, providing you find yourself in the right pair of hands.

Masseurs usually use a 100-year-old Swedish method, created by Per Henrik Ling, a Swedish medical gymnast, which involves working from toe to top. The masseur uses *effleurage* (stroking), friction (rubbing), *pétrissage* (kneading) and *tapotement* (tapping), all to increase blood and lymph flow through vein and lymph vessels, rather than through the arteries.

Some masseurs prefer to work with rubbing alcohol, talcum powder or even salt – which feels coarse but gives the body an extraordinarily clean, smooth feeling once it's washed off with a warm fragrant cloth.

PRESS FOR HEALTH AND STRENGTH

If you meet someone whose thumbs are insured, you may be meeting a special Shiatzu expert, who uses the thumbs to relieve the tensions and traumas of the rich. The names of the best practitioners of this 4,000-year-old art travel first class from client to client, from capital to capital. This is because, unlike Swedish massage and the like, Shiatzu is known to have extraordinarily curative powers.

Shiatzu, like acupuncture, is applied to the relevant pressure points of the body – 360 of them based along one of the twelve meridian lines that run vertically through us. No needles are used, but generally thumbs and sometimes fingers apply the pressure in an expert manner to reduce muscle tension and aches and pains, especially of the head and back. The underlying purpose is to activate organs that are not working correctly, to help them behave in a 'younger' way, to be more active, and to correct faults in circulation.

Shiatzu devotees believe it helps the condition of their skin as well as their shape. As one masseur explains, 'Skin is one of the best indicators of intestinal and respiratory health. If it looks drab, the intestinal muscles are tired, but a change in diet won't always help because food isn't being digested properly. Shiatzu massage can help correct this.'

Although do-it-yourself treatments can never equal those given by the experts, Shiatzu does have distinct go-it-alone possibilities. Even better, you can exchange pressure point information with your partner and take turns at relieving each other's anxieties or whatever else you happen to have on your mind (achewise, that is).

I was told in Tokyo (at the Founder's Institute) that Shiatzu can be self-administered if the subject takes the time and trouble to find out what goes with what.

If you want to improve your skin tone (colour, texture and overall look) use the ball of your thumb to apply light pressure along the brows and out to the temples, a heavier thumb pressure along the sides of the neck and in a V line from chin to throat base. Continue pressure from the centre of the rib cage straight down to the abdomen and to the pubic bone, then increase pressure on both sides of the body just above the buttocks. All this stimulates the adrenal glands and kidneys to help the skin from within.

If you have a headache you can't shake off (see page 296), try a spot of Shiatzu. Find the centre spot of your skull, where you had a 'soft' spot as a baby, and apply thumb pressure there steadily. Move to the area on top of the foot between large and second toe and press there for several minutes before going back to the skull.

The Japanese much prefer Shiatzu to aspirin and believe our hands and feet can literally reveal our innermost problems. Much of Shiatzu is carried out on the hands and feet, the treatment manifesting itself on the pressure point of the meridian activated by the reflex points on each hand or foot.

Pressure applied from one thumb to another (on the thumb tip) is, according to the experts I talked to, beneficial to the entire head. Pressure on the side of the index finger can settle an upset stomach, while pressure on the ring finger is directed towards helping liver problems.

If you're a foot person, apply thumb pressure to the centre of the upper and lower arch and you could be influencing your colon to be healthy. Pressure applied to the side of the heel apparently stimulates the ovaries.

There's no end to the marvels of Shiatzu. I don't pretend to understand it, but, judging from what I've seen and heard, I'm not about to dismiss it either.

ACUPUNCTURE – MYTH OR MAGIC?

One of the most fascinating things I ever learned about acupuncture was that in the old days in China (when emperors dozed on golden thrones and Chinese baby dolls had their feet bound tight to ensure they'd only wear size two slippers as debutantes), the acupuncturist, a revered member of the medical profession (then as now), was a regular visitor – three or four times a year to rich households – but *he was only paid for those visits if members of the family stayed well*. If, in spite of his regular calls, a client turned into a patient by falling sick, he was obliged to treat for free.

From this it's easy to deduce that in China acupuncture was – and still is – used to *maintain* health rather than to *retrieve* it. In the East, unlike the West, the attitude towards medicine and medical treatments is to use them to *prevent* the appearance of symptoms, rather than to fight them when they appear. Perhaps this deep-rooted difference in attitude explains a great deal about the present controversy regarding the value of acupuncture. It's hard for many of us to accept that merely through the correct placement of needles in the skin migraine headaches, slipped discs and even arthritis can be alleviated, if not cured – particularly when the needle that apparently works the magic isn't even inserted where the pain is!

'Ha, ha, ha, but that's the whole point of the story,' as the comic said to the straight man. In the East, it isn't only the acupuncturist who believes the human body is an electro-magnetic field, forever vibrating and responding to outside stimuli, it's the entire medical profession.

The traditional acupuncturist taps that field, releasing the body energy that he believes is continually circulating through twelve connected pathways, or 'meridians' as they're called. The needles, no thicker than a heavy hair, are inserted at points along these meridians where electrical resistance is lower than normal. When a needle is inserted at one such point, it supposedly delivers a minute electrical charge which increases the quality and concentration of energy all along the meridian on which it lies, eventually leading to the area in trouble.

If, for example, someone is suffering from an attack of food poisoning, which can happen in the nicest of families, the acupuncturist might insert one needle on the inner side of the big toe and another somewhere on the foot, because this is where the route to the liver meridian begins, running from the foot along the inside of the leg, across the abdomen to the thorax with branches spiralling off deep inside the body, one leading directly to the liver itself.

The minute electrical charge apparently releases enough extra energy to re-establish a proper energetic balance in the body, so that almost before the patient realizes it the liver is feeling in good shape again and food poisoning is a thing of the past.

Intriguing, and I know from past experience that acupuncture can most certainly alleviate.

It isn't a universal panacea and it can't patch up broken bones, but, as Einstein said and proved, 'energy is the essential factor in life', so why shouldn't a lack of it be a motivating factor in what makes us sick? It's worth thinking about.

Has She or Hasn't She . . .

HAD HER FACE/BOSOM/THIGHS LIFTED?
HAD A NOSE/STOMACH/CHIN JOB?

THE question is still not asked directly – but the conjecture never stops. More significant, every day, all over the world, the number of plastic surgery operations taking place for cosmetic reasons grows, while the age of the patients is getting younger. For those who care, it's London, Miami and New York for face lifts, Tokyo for nose jobs and eye openers, Moscow for hair transplants, and Rio de Janeiro or Buenos Aires for thigh lifts in particular, body tucks in general. This is sometimes poetically described as body sculpting, but it is a poetic description, for it is the most painful of all plastic surgery operations.

All over the world the traffic in clients in search of the right plastic surgeons grows, as the need to look younger becomes greater. The plastic surgeons say that forty now seems to be the average age women begin to want a fresh start.

Once magisterial towards purely cosmetic jobs, more and more plastic surgeons are now exchanging views and holding worldwide seminars to discover how best to correct or improve on nature, while more and more articles are 'disclosing' facts about the famous and their various lifts.

When Vidal Sassoon revealed he'd had the bags beneath his eyes removed, he told me he thought he had the best possible reason for having done so. 'I go to a gym every day to keep my body in top shape. Why shouldn't my face match up? I may be over forty, but I feel like twenty-five. My body looks it. Now so does my face.'

As Vidal now lives in the U.S. this makes him typical of the million *younger* men and women who annually undergo some kind of surgery for the sake of their looks. Since 1949 the number of operations

Beautiful Luciana Avedon, one of the first 'to tell'

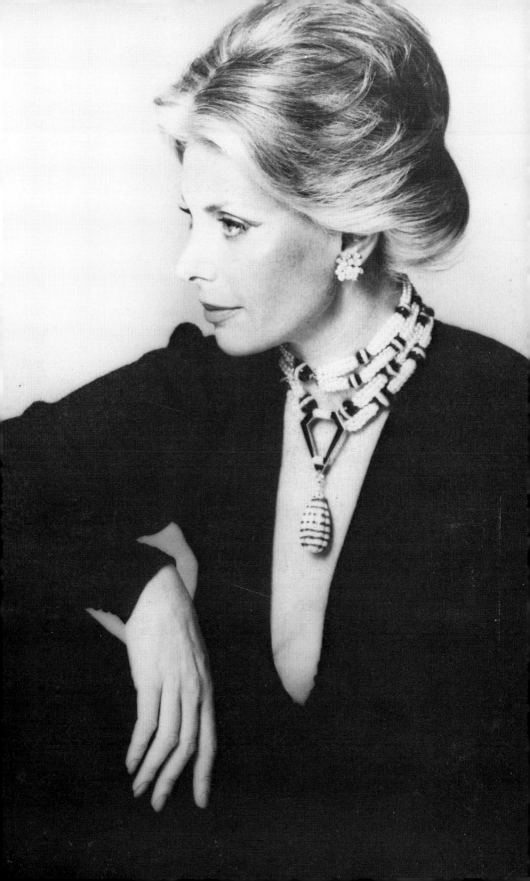

has rocketed, in the last decade tripling for women and doubling for men, and these operations all involve what plastic surgeons call 'surgery performed in an attempt to improve the appearance, not necessary for physical health or safety, but desirable for emotional and/or psychological benefit.'

A typical plastic surgeon's year will include at least fifty breast operations (mostly to reduce size rather than increase it), 100 face lifts, 150 nose operations, twenty chin corrections and seventy-five ear operations.

In France and Switzerland, husbands and wives go to clinics together, with the intention of regaining lost looks, while in Rio de Janeiro, Brazil, the celebrated Dr Ivo Pitanguy is booked from one year to the next for his equally celebrated body lifts, particularly the operation for removing what he calls 'riding breeches', ridding the thigh area of excess flab, which is as distressing to women over thirty as is the deadly, if controversial, cellulite (see page 280).

TWO SCHOOLS OF THOUGHT

Despite the huge increase in the number of patients, there are still primarily two schools of thought regarding cosmetic plastic surgery. On the one hand, there are those who unrealistically expect it to be the answer to everything; they can't wait to try it as soon as make-up fails to cover up all of nature's inadequacies.

On the other hand, there are those who are scared to death of the whole idea; they brainwash themselves with the thought that once past forty-five or fifty they shouldn't expect to look unlined, let alone attractive.

What are the real facts? Viewed in the most matter of fact way, cosmetic surgery is not a cure-all. It is simply a question of cutting away from or adding to the face or body to improve it. A new nose is precisely that – a new nose; it will not turn a plain woman into a stunning one overnight. Neither will a face lift, a body lift or a different set of bosom measurements.

Once a patient realizes how much mileage she's going to be able to get out of the surgery she's contemplating, much more can be accomplished. As Dr Pitanguy reiterates, 'Arriving at the surgery with the wrong size dream causes the most problems for patients, not the actual operation itself.'

One of the most commonly dreamed 'wrong size dreams' is that the results of plastic surgery will last forever. In the majority of operations that is just not so. Only those operations that change bone structure or deal with areas uninfluenced by muscles or fatty deposits (such as noses, ears and chins) give enduring results. Otherwise, as any respected plastic surgeon will tell you, 'A woman's face continues to age at the same rate the second after the face lift has been carried out. Plastic surgery puts the clock back, it doesn't stop it.'

One aggravation that many plastic surgeons complain about is that after a successful face lift a woman is apt to give her face no special post-surgery care and, worse, tends not to realize that as she possesses a younger looking skin, she needs a lighter make-up.

Women with heavy bags beneath their eyes may have tried to cover them up, usually in vain, with false lashes and a heavy eye make-up. If surgery to remove the bags is successful, the last thing the patient should do is to continue with the same false lash/heavy eye colour routine. Yet nine times out of ten she will, unless she's lucky enough to run into a surgeon who explains to her *at the beginning* that his work will make her look younger, so she should switch to wearing mascara and use a lighter hand in applying eye shadow.

Post plastic surgery skin (see page 316), needs extra help in the easy form of moisturizers day and night. This helps to fight the ageing process by keeping the skin in optimum condition, warding off the dryness that will encourage the return of tiny lines and crevices.

Once cosmetic surgery is approached the right way, with the knowledge that much can be accomplished in a reasonably short time, but that no miracles are handed out with the anaesthesia, then most can benefit. If you feel you need a few facial revisions or an ironing out of an over-wrinkled skin, don't hesitate to consult a reputable plastic surgeon. It's a perfectly healthy, normal thing to do, once your mind is made up and your attitude is the right one.

LIFTING THE FACE

There's more than one kind of face lift. The basic version only takes up the slack in the cheeks and upper jowls, while the radical kind means cutting around the entire hairline to the nape of the neck. Even the average lift takes about four hours, but if all goes well the patient should be able to face the world happily within three weeks. As far as scars are concerned, the better the surgeon the fewer the scars, and they are usually concealed in the hairline.

Most surgeons agree a face lift should give a fresh approach for at least *five to eight years*, but it all depends on the skin. Some react better than others, so some last longer.

How old should one be to contemplate a face lift? Princess Luciana Pignatelli, one of the first to 'tell it all' about her silicone injections, nose job and eye ops, says, 'I prefer not to wait until something drastic has to be done. There's no sense in trying to come out as smooth as a baby when you go in looking like an old topographic map.'

Most surgeons would agree with her, although many try to dissuade the forty-year-old patient from having a total face 'job'. The best deterrent: the news that the earlier the visit, the more return visits will probably have to be made.

At Your First Appointment

When you make up your mind that something has to go – whether it's eye bags, cheek droops, or just a baggy old face, you may have different ideas from the surgeon you select.

At your first interview he will examine you and ask for your medical history, just like any other doctor would do before an operation because – make no mistake about it – *this is an operation*, not a lark, however frivolous your reason for the visit. The surgeon may show you before-and-after photographs to demonstrate his work, and he will certainly photograph you for planning and record purposes.

The surgeon's main challenges in a face lift are: how far he can separate the skin from the fat and muscle beneath, how much excess can be excised, how far it can be stretched, and in which direction. A woman may arrive at the surgery thinking she needs the 'works', a standard face lift called a *rhytidectomy*, whereas the surgeon may point out with pictures and demonstrations on her own face that only a *blepharoplasty*, removal of eye bags, is needed.

For a full face lift job, the surgeon usually starts with an incision in the scalp about midway along the forehead, back from the hairline, continuing down on either side to the point where the ears are attached to the head. From there the incision proceeds in front of the ears, curving around them, continuing upwards and sharply backwards, finishing at the back just above the nape of the neck.

Once the skin is separated from the underlying tissue, the surgeon's most delicate job is to gather the tissue upwards and backwards on either side towards the ears, suturing it firmly to the fascia (which protects the facial muscles) and tightening it, so providing a smooth surface over which the ageing, inelastic skin can be 'stretched', any excess being cut off. A local anaesthetic, combined with intravenous analgesia, is often used for this op, because a general anaesthetic tube can obscure the face's overall condition and shape. Some sutures are removed after three to five days, those behind the ears not for ten days. With lines 'ironed' out, skin stretched but not too taut, the face in the right surgeon's hands will inevitably look smoother and so younger – for a few years at least.

AWAY WITH THE BAGGY EYES

The older the eyes, the more beautiful they often become, with experience showing in their expression. The skin around the eyes is not so pretty. This is where the *blepharoplasty*, eye wrinkle job, comes in, in which fat and excess skin are removed from the upper or lower lids or both. Rapidly becoming top of the pops in plastic surgery ops, the number being carried out nowadays approaching that of the number of nose jobs, blepharoplasty is even sought by model girls in their late twenties who want to cover all markets and not lose their lucrative 'teen look'.

To smooth out bags, the surgeon starts by making an incision just beneath the lower lashes, angling downwards at the outer corners, drawing the loosened skin upwards, trimming, then stitching. To correct a sag on the upper lid, an incision is made at the eyelid's crease; again, off comes the unwanted skin and fat, then a fine seam is angled upwards.

Most operations take place under a local anaesthetic. Many surgeons like patients to be *awake enough* to cooperate when asked to open or close their eyes.

If it sounds simple, it isn't. The surgeon has to be able to measure exactly the right amount of skin to be excised. Too little, and it would all be a waste of time. Too much, even by a fraction of a millimetre, and the eye will look distorted or, worse, not be able to close properly. The surgeon also has to decide whether the ageing look comes from sagging lids or drooping eyebrows. If it's the latter, he elevates the brow by excising skin above the browline, with the suture line buried in the upper hairline.

Step-by-Step Anti-Bag

One editor I know went into a clinic at the beginning of the week for an anti-bags job. The first morning she was given a blood test, coagulation test, and urine analysis and after about twelve noon she wasn't allowed to eat or drink anything, not even a glass of water.

At about 1.30 the surgeon came to explain exactly what he was going to do, demonstrating by drawing on her eyelids with an indelible pencil to show her exactly where he intended to make his cuts. She had to look up, down, right, left, smile, frown, and make as many expressions as she could think of that she regularly made during the day – surprise was one of them – so that he could see where she 'made' her wrinkles. The idea behind it was very practical. He explained that he intended to make incisions, where possible, where there were wrinkles already so that each tiny scar could be hidden there.

At four o' clock she was given an injection to make her drowsy and an hour later she was taken to the operating room for a second injection. The operation took about two hours, and in this case (although it certainly doesn't always happen) a nurse sat with her from 8 p.m. to 8 a.m. putting pieces of ice wrapped in little squares of gauze on her eyes all through the night. Later, she told me she thought this was invaluable, as she never did go black and blue, which can happen.

The next morning she felt fine, althought the first sight of herself was a shock – tiny black stitches surrounded little slitty eyes, while her eyelids were very red and swollen. The nurses were helpful as they kept saying what a marvellous job it was, so she wasn't as depressed as she might have been. Two days later she went home under dark glasses, the underneath stitches completely out, the top ones still in.

By the end of the week, her eye lids were much less swollen, although the skin under the eyes was turning slightly yellow and itched. By the end of the weekend her eyes were even less swollen and all the stitches came out.

A week from the day of the op the upper lid looked perfectly normal, the under one a little red. At the end of the second week, twelve days after the operation, she started to put on normal eye make-up. She waited that long not so much because it would have bothered her eyes, but because the thought of *taking it off* was unbearable. The result? I and many of her friends told her when next we saw her how very healthy and well she looked – which is how I came to hear the story.

GRANDMA, WHAT A BIG NOSE YOU HAVE

Plastic surgery, and nose jobs in particular, were mentioned in early Sanskrit literature in 600 B.C. In the Middle Ages, when nose slicing was a regular punishment, nose mending became a lucrative, if rather inept, job.

Rhinoplasty, as it's called today, is now so refined that surgeons can shorten, lengthen, tilt, straighten or do almost any other shaping on a nose.

Surgeons say the hardest part of the job is to convince someone who wants a new nose that the one they've chosen isn't necessarily the right one for them.

The decision as to how much to remove and how much to leave behind is what makes rhinoplasty still one of the most delicate, complex and unpredictable plastic surgery operations, despite the enormous advances that have taken place. The reason? The slightest fraction of an inch more or less at nose level can make or break a face. Sometimes a surgeon has to make a patient realize it's not her nose that's at fault, but rather her chin that needs augmenting with a slice of silicone (see page 312), so that her proud nose no longer appears to protrude like a beak, but instead adds character to her looks.

The best surgeons know how to minimize or build up a slightly faulty nose without losing its 'character', even the ancestral quality that sometimes gives a face drama.

As one famous surgeon wittily pointed out, 'The nose is a peninsula, not an island. *It makes no sense unless considered in relation to the mainland – the face.*'

What Goes on in a Nose Op

Surgery is generally performed from inside the nose under a local anaesthetic, to prevent the patient from bleeding as much as he would under a general anaesthetic, keeping the face as natural looking as possible while the operation is in progress.

Generally, to make smaller takes about forty-five minutes with seventy-two hours spent in hospital and one week in bandages. The black and blue eyes generally associated with this operation vary according to the patient's skin, its healing capacity and the surgeon's skill. If the object is to narrow the nose, a knowledgeable handling of the delicate bones is vital to avoid bruises and, as nose bones have a good memory, to prevent them from resuming their previous position.

Where there's not enough nose, *profile* is often built up utilizing the body's own resources, a sliver from the hip bone or from the rib cartilage being used as an implant. Otherwise a piece of silicone is sometimes shaped into place.

Because of the skin's astonishing resilience and elasticity, it will stretch over the new more substantial 'nose' with ease. After a few days on antibiotics, five days to a week in hospital, and regular checking of bandages, in three to four weeks, when the incision has healed, the new profile looks as if it has always been in residence.

CHINLESS WONDERS CAN BE BUILT UP – AND SOME DOUBLE CHINS 'TRIMMED' DOWN

It's been reported that until Marilyn Monroe had her chin built up, she was known as a chinless wonder – and her career was chinless, too.

Silicone is regularly used to build up, but when *reduction* is needed, in the case of the iniquitous double chin for instance, the best solution is a matter of controversy, for this is a job that can leave noticeable scars on the neck.

Where does the double chin come from? As Dr Ralph Millard, M.D., Ronald W. Pigott, F.R.C.S., and Abdulhamid Hedo, M.D., from the Department of Surgery, University of Miami School of Medicine, explained in a paper, part of a panel discussion on facial rejuvenation: 'Increasing age, loss of skin elasticity, and repetitious stretching of the neck finally end up in loose excess. This excess tends to make the jowl sag. *Repeated gains and losses in weight* over the years also effect the stretching of skin. This can be accommodated in youth but droops in dewlaps in later years.' Descriptive and telling.

In a paper presented in Australia at the Fifth International Congress of Plastic and Reconstructive Surgery, it was put another way:

> The loss of youthful profile of the neck is caused by the widening of the cervico-mandibular angle. This presents a puzzling thera-peutic enigma. It may be manifested by the double chin, with an accumulation of fat but with little or no excess of skin beneath the neck except that which encompasses the heavy fat pad. Such patients may be obese, have short necks, recessed chins, and an inclination to deposit fat beneath the skin. Due to ageing and stretching of the skin and *repeated gains and losses in weight*, the neck may develop a 'turkey gobbler' deformity.

One specialist opinion on what age, the gradual drooping of the skin and additional fat deposits can produce.

What Can Be Done about the Double Chin, If Anything?

The best method of erasing this age telltale is called *lipectomy*, and it is generally carried out in connection with a face lift.

As Dr Millard explains, various techniques have been used to remove fat from beneath the chin, leaving criss-cross scars which are often quite noticeable. Lipectomy involves making only a small incision under the chin for removal of fat and muscle, then a face lift gives access to further removal of fat along the chin line, 'lifting' and 'tightening' the skin all around. Dr Millard further elaborates by stating that out of the last 100 face lifts he carried out, sixty-three had had this combined procedure, the majority ending up with a better neckline than they had possessed when younger.

THE BIG PEEL

While the face lift takes care of face sag, it doesn't necessarily remove *all* the wrinkles on the face, the fine kind that corrugate foreheads, the frown lines we make between our eyes, the fine wrinkling often found between nostril and upper lip.

We spend our lives making these wrinkles, publicizing our emotions in the same way again and again, although we rarely realize it. These expressions are the habitual giveaways that secret agents have to learn to iron out before departing disguised on a mission.

If we could see ourselves through the mattress when we sleep on our faces (about 75 per cent of people sleep this way during some part of the night), we would *pin* ourselves *down* on our backs rather than ever do it again. Think of how you look when you press your face against a window or mirror and you will get the general idea of the mattress picture, one that we press in a little more every night of our lives.

Before twenty-five, our natural expressions come and go as swiftly as the emotions that cause them, leaving no trace, the skin's early and lively elasticity snapping the face back into place (see page 25).

Once the subcutaneous fat beneath the epidermis starts to dissipate with age, there's nothing there to do the 'snapping,' and so the patterns we've been making for a lifetime start to settle in for good in the form of wrinkles.

313

An article in the *British Journal of Plastic Surgery* stated,

> The disfigurement of the ageing face is a triad of *hollow*, *sag*, and *wrinkle* and should be dealt with as far as possible in all its triplicity. A surgical face lift in hands experienced in shifting skin is an excellent operation. Only if claims are extravagant is there disappointment – usually the basis for dismay lies in the *persistence of fine wrinkles*. For the fine wrinkle there is the acid peel.

Since this endorsement, peeling with chemicals, called facial chemosurgery by the medical profession, has become generally accepted as the best method for removing the tiny lines that still give the age game away.

Dermabrasion is another form of peeling, carried out with a fast rotating wire brush that literally scrapes the skin's top surface away; it is used by expert dermatologists and plastic surgeons to remove acne pits or traumatic scars rather than the everyday sort of wrinkles.

Controversy still exists about chemosurgery's limitations, though there's general agreement that it works well with a face lift, expelling the fine wrinkles commonly left around upper and lower lip and forehead.

The treatment should be clearly defined as *a chemical burn*, using phenol to destroy the epidermis (skin's top layer), significantly altering the dermis beneath. This 'burns out the wrinkle' by changing the cellular construction and collapsing vertical age lines to make them horizontal, so tautening the skin. In other words, *wrinkles are straightened out*.

As acne is already taut and fixed in its furrows and mounds, burning with chemicals can increase this immobility, which is also the case with deep scars. On the other hand, as far as fine wrinkles are concerned, peeling does seem to produce a relative permanency in dermal changes, and it's been proved that in most cases there's far less tendency for the wrinkles to re-occur.

Fair complexions react better than dark, for following chemo-surgery a certain 'pinkness' can persist for some months. It fades in time, but perhaps pinkness is a small price to pay for a no-wrinkle, smooth texture.

The right make-up is adequate camouflage, but one thing to remember is that sunbathing is ABSOLUTELY OUT FOREVER (see pages 51–55).

What Happens in Chemosurgery?

Following a local anaesthetic the skin site is cleaned with ether, then a phenol-based solution (phenol, croton oil, liquid soap and distilled water) is painted on with a cotton applicator until the skin is uniformly white. Particular effort is necessary to get to the bottom of deep crevices, frown lines on the forehead, the network of fine wrinkles between nose and mouth, the lines stretched from mouth to chin.

Application encroaches on the hairline, to avoid a visible margin, and around the lips the acid is painted up to the skin's vermilion border. The face is then divided into natural sections, and on most skins, except the very delicate, each section is immediately covered by tape following the 'painting' to increase the action of the acid. After forty-eight hours the tape is gently eased off to expose flaking flesh – the debris of the burn.

Antibiotic dusting powder is applied frequently for the next twenty-four hours, then an ointment is used to help soften the crust, which can be taken off the next day.

Beneath lies a new skin, pink and shining, that can be washed immediately with ordinary cleansing methods, mild soap and water being recommended, followed by a very emollient cream if the skin is dry and scaly.

Make-up *is* permissible after a week, but it's more often two, three or four – for a peel job means you're likely to consider yourself unpresentable for at least that length of time.

What Happens in Dermabrasion?

This surgical procedure is also called skin planing, for, as the name suggests, the skin *is* planed mechanically. First, the skin is frozen, then a rotating wire brush is stroked rapidly across to remove the surface layer of skin. Scabs that develop are shed within two weeks, when the skin swells and appears pinker than usual.

It takes quite a few weeks for the face to return to normal in terms of swelling and colour, but some dermatologists prefer to work with dermabrasion than chemosurgery because they feel there's less natural colour destruction.

To sum up, while chemical peeling works by burning, mechanical peeling works by scraping. As one eminent doctor put it, 'In nature a scrape among animals heals faster and more accurately than a burn. It's a more natural procedure.'

It's also a highly skilled one, which means dermabrasion should

315

only be contemplated if it's certain a doctor with high credentials is behind the brush. In under-qualified hands, dermabrasion can be highly dangerous – for the face can be planed to the point of no return, where only the epidermis around the hair and sweat glands remains. If the epidermis were to be destroyed also at those points, there would be nothing left to regenerate the skin. Because the brush works so fast, unless the hands operating it are extremely qualified it can catch the lip or nose, leaving behind a scar instead of taking one away.

Because of all these horrifying dangers, check and check again on credentials when choosing the man to do the job. *Peeling or 'brushing' can work wonders, but only when the peeler knows his business and has several medical degrees to prove it.*

POST PLASTIC SURGERY MAKE-UP

The part make-up plays post face lift or skin peel is recognized today as vitally important.

One of the most important things patients should know is to avoid the use of the wrong colours post peel – colours that can permanently stain the ultra-sensitive new skin. For this reason all gel make-up should be avoided. Instead the more old-fashioned bases with sediment, coloured through powders, not pigments, should be used. A light tan to warm beige is the most flattering shade for most skins, worn over a *very* emollient moisturizer.

Many post plastic surgery clients are successfully introduced to dyed lashes (black), extra eye make-up (blue pencil above lower lashes, brown beneath the brows) plus a touch of brush-on rouge over cheekbones, bridge of nose, and forehead.

Once you've had your face lifted, it should stay lifted, and make-up can help create this impression, giving an illusion of brightness and well-being.

One last word of advice on Post Plastic Surgery make-up: *pat* in everything you put on your face. Never, never rub.

THE BOSOM AND HOW TO WEAR A SEE-THROUGH WITHOUT COLD FEET

Revolutionary techniques in breast surgery have occurred during the last two decades. This, combined with the acceptance of the no-bra, see-through, streaking era, has sent many under- and over-endowed women scurrying to see a plastic surgeon. Statistics say that most of these women are between eighteen and thirty, but this is not to exclude a very interested over-forty group. I know several who have revamped their bosom shapes in the last few years.

When a woman looks down and sees her front is as flat as her ironing board, her confidence often begins to crack. Until 1950, if she felt she couldn't go through life without a lovely pair of bosoms she had to be prepared to relinquish part of her buttocks. It was a difficult and not too successful operation.

'So Flat Chested I Could Cry'

I have received many readers' letters over the years with the above sad complaint, and I'm happy today to be able to write back to tell the deprived ones that their breastlines can be filled out with implants of fluid silastic encased in plastic bags, inserted through incisions at the base of each bosom, and tucked neatly behind the mammary glands for life.

The implant is in effect a 'falsie', filled with a silicone gel, that comes in eight sizes ranging from petite to extra-full. This is not to be confused with the *direct* liquid silicone injections for extra inches, which is no longer used. Dow-Corning, the first company to manufacture silicone in the United States (and the only one to produce a medical variety), discovered in the mid-sixties that it was being used far too generously and haphazardly by certain doctors. Alarming cases came to their attention of the silicone moving about in the body unchecked, disappearing in one place to reappear somewhere else in alarming lumps under the skin. At that time Dow-Corning immediately and voluntarily listed it with the Medical Authorities, so that their medical silicone ceased being an 'implant material' and became a drug available only under the strictest medical supervision.

The silicone used today is a specially tested gelatinous silicone, always sealed in silicone rubber envelopes shaped like breasts.

There's also another type of insertion, sometimes referred to as the 'balloon' implant. Again, this implant is slipped behind the mammary glands in the form of a balloon-like empty envelope made of silicone. This is filled with a sterilized saline solution (pumped through the balloon's valve) which, when full, is sealed off, the valve packed beneath the balloon to avoid leakage. This method delivers a softer, more mobile looking breast and, because the liquid can be carefully measured, in cases of breast asymmetry it's easy to match the two by filling one balloon a little more or less as the case requires.

For the augmentation process, general anaesthesia is usually used, the stitches and brassiere-like bandages being removed after about a week, while convalescence lasts about a month to six weeks during which time the patient wears a special stretch bra.

Top-Heavy and Awkward – What Can I Do?

Breast reduction, alas, is hard work, say the surgeons, who've been working at it in different ways for the last four decades.

Fat deposits can be removed and nipples relocated, but no matter what technique is employed reduction *mammoplasty* does usually leave scars. If the patient heals well, the scars fade to a discreet pale colour and can be partially disguised by the breasts' natural folds, but they are permanent, and depending on the skin very visible to slightly visible.

However, women who have unusually overdeveloped breasts – called macromastia – usually happily trade in this condition (which can cause chronic exhaustion, arthritis, or even a curvature of the spine, let alone embarrassment) for a couple of scars, pale or not.

BODY DARTS, SEAMS AND TUCKS – NO PLEATS WANTED

With the continual – and sensible – emphasis on dieting, many people's weight fluctuates for years. Even when the right weight and shape is maintained, the skin isn't always accommodating, so that flab ruins the effort, bubbling up on the seat, stomach, thighs, and/or upper arms.

Abdomen Tightening

A frequent victim of unattractive fat is the abdomen, which resists all attempts with massage and exercise to return to its original taut state. An operation to excise excess flab, tightening and realigning the muscle fibres, is the plastic surgeon's way of coping with this problem. One plastic surgeon told me that in a recent abdomen tightening op he removed 20 lb (9 kg) of skin and fat, then transplanted the navel back to its proper position.

A stomach reduction works on the same principle as a face lift, in that it is not just a matter of removing excess fat and skin but of controlling underlying muscles to help the new 'stomach' stay in shape.

More and more women are using this type of operation to smooth out stretch marks left behind by pregnancy. The major incision is usually made low on the stomach, the fine scar coinciding with the pubic hairline, so that it's virtually invisible, even in the smallest bikini.

The operation takes two to three hours, depending on the amount of excess skin to be removed, and the hospital stay varies from five to eight nights. Sutures are removed after ten days, when the patient is advised not to engage in any hectic sport – or sex – for at least six weeks.

Bottoms 'Up'

The celebrated 'riding breeches' operation, pioneered by Dr Ivo Pitanguy in Brazil, now plays a part in a surgeon's day in other parts of the world, too. 'Riding breeches', as Pitanguy calls the fat jutting from the buttocks on to the thighs, spoil the line of jeans and skirts alike, and it's often obstinate fat that won't go away however stringent the diet, or rigid the exercise routine.

In the surgeon's operating room, the quantity of tissue to be cut away from the thigh area is measured. Two lines are drawn on the buttocks – the upper line establishing the first incision, the lower indicating the second. When the patient is anaesthetized, obviously lying on her stomach, the cuts are made along the tracings to remove the skin and fat tissue. Several pounds of lumpy fat can be removed from each thigh with this operation, so of necessity it's a lengthy job, lasting anything from two to four hours.

Recovery is also slow. The first few days the patient must stay wrapped in elastic bandages from the waist down to the knees, and although most patients can leave the hospital after eight to ten days normal activity is impossible for at least two weeks after. Even sitting down is uncomfortable, which makes the plane ride home to New York or Europe almost as bad as having another op. Depending on the patient, normality returns in about six to eight weeks, when I've heard it said that the new silhouette makes everything worthwhile – and memory is short, after all. Again, as with all plastic surgery operations, the better the surgeon, the less visible the scar!

SUMMING UP THE COST OF THE KNIFE

Plastic surgery costs money, big money – first there's the surgeon's fee, then the anaesthetist, then the cost of the hospital room. All these have to be taken into consideration – plus the amount of time you'll be out of circulation.

The saddest story I heard was about the woman who found she couldn't live with her new nose and had to have her old one back – expensive, frustrating and time consuming. But I'd say she wasn't lucky with her surgeon, or else she didn't listen.

The only way to commit yourself to any plastic surgery is, as Dr Pitanguy advises, to have the right size dream in the first place – then the right surgeon will do everything in his power to make it come true.

WAYS TO AVOID THE NECESSITY FOR PLASTIC SURGERY

'Don't smoke. It constricts the blood vessels, encourages pasty looking skin and extra wrinkles around the eyes. Drink a couple of martinis a day – that will dilate the blood vessels and help the skin look younger. Take lots of vitamin C and E.' That uncompromising advice, whether you believe in it or not, came from a well-known plastic surgeon, surprisingly intent on *warding off* patients by helping them stave off the all-too-obvious signs of an ageing skin. Frequently, you will find a conscientious plastic surgeon not only refusing to carry out a face lift operation, but actually trying to teach his would-be patients to live differently in order to avoid facial surgery for at least a few more years.

I know one who regularly sends the patients he considers have come to him 'too early' to make-up experts, to show them that in many cases they look 'older' not because of nature but because of badly applied make-up and the wrong hairdo.

Eyebrows, for instance, often add years to a face – because they are too thick and the wrong shape. Hair that is worn too long or too short – in other words a 'dramatic' length – also is ageing, not to mention mascara that looks as if it were put on in the dark like 'pinning the tail on the donkey'.

In short, before making the final decision to seek the help of a plastic surgeon, a woman should first minutely examine her make-up and her approach to grooming. There's a strong possibility that she will learn she doesn't need a face lift or even any eye work for at least ten years! Over-dark make-up colours are too harsh for most over thirties to handle – just as too dark a hair colour can draw attention to the fact that the skin tone is faded.

A light hand with make-up is essential. Anything that looks

'plastered' is ageing, and probably can harm the skin as it's doubtful whether every iota comes off. Unless skin tone is really dark, the light shades of base usually achieve the most youthful impression. 'Up' is the mood to aim for, which is why a light brush of pink or light brown *above* the temples (especially if you wear glasses) or beneath the hairline can lift the face 'up'. Blusher is useful and shouldn't be feared, because when correctly blended, it ends up looking like a natural blush on the cheek. The best colours to achieve this are the cinnamons and coppers, because they resemble the colour of our own blood. Always smile when applying blusher (see page 107).

If you fight the downward pull of gravity, don't lose points with a hairstyle that's strictly 'downhill'. When hair hangs around the face, below the chin line, it creates a downward movement, and long earrings don't help. A chin-length hairstyle is the best length for most women past forty, for even a chignon for long hair can be ageing. It takes a very special set of features to wear a chignon day in, day out.

If you're not sure of your hairstyle, check out a new one by trying a few wigs. You may find you don't even *notice* any wrinkles once you have found a different look, with a new, snappier make-up.

17

Sleep Tight

WE SLEEP through howling gales, crying babies, and barking dogs, yet the slightest whisper from the mattress at a certain hour of the night has us wide awake and mad at the world. Why is it that most of us can sleep through the most fearful hullabaloo in the middle of the night, yet, just when we want to sleep late, get disturbed by something as light as a mouse step?

THE FOUR SLEEP CYCLES

Recent studies show it all depends on how much time we happen to give to each of the four sleep cycles we all travel through at different speeds. Each cycle has its special characteristic, including the cycle (called Delta) which is the deepest of the lot, the cycle when it's a hard job to wake anyone up.

What happens to our bodies when we sleep? Our body temperature drops slightly, our metabolism slows down (so that we only spend about 10 calories (40 kilojoules) an hour keeping our body machinery working), our muscles slowly relax (even the chin muscle, as some of us may know if we have a 'darling little relation' who once photographed us asleep 'catching flies').

Our heart rate slows down, too, and, as the body sleeps, the largest organ of the body – the skin – appears to rest. Our skin-making machinery, however, still sloughs off dead skin cells, while new ones are on the way up from the sub-dermis below. This is why 'beauty sleep' isn't a misnomer. It's a nifty little phrase that means exactly what it says. Your looks improve with sleep, can disappear without it, because sleep is a vitally important cog in the skin-making machinery. Skin cells divide and make new cells twice as fast while we're asleep as when we're awake. When replacement falls behind loss, those all-too-obvious signs of ageing begin to appear.

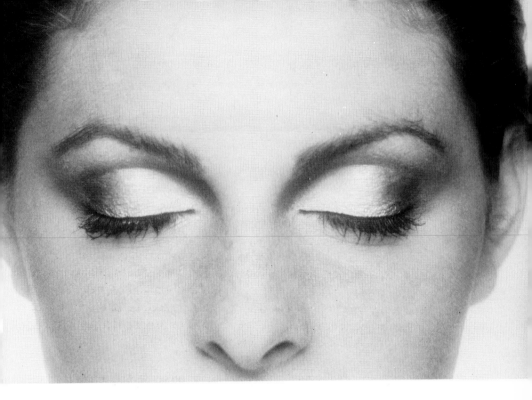

The last phase of sleep, experts agree, is the most important. Without it, our waking hours aren't as vital and productive. It is the deepest part of sleep, and when we dream during this period it's rare to be able to remember any details. If suddenly awakened from this phase, we feel confused and disorientated, and this feeling can persist throughout the day, because, to quote the experts, 'phase four has not been completed'. The deep dreaming that goes on then is important, and if we could see beneath our eyelids we would observe, I have it on good authority, what is known as our R.E.M. (rapid eye movement), which is the body's giveaway clue to show we *are* dreaming *and* sorting out our problems, without being aware they were even on the agenda. Many doctors feel that the phase four dreams clear the brain of one day's input, then get it ready for the next. If you feel you've never had a dream in your life, yet have never really had a sleepless night either, I think you're proving my point. You sleep healthily and every night, phase four – during which the deep dreaming we can't remember takes place – is part of your sleeping pattern, which is as it should be.

Before phase four is reached we all have to go through the other three, but they aren't as important. There are many people who find it difficult to 'sleep' well on a night flight and they are the ones who experience only three phases of sleep. I'm certainly one of them – I seem only to be able to experience phase four in my own bed.

Phase one is the lightest sleep of all, when even a leaf crossing the lawn or a stair creaking can wake you. In phase two sleep is deeper, when perhaps an outbreak of snoring or a gentle shake or a kick or two will disturb you. Phase three is getting nearer to the healthier sleep and definitely does include one or two dreams, the dreams that you can remember vividly if you happen to wake up then.

How Many Hours Should You Sleep?

Towards dawn, like all animals and birds, human beings, whether they like it or not, are being prepared for the day ahead. Body temperature is rising from the sleeping night's low. Blood chemistry changes, and except for those of us who went to bed at 4 a.m. most of us are entering the lightest sleeping cycle, which ironically usually follows the deepest phase four.

Just as we differ in the amount of time we give to each phase of sleep, we obviously differ in the amount of sleep we need. It isn't so much the hours we sleep at night as how we operate during the day. Many tycoons like Sir Charles Forte and Sir Charles Clore seem to flourish on an extraordinarily little amount of sleep, three or four hours at the most, whereas superstar Liza Minelli, for example, who pours out a similar amount of energy in her stage appearances, needs plenty of sleep, at least double the amount of the two Sir Charles's, to be able to keep up the pace.

Studies carried out on volunteers who went clockless in a deep cave for a few weeks seem to point to the fact that there is no set pattern for sleep. One man had a sixty-five-hour day followed by an eighteen-hour sleep period. Many under observation would have a twenty-four-hour day followed by a five-hour sleep, which they mistook for a short afternoon nap, before following more or less an extra long day, followed by an extra long night pattern.

It has been proved again and again that the amount of sleep each person needs is highly individual, and it can change without causing any harm. And just as there are 'night people' who come alive after dark, there are 'day people' who start stifling yawns around 11 p.m. The owls rarely change into larks or vice versa. Our pattern of sleep is generally set in our twenties, and although the actual hours spent sleeping usually lessen as we grow older, the moment when people most feel like sleeping usually doesn't.

Lack of sleep in itself is not necessarily harmful. It all depends how the non-sleeper feels during the day. If little sleep means that little work gets done and life itself becomes a drag, then lack of sleep is a problem and the insomnia has to be tackled.

At the other end of the scale, there are people who crave too much sleep – a ten to twelve hour withdrawal from the world – because sleep is what we all crave when being awake, in other words *living*, gets impossible to bear ... then that length of sleep does occur, but it shouldn't be a regular occurrence. If you find you keep clocking a lengthy time up, it's time to check out the reason with your doctor. After all, you never know what you may be missing.

HOW TO SLEEP YOUR CARES AWAY

As I have mentioned, we all need a good R.E.M. sleep period during the night, R.E.M. standing for Rapid Eye Movement. Unfortunately, for the insomniacs, sleeping pills and alcohol almost certainly blot out the R.E.M. periods, or at least greatly shorten them. This is the first disadvantage that sleeping pills present, and while the occasional pill to help induce sleep doesn't present a hazard, regular pill taking for this purpose most certainly can.

Instead, there are many non-addictive tricks to help sleep along. The first one is so non-addictive it's hard to get anyone to try it, but it does work, believe me. I'm referring to that leisurely walk you should take after dinner and before bed. It's a perfect way to get home if you've been eating out, and if mileage is a problem leave the transport of your choice about a mile from your front door, so you can walk home, then rush grumbling into your bathroom to take a warm to medium hot bath before tumbling between the sheets.

Renewing the air in your lungs helps sleep along, too, ensuring the best quality kind of sleep, the only kind to have. Providing you're in an unpolluted area – the deep country is perfect – stand by an open window (even a crack will do, if the temperature is low) and inhale and exhale deeply to the count of ten about ten times.

Cocoa is also good for soothing you to sleep. It's also pretty calorific, so if you worry about putting on weight one idea might cancel out the other.

Preparing a night-time ritual for yourself, one that you follow every night so that it's intimately related to the idea of going to sleep, is particularly helpful. One ritual might be to take a long, leisurely, warm (never hot) bath, preferably as fragrant as a honeysuckle patch. Turn the bed down before this and put a sweet smelling soft pillow on the sheet, one you can hold to your cheek as you close your eyes. Make sure the lighting is soft and not too harsh – a 100-watt bulb is much too high for soothing you to sleep. Read a little, making sure you're not just comfortable, you feel cosseted. Don't read anything too thrilling, unless it's a letter you've been waiting for. Don't switch on the T.V. You could easily end up with a mind full of confused plots and characters when the light's finally out. Make sure your bed is not too cold. Cold sheets can shock all idea of sleep out of anyone. Wear a soft cuddly night-dress, and if cocoa's out for avoirdupois reasons sip warm milk and honey. If for some reason you don't feel safe, don't fight it and say to yourself how silly you're being. Lock yourself in or do whatever you have to do to feel totally safe and sound.

If you have any sort of sinus or respiratory troubles, be greedy and take at least two pillows, to discourage any sort of congestion from developing in the night.

Never eat a large meal anywhere near the time you're planning to go to bed – always eat several hours beforehand.

Never carry out any strenuous exercise regime just before going to bed. This is not the time to try a change of furniture. Don't carry out an exercise session before bed either, even if your exercise mat is next to your bed. You don't want to rev up your circulation, you don't want to make your muscles tingle. You want to relax your muscles, especially the muscles of your head.

If you're working against the clock, discipline yourself to stop the job in hand at least an hour before bedtime, then set the alarm early to compensate. Exercising your brain too strenuously before sleep is a sure route to insomnia. If, when the lights are out, you've kept your eyes closed for what seems an eternity without a wink, try a sleep-inducing exercise told to me by one of the best looking girls in France (who swears sleep is her route to beauty).

Using the base of your palms start stroking movements between the brows, out on each side, across the forehead to the hairline slightly lifting the skull above the ears. Start slowly, then move even more slowly still, until the strokes become almost weary, until you fall a-s-l-e-e-p. Or lie flat on your back and relax your body one tiny piece at a time, starting say with your big toe, working up to the top of your head. With luck, by the time you get to your waist you'll have forgotten why you started. Tip for those in love: love making is just the right amount of exertion, perfect for inducing beauty sleep.

According to some pretty hefty medical minds, insomnia does no known *physical* harm, but it is pretty disturbing for one's poor old mental state. Thinking about one's income tax at two in the morning is nobody's idea of a good time. There are many sleep clinics in the United States and France where doctors observe the patterns of sleeplessness. Ironically enough, they have found that worrying about getting to sleep is one of the main culprits in producing insomnia. After tossing and turning for hours, patients are encouraged to get up and settle in an arm chair, to be covered with a blanket by an ever attentive nurse. We can all do that for ourselves. The point they are getting across is not to spend hours in bed worrying about lack of sleep, but to get up and settle yourself in a favourite place where it's quite likely you'll begin to feel drowsy – and sleep will follow. It may be you will wake up with a crick in your neck, but then you can stumble back to bed to stretch your muscles and relax in a more natural sleeping position.

Deep breathing is another key. Inhaling and exhaling deeply and being conscious of every breath. This is something that you can do together if you have a partner in bed, inhaling and exhaling to the same count as if you were walking in step down a long leafy road. It beats counting sheep.

If you sleep well, but sleep with an insomniac, try not to relay any stimulating news too late at night, and that means the good variety as well. Keep it for the morning – unless, of course, you know that what has been keeping your nearest and dearest wide awake for nights is the delay in receiving good news. Then obviously tell it when you receive it. Mental anxiety is obviously a major culprit. Take the problems away and many times you've taken the insomnia away.

The Anti-Snoring Device

Are you one half of a twin-bedded couple or part of a double-bedded pair who constantly loses out on sleep because of your partner's (a) snoring, (b) teeth grinding or (c) a maddening combination of both?

There is something that can be done about it – if you make use of tricks that some French aristocratic ladies devised so as to be able to continue sharing their beds with snorers and/or teeth grinders, tricks that have been handed down from generation to generation. You have to hand it to the French. They never waste a thing, and sharing a bed for life is one sure way of keeping your mate, of that I'm certain.

To cut down on snoring: relax the head and neck completely on the pillow. The fastest way to do this is to tense up deliberately, then just as quickly 'let go'. As you close your eyes, smile to yourself then roll your closed eyes up as though looking at the deepest, darkest sky and keep them raised. Next on the anti-snoring agenda, inhale and exhale in perfect rhythm, always aware of your breathing, never changing the amount of air inhaled or exhaled.

The best way to introduce this to a snoring partner is to suggest that you follow the regime together, keeping your bodies touching as closely as possible. There should only be two pillows and the bed should not be too soft. There should always be some air circulating throughout the room.

If this doesn't work, and one of you wakes up in the same old irritating way, to that special serenade, try rubbing a heel *gently* over your mate's feet, or with the ring finger gently trace along his or her cheekbones. This should stop the 'music' short without waking him. Then you have to go through the same sleep exercise again.

Too little exercise and too much food just before bedtime, aid and abet the snorer, so forget about the little à deux supper at 11 p.m. Light the candles four hours earlier, so that you can take each other for a short walk around ten, before lights out.

To help the teeth grinder cut down on his or her grinding the French have another remedy, which for the sake of camaraderie I suggest you also do together. Lying on your back, close your mouth lightly and start to swing the tip of the tongue back and forth across the outer surface of the upper teeth as far as the tongue can reach. If you keep it up for more than twenty times, you will feel your head tingling, as the brain is refreshed with a rush of fresh blood, while the inner throat is exercised. The gums are toned up, while taste, smell and hearing feel sharpened. If this is done regularly, teeth grinding does come to an end.

My same French informants tell me that the more love making carried out before sleep, the less likelihood of snoring or teeth grinding, which can be signs of frustration and hidden anger.

ONE WAY TO BEAT THE JET LAG

I often have to cross the Atlantic for short trips of between four and five days, and usually, because there's never enough time in my day, I choose a night flight leaving New York at 10 p.m. and arriving in London in the early morning. Even if I catch a couple of hours sleep on board, those four or five days still pass fairly groggily, and I never feel totally myself until it's time to catch the plane back.

Once, knowing that I had a particularly packed and important schedule in London, I decided to indulge myself and fly during the day, catching the 10 a.m. British Airways flight from Kennedy to arrive at London Airport a few minutes early at 9.30 p.m. local time – 4.30 in the afternoon as far as I was concerned.

I'd forgotten that in high summer London stays lighter for much longer than New York. On this particular night the sky was still blue at 9.30 and there was a sense of there being plenty of time left in the day, but by the time I reached my hotel it was nearing 11.30 so I couldn't expend any of my pent-up energy making telephone calls. I soon found I couldn't sleep either. Nor could I sleep the next night, which was more of a nightmare than any bad dream. By the time I caught the afternoon flight back to New York, I was groggier than ever before. There was a sense of unreality about everything I did and said, and I even found myself groping for the most common words. It took me at least a week to recover – the worst case of jet lag I have ever experienced.

In fact we know that our ability to function *well* is severely challenged when we make frequent changes in longitude. Generally speaking, doctors and psychologists have found that swiftly switching from one timespan to another can impair man's memory, judgement, mood, and even sexual ability. Some regular jet travellers experience jet-style fast changes of mood, switching from irrational depression to equally irrational feelings of excitement and hilarity.

Over the years I've often heard T.V. announcers blaming heavy travel schedules when various players in major tournaments appear to be off form. To overcome jet lag, racing drivers, for instance, always arrive at the place where a race is going to take place at least a few days before the event. Doctors have pointed out that it's possible some of the fatal crashes that have occurred among healthy, top-class racing drivers could have resulted from a lack of co-ordination and judgement due to jet-lag problems.

Travelling longitudinally doesn't present the same sort of problem as travelling latitudinally because the sun rises and sets at the same time, no matter how far we travel.

This leads us right into the heart of the matter. From research

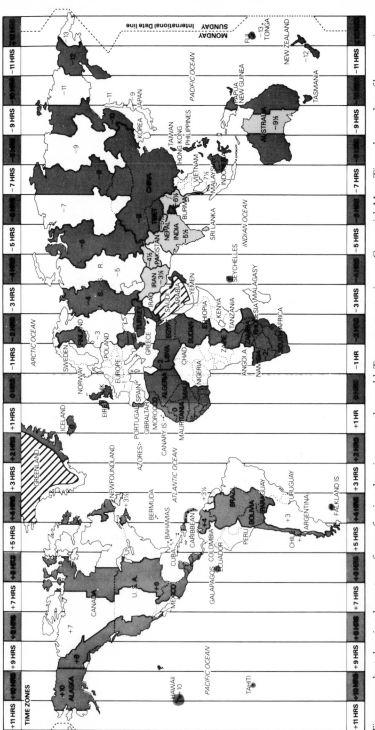

Time zone chart showing the system of zones for time-keeping across the world. To convert zone time to Greenwich Mean Time, the number of hours as given by the zone number is added to or subtracted from the zone time, e.g., in Zone –4 the time is kept 4 hours in advance of Greenwich Mean Time. In most cases, Standard Time is that of the zone in which the country mainly lies. Countries having the Standard Time of an even-numbered zone are shown in light grey shading. Countries having the Standard time of an odd-numbered zone are unshaded. Countries in which Standard Time differs from zone time by a fraction of an hour are in dark grey, and those in which standard time is not fixed by law are shown in line shading. The International Date Line is shown by a dotted line. *(Chart by Ed Stuart, from information supplied by the Ministry of Defence)*

carried out in connection with the oral contraceptive pill, it has been learned that the glands in our body are very much influenced by the length of exposure to daylight and its brightness. In other words, our reactions, moods, successes and failures are far more geared to our longitude and environment than we ever realize.

The only solution I've found to the problem of coping with jet travel is to give more time between arrival and departure. When that isn't possible, doctors have suggested that it's best for the first twenty-four hours to live at the time just left behind. In the circumstances just described that would have meant continuing my work on arrival at the hotel in London just before midnight (6.45 p.m. in New York), going to bed at about 3.30 a.m. in London (10.30 p.m. in New York), getting up at my normal time, which would have been noon in London (7 a.m. in New York), then playing it by ear from then on.

Doing this helps the metabolism become adjusted – and there's nothing wrong with having an English-style breakfast at lunchtime in London, when it's still the breakfast hour in New York, and eating dinner in London when it's time for a late lunch in New York. It's the only way to beat jet lag as far as I'm concerned – if the duration of the trip is less than a week.

Scent and its many Applications

THERE'S MUCH MORE TO IT THAN MEETS THE NOSE

AREN'T you glad you're alive and well in 1978 and not 1400 B.C. when beauty was such a bothersome business? Way back then, in order to make a scent-sational impression on her subjects, even the likes of Queen Nefertiti had to go to the trouble of making little wax balls impregnated with flowers, full of natural fragrance, which she planted in her intricate hairstyle, knowing that as the day went by the wax would gradually melt leaving behind – hopefully – only the sweet aroma of the flowers. What a mess for the shampoo slave to clean up, and she didn't even have a bar of soap.

Now to make a fragrance last all day and night wise girls know to spray themselves liberally when still wet from the bath or shower. It's a fact that scent doesn't last anything like so long on dry skin as on oily, so as 90 per cent of us are in the 'dry' category, this is one good tried and true remedy.

One of the most important decision makers in the cosmetics industry I ever knew was a man who was crazy about scent. Crazy in the colloquial sense, for he was always overly anxious for women to wear it – providing his company created it, of course. He was also crazy with frustration that he could not come up with a scent that was as irresistible as the 'chemistry' Mike Todd once described – the invisible attraction that pulls one woman to one man, one man to one woman, as surely as a magnet (frequently mystifying the onlookers).

Although perfumers usually skirt around the idea that sex could be the undercurrent they're trying to evoke when creating a perfume,

332

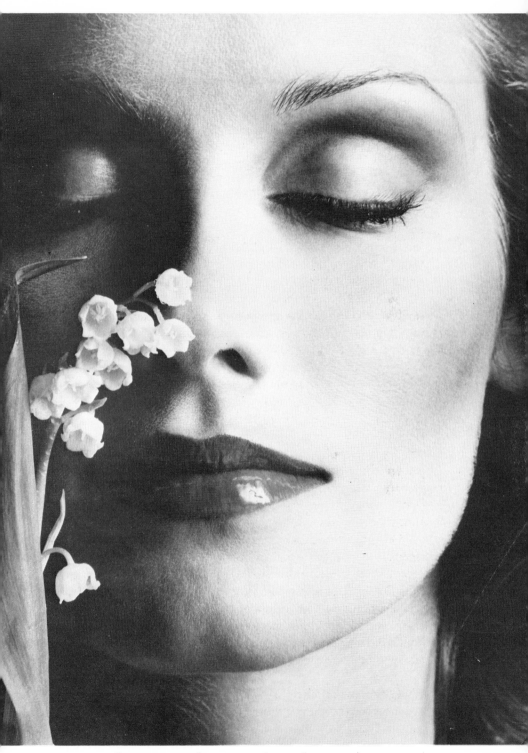

**Fragrance and a woman's psyche –
intimately related**

this tycoon made no bones about the fact that to be able to create this 'instant chemistry' would be the crowning achievement of an already spectacularly successful life.

CREATING A NEW FRAGRANCE

The sense of smell plays a greater role in human activity than most people realize. It's at least a thousand times more sensitive than the sense of taste, one reason it can be a penance to sit in a restaurant next to somebody wearing a perfume that acts like gunpowder on the senses – so strong, the smell can *annihilate* the taste of anything, even steak au poivre.

In the perfumery business a 'nose' is the name given to a top perfumer, the one who instinctively knows when a *mélange* of ingredients have come together to create a great fragrance (often after years of trial and error).

A 'nose' is in 'training' for most of his life, in the dedicated way that an athlete, opera singer or record breaking mountain climber is in training. Usually, he's born not made, and he or she (usually he) never smokes, because it could affect the smelling cells of his nose. He rarely eats spicy food, or even food we would describe as tasty, because any piquant or special taste can also have a special smell which can interfere with his work.

All the 'noses' I've ever known have admitted that studying women in all their glorious complexities is very much on their agenda. It's important that the great perfumers understand women and have an appreciation of them, because they're trying to create scents that women will love so much that they're accorded as much praise and glory as works of art – scents that will then bring in tremendous financial rewards.

Competition is fierce and the top 'noses' work in a world of secrecy, often behind locked doors – and yet it takes years to create a great new perfume. One of the main reasons is that the 'nose' can't keep on sniffing something he's working on day after day hoping to reach perfection. He has to leave one job for another in order to get a new perspective, sometimes not returning to a venture for a year, when, sniffing again and again, many subtle (usually one drop at a time) minuscule changes are made.

A 'nose' can instantly detect one single aroma in a fragrance and label it. He has firmly memorized at least a thousand individual essential scents, just as a musician has countless notes stored in his head.

When a new perfume is being created, he can begin to put together an outline of the new perfume by bringing to mind certain of these essential fragrances, without going near a vial or test tube. It's this ability to add one essential oil to perhaps 300 others (in the right order and amount to create a perfume masterpiece) that makes a 'nose' as opposed to a good technician. Many of the fragrances we hold so dear today may easily have taken from five to fifteen years to develop. The major problem is one of communication – to express in words what we conjure up as a scent in our minds. So far the language of fragrance is still underdeveloped. Green, musk, amber, warm – these words are expressive but don't really indicate any particular scent.

Time has no effect on a great perfume – it goes throbbing on, as popular one year as the next. Chanel No. 5, Jicky, Emeraude, L'Heure Bleue and Shalimar are all over fifty years old, while Arpege was created in 1927, Joy in 1934, and Heaven Sent in 1941 – all perfumes that are instantly recognizable.

All our noses accept, analyse and identify odours – as different as chocolates from cheese, onions from oleanders – with a speed that no laboratory instrument can duplicate. A chemist or beauty expert who is labelled a 'nose', however, can also immediately pick out the jasmine from the Bulgarian rose in the formula, however deeply it's buried. Some of the most expert can also smell the differences in skin and hair colour, red-headed women apparently possessing uniquely pleasant smelling skin (see page 345).

Sexual Urge in a Bottle

Twenty to forty million olfactory receptors are at work in the nose telegraphing, by electrical impulse, odour information to the brain. Because of this brilliant system, it isn't exaggerated to claim that

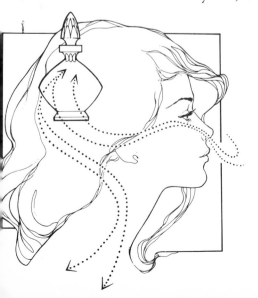

certain fragrances do send impulses to the part of the brain in charge of sexual urges. The strangest thing about this is that what turns one man on will have nil effect on another.

The musk-like synthetic called *exaltolide* used frequently in perfume is similar, I'm told, to the *signal* scent produced by the human male. Apparently, it can be smelled most easily by women between the ages of fifteen and forty-five, but, although I'm glad to say I fall in that category, I've never been aware of smelling it. That doesn't mean my olfactory system isn't working, however. I'm told by the experts I could be picking it up without ever realizing it, reacting to his 'signal' instead of, say, his dark brown eyes.

We accept without question the fact that our body chemistry makes the scent we choose smell differently on us than on others. Our *skin* makes the difference to the alchemy in the bottle, not necessarily lessening or increasing its effect but definitely making it *different*. In fact, it's rare for the same scent to smell the same when worn by a redhead, blonde or brunette. Skin oils vary, and it's the relationship of skin oils to fragrance that makes the whole subject so provocative and mysterious.

Not only does body chemistry affect the final result of the scent worn; the scent that emerges is also going to affect the body chemistry of the person who smells it.

Studies are now going on relating to 'chemical substances produced by one individual that affect the behaviour or physiology of another'. They pose the possibility that marital, social or even professional discord can be worsened or mediated by people picking up subconsciously irritating or, on the other hand, *provocative* scent signals from each other.

Whatever develops with 'pheromones' (the term given to these chemical substances), biological phenomena are always there for a REASON.

One of the big 'noses' in the beauty industry told me that although it's been known for years that human beings produce pheromones like animals do, until now it hasn't been documented that human beings, may provoke reaction in others because of their natural scent without being aware of it. In other words, we may use pheromones as animals do, as come hither or stay away signals . . . totally unconsciously.

Where is all this leading? Hopefully, said the 'nose', to perfumes beyond our wildest dreams, irresistible, exotically fragrant lures turning every woman into an instant Salome.

There *is* a snag and one that the perfumer has to be aware of, even if he's not admitting it. As I've told you, scent in a bottle can and often does smell totally different once it's on the skin, and each skin reacts differently, so that while this perfume of the future may well turn one woman into a Salome it's quite likely to make a wallflower if nothing worse out of her neighbour. As the chairman of one of the largest flavours and fragrance houses in the world puts it, 'The ability of any human being to perceive the environment is directly connected with the five senses of which smell is one, but we are all divinely different with different odour receptors, so when we see or smell the world around us, we are experiencing something unique. Every fragrance smells differently to different people.'

Even if so far perfume can't be proved to be an aphrodisiac, it is still the most satisfying, extraordinarily mind boggling booster for a woman's morale, linking her to the past, encouraging her to enjoy the present, ensuring she has a future.

One fact is established for all: perfume can affect the psyche faster than a glass of champagne.

WHERE ARE THE BEST PLACES TO PUT SCENT?

Starting at the toes, hit all the pulse points on the way up – backs of knees, on the soft skin between the thighs, above the heart where the heartbeat warms it, backs of wrists, inner arms, bosom, throat, nape of neck, temples. Not so much behind the ears, although it isn't a crime if it goes there, but in such a concentrated area fragrance can mix poorly with perspiration and so negate its effect. The temples are better scent spots.

Scent application should actually start in the bath – particularly if skin is dry – to ensure it lasts as long as possible. Use bath oil or bath milk that attaches to the skin, the globules getting towelled into the pores. Spray on a cologne or toilet water before dressing, then use a final touch of real perfume before going out; all this ensures fragrance will last at least half the day.

If perfume refuses to stay put on your skin, choose one without alcohol, in cream or liquid form.

When asked what she wore to bed Marilyn Monroe's famous reply was 'Chanel No. 5', and it's not a bad idea. If you'd prefer to combine it with a pretty nightie, sprinkle cologne or toilet water on your pillowcases and sheets. Keep cotton wool balls soaked in fragrance

Pulse points of the body for applying scent

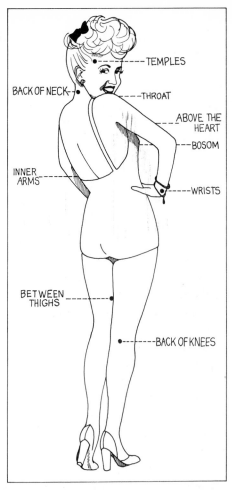

TEMPLES

BACK OF NECK

THROAT

ABOVE THE HEART

BOSOM

INNER ARMS

WRISTS

BETWEEN THIGHS

BACK OF KNEES

in your linen cupboard and lingerie drawers. Have a fragrant welcome ready for guests by spraying fragrance on your light bulbs. Just like your heartbeat, the wattage will warm up the scent, and its insistent fragrance will pervade the house – better than scented candles, although they're good to have around, too.

Use a drop of fragrance in the rinsing water when you're washing through tights or lingerie. Add another drop to your comb or brush, but don't add it directly to your hair. It could be drying, and dryness is something hair does not need.

If you like one fragrance tremendously, develop that 'identity' by keeping the message coming through loud and clear with bubble baths, dusting powder, soaps, sachets and the good old portable spray. Spray the hem of your skirt to spread your scent message. Sprinkle a few drops of toilet water in your handbag so you get your own message back every time you open up.

Spray cologne on tired feet, it will un-tire them. Pour cologne into palms and inhale for a quick pick-me-up – but *don't drink* it. Spray cologne over ice cubes, then saturate a cotton pad in the icy mixture and place it on your forehead for a few minutes. It will not only cool you, it will calm you.

Keep your cologne in the fridge, so it really refreshes you after a fast game on the tennis court.

BUYING SCENT

A woman's sense of smell is stronger than a man's. It's also keener when she is approaching menstruation, waning when it's over. For this reason, when you feel it's time for a new scent, choose that 'time of the month' to buy it, when your olfactory senses will be working full strength. Because research has proved our sense of smell is less acute in the morning than it is later in the day – from 9 p.m. to 3 a.m., if we're not snoozing, tests have shown our noses are at their most super alert – go shopping for scent in the afternoon not the morning.

Never buy a scent solely because you like the way it smells in the bottle. Always test it on your skin – preferably on a pulse point (so your heartbeat can warm it up). Don't inhale until a few seconds have passed – that way you will get the full thrust of the effect as it works for you, skin oils and all.

The reason it's best to wait a while is that all perfumers work to establish 'notes' in perfume: the top notes are the ones that hit you first when you lift out the stopper; the middle notes relate to the main body of the scent, and the bottom notes to the fragrance base. The more creative the perfumer, the more a 'melody of notes' will suggest itself to you, lingering, working on your psyche to evoke more and more suggestions. Remember, the sense of smell scores 100 per cent in evoking memories, happy and unhappy. Ironically, if a situation changes from happy to unhappy or vice versa, the same scent can immediately switch sides and accommodate the current mood.

Never buy a perfume because you like it on your best friend (or worst enemy). *It won't smell the same*, because the chemistry of your skin affects it considerably. Test a new one in a bath form product, less expensive and still effective enough for you to know if you're going to like the real McCoy.

If you think you're allergic to scent you may still have a chance with a few. Spray a little on your wrist just under the curve of your thumb and wait a few minutes before sniffing to let the full bouquet strike. If you don't sneeze or scratch and you like the effect it probably means it likes you, too, and you'll achieve wonderful things together.

Keep perfume in a dark, cool place and it will stay in great condition for a long, long time, *but don't hoard it.* The fragrance may change, which is a terrible waste. Don't pack perfume in your suitcase when you travel. Hand luggage, held in your hand, is a safer place, ensuring perfume isn't subjected to extremes of temperature or too much tossing about. Think of it as fine wine – they have a lot in common.

Don't forget to encourage your man to wear fragrance, increasingly important in this hostile world. It's good for his psyche, too . . .

A herbal manual of 1447 advised, 'Ye will by smelling learne . . .' That still makes a lot of sense when it comes to choosing your perfume.

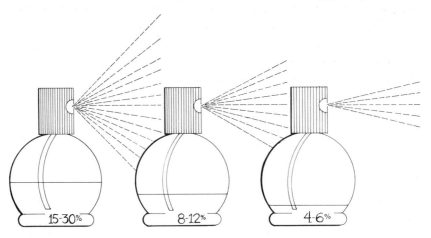

Different Forms of Scent

Scent measures like this:

Strongest: the real McCoy is *concentrated perfume,* made of perhaps a few hundred ingredients, including flower and plant oils from all over the world – lilac, honeysuckle, lavender, rose, patchouli, fern, jasmine – rare and lovely and part of nature. Apply real perfume via an atomizer to diffuse the alcohol content while the true scent clings to the skin. The amount of alcohol added to the formula determines the perfume's strength. Real perfume usually contains 15 per cent to 30 per cent of concentrates.

340

Strong: eau de toilette, toilet water, eau de parfum, or parfum de toilette – all these contain no other fragrance note than that of the true perfume but they have less concentrates of the many ingredients, usually from 8 to 12 per çent.

Less strong: cologne is the lightest form of fragrance, containing only about 4 to 6 per cent of concentrates, beguiling, but so light it can be rubbed on hands to keep them cool and dry. Cologne also relieves aching muscles when used as a rubdown after a strenuous day.

CHARACTER IN PERFUME

The sign of a great perfume is its character, one that never gets overlooked or accidentally mistaken for something else – just like an outstanding human being. That character can be *sultry* (also described as oriental), blending together ingredients such as musk, ambergris, civet and other exotica. It can be *green* and *woodsy*, a clear composition of sandalwood, rosewood, oakmoss or ferns. It can be essentially *floral* like an English garden, full of roses, lily of the valley, delphiniums, tuberoses, honey-suckle. A newer note is woody, *not* woodsy, and not at all green, but an unusual blending of floral and wood bark notes, while the newest of all delivers unusual perfumes with full fruity notes (Hermès Amazone is a good example).

Who Wears What

One of the highest paid models in the world, *Lauren Hutton*, likes the musk she bought in Ethiopia, and frankincense from Egypt. She also uses fresh mint on her hands and oil of rosemary as a rinse and light scent for her hair.

Opera star *Beverly Sills* has used the same perfume for years – Piguet's Fracas. 'The men I sing with say it turns them on, and my husband always knows where I am just by sniffing the air.'

Lady Sassoon (widow of multimillionaire industrialist, Sir Victor) is an inveterate traveller and friends know when she's in Customs, about to emerge, for Shalimar is always with her.

Mrs Harold Robbins, wife of the best-selling author, wears Weil's Secret of Venus, but in bath oil form for maximum impact. She buys several colognes for her husband, which he uses when the mood strikes.

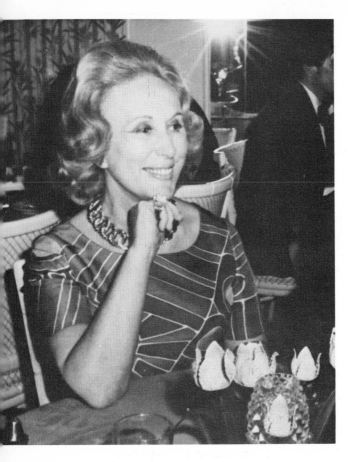

**Estee Lauder,
creator of great perfumes**

Jackie Onassis changes her own perfume constantly but is faithful to cinammon sticks in the fireplace, burning them with the logs in winter to create a fragrant aroma throughout the house.

Greta Garbo is addicted to Vetiver, *Ali McGraw* to a man's scent, Dior's Eau Sauvage, *Liza Minnelli* to Vivara by Emilio Pucci, which she sprays on while she's in the shower. She knows that 'wet skin makes perfume last longer'.

A TO Z OF PERFUME

AMBERGRIS stands for grey amber, an odourless fixative that blends
ingredients together to ensure they last. It's difficult to find, so it's
expensive. In actuality, ambergris is the spew of the sperm whale
that's goaded by indigestion, in the same way that an oyster,
maddened by a grain of sand, makes a pearl.

BERGAMOT is the small fragrant fruit of a citrus-type tree, flourishing
only in Calabria, southern Italy. The fruit looks like a green
orange, but it's inedible, bursting instead with an oil that's
essential to making zippy, tangy perfume. Bergamot is tricky,
however, because it can cause a phototoxic reaction on skin (brown
spots) when exposed to too much sun. For this reason Bergamot
is now often synthesized.

COLOGNE is the lightest form of scent, originating in France in the
eighteenth century.

DIVISIONS are categories into which the perfume pros grade scent
types, such as Floral Singles (one-note perfumes such as gardenia,
violet, lilac), Floral Bouquets (a medley of flowers), Spicy
Bouquets (including cinnamon, ginger, clove), Green Scents
(mossy, grassy), Musky Blends (made with musk, amber, sandalwood, civet and patchouli), Citrus and Modern Blends (man-made
synthetic departures and innovations).

EROTIC is the description given to any scent that chemists believe is
capable of arousing sexual desire or any scent that makes itself
felt sensually through the olfactory senses.

FRAGRANCE FATIGUE means it is possible to become so accustomed
to a particular scent you can no longer smell it. Short term, it
means your nose is 'descenticized' to the odour of a room you've
been in for a long time. Long term – after fifty, for instance – our
olfactory senses change, which means even if a woman has been
faithful to one perfume for years, she may find herself reacting
to it differently and may even think the perfume has 'changed',
or at least deteriorated. When buying scent never try to evaluate
more than three at once. The olfactory nerves overload and
become unable to give you the true expression of each scent.

GRASSE is the perfume capital of the world, a charming eighteenth-century town in France's Alpes Maritime. Flowers grow there in profusion, and no sooner are they plucked and stripped of their perfume-producing petals than more crowd the slopes to take their place. Their valuable oils – from roses, orange blossom, violets, jonquils, acacias, mimosa and jasmine, to name only a few – are shipped all over the globe. No well known perfume is made in Grasse, but it's the chief supplier of the main ingredients to perfumers everywhere.

HEAT makes fragrance move faster, so on hot days in summer scent dissipates easily out of doors, therefore needs re-applying frequently. Indoors, fragrance stays longer on the body. The point is to use only a light fragrance in the summer in order to be able to re-apply frequently without causing offence.

INCENSE is the perfume that has been burned through the ages to create a fragrant atmosphere. Offered to the gods in ancient Rome, then as today the most aromatic incense came from China – to the Chinese perfume means incense and nothing else. They divide it into six types: Tranquil, Recluse, Luxurious, Beautiful, Refined, and Noble, each of which is meant to induce a corresponding mood. In the West, we try to create the same atmosphere with perfumed candles.

JASMINE is the most rare and so the most expensive perfume ingredient – about £3,000 a pound ($\frac{1}{2}$ kg)! White, and intensely scented, jasmine reaches its peak at dawn, when anyone who can get up in time is rewarded with its full sweetness, even voluptuousness. Every classic perfume – like those mentioned that are at least fifty years old – contains at least a pinch. So far, man has not been able to synthesize jasmine.

KEY NOTE is the first expression of a perfume, the top note that attacks your senses before you absorb the whole. It has been described lyrically over the centuries, the most frequent description likening it to the excitement of a supreme solo voice that first carries a musical message and then recedes to let the full orchestra take over.

344

LINGER. In the professional language of the perfumer, this relates to the cling or persistence of a scent. Perfumes that use musk or civet as a fixative are very clingy, and it's a fact that all perfume lingers longer when sprayed on to wet skin.

MUSK used to be used only as a fixative. Found in the glands or pods of the male musk deer, it gives off the strongest fragrance during the mating season. The dried pods are nearly odourless, but when moistened they become ambrosial to some, overpowering to others.

NOSE refers to the perfumer, a man who possesses an extraordinary and creative sense of smell. The 'nose' is the one to cry 'eureka', sometimes after five or six years, when he recognizes with one sniff that he has at last created a great scent. There are very few great 'noses' – but they've all usually had a training stint in Grasse.

OILY SKIN 'grabs' perfume and 'holds' it on the skin far longer than dry skin can. This means oily skin should stay away from the heavier perfumes, should choose instead colognes, eau de toilettes or lighter derivatives of real perfumes. Otherwise the combination of oily skin, body heat and heavy perfume can be too much.

PATCHOULI has a wild, haunting odour, possibly the most intense in the whole plant kingdom. It's used mainly in exotic perfumes that seem to carry a touch of the East.

QUASI are what many perfumes set out to be – *direct* copies of a celebrated scent, with some slight amendments, so the sweet-smelling public never usually realize a 'scent steal' is going on. In fact, most copies lack a lot, as most 'quasi' things do.

REDHEADS. As mentioned on page 335, a perfume will smell different on the skin of a redhead, blonde and brunette. But redheads have problems retaining fragrance, because they're usually emotional, excitable people. High emotions produce body heat, and as just mentioned heat makes fragrance move off the body fast. This means redheads need to re-apply fragrance constantly throughout the day, so they should choose a light version of their favourite scent.

345

SYNTHETICS relate to the fragrant inventions of man, born in a test tube, but often formulated to resemble the fragrance of real flowers. They produce en masse what nature does a drop at a time, so making the perfume operation a far more economical one. Synthetics have introduced a more lasting quality to perfume, too, as well as, in a few cases, introducing a totally new type of smell.

TEMPERATURE. Cold and heat affect the strength and life of a perfume. To help perfume travel through the air, a warm humid atmosphere is best. Conversely, if you want to avoid a certain smell in the house, cold air cuts it down. Example: to slice an onion without tears, freeze it first – odour molecules are sluggish when cold – or cut it under cold water because, again, odour molecules don't travel through water. For this reason, it's not wise to keep real perfume in the fridge. Chilled perfume is refreshing, but invariably loses much of its clout.

UNISEX. More and more this description is given to new scents that seem to 'fit' both a male and a female personality, providing a source of pleasure to both sexes.

VETIVER is an essential oil derived from the roots of aromatic grasses, growing in Java, Haiti and South America. Intense and smouldering, it's a memorable part of many perfumes you know and love.

WEATHER. It makes sense to change your perfume from season to season, because the temperature outside affects a perfume's performance. In cold weather fragrance molecules 'lift' slowly, and even our own ability to smell is diminished. This means a strong perfume will not smell so strong in winter. With more moisture in the air, fragrance is intensified, so spring is the time for a lighter, fresher version of your favourite scent, or a totally different lighter mood. The warmer the weather, the lighter the fragrance should be, as warmth boosts the entire effect.

X is the unknown element in perfume, the mysterious X factor that relates to *your* skin and your skin alone, adding an intangible note that either makes it special to you or turns it into an also-ran you won't try again.

YOU make the perfume. It is *your* skin oil that mixes with the perfumer's magic and produces the final result. *Your* perspiration doesn't directly alter the fragrance, but it does change its background. If you're fond of eating spicy, garlicky foods, this can affect your skin and disturb the true fragrance of the perfume. Remember, never buy fragrance because you like it on somebody else. It will invariably smell differently on you. Use a tester, try it on the back of your wrist, wait for a few seconds and then make your decision.

ZANZIBAR is an island where the air is thick with the spicy breath of cloves, an essential part of many floral scents.

19

Voicing Your Beauty

JUST as our private scent can turn people off and on, so can our own set of decibels. We all know the person we try to avoid simply because his or her voice tears at our senses – as the experts describe it, 'causing a fright or flight syndrome, *repelling* through stridency and shrillness'.

Obviously, the most important thing about a voice problem is to acknowledge that you have one. Once that step has been reached, it isn't that difficult to solve. If you've never heard yourself on tape, the time to do so is right *now*. I bet 100 voice lessons you will be surprised at how you sound – in fact, some people have had to be introduced to themselves. Listen to yourself read the front page of your local newspaper on tape. If you find you talk at the rate of knots, try to remember to use your tongue every so often as a reminder to yourself to slow down, touching the roof of your mouth every so often, like tying a knot in your handkerchief.

If, on the other hand, you start nodding with boredom at the slowness of your speech, practise speaking faster by reading out loud whenever you get a quiet minute alone with a book or a newspaper. Concentrate on getting words out at about 150 words a minute. Don't kid yourself that 'too slow' can be 'too seductive for words'. It's as seductive as a dripping tap.

One of the best ways to start practising voice improvement is to look in a mirror as you are speaking. The way you look has an effect on the way you sound. You will try harder when you see your image looking back at you – even if you haven't combed your hair. If you

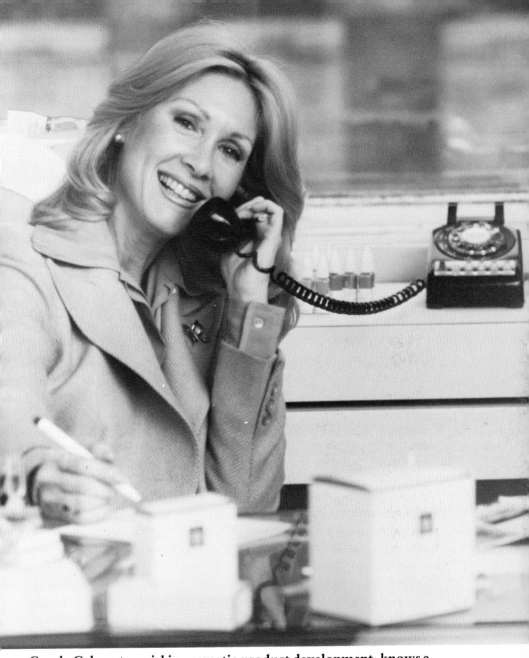

Carole Gabay, top girl in cosmetic product development, knows a
smile can be 'transmitted' by the voice

really don't like your *sound*, start thinking *lower*, not higher. Chances are you're up there already. Lower means automatically the amount of shrillness in your voice. You can check out your pitch easily by matching it to a few keys on the piano. Speaking quietly and clearly is always more effective anyway than raising your voice – whether in discussion or disagreement and certainly as far as a tête-à-tête is concerned.

Correct breathing is part of being able to communicate attractively. Try contracting your diaphragm as if to get back to your solar plexus while exhaling. This amplifies the voice in the chest, leading to better control when the words start coming out. Many speech therapists encourage their patients or clients to yawn widely in order to give them the sensation of an open throat for greater clarity, and so the ability to be heard without yelling. Many stars have already related the yawn to relaxing the throat muscles and so calming stage fright.

Apart from too much sound, (or too little – mutterers and swallowers of words are in as much trouble as bellowers and those who always sound belligerent), speech patterns have to be carefully watched. The number of otherwise articulate people addicted to 'you know' and 'er' and 'um' is incalculable. Many blame the mindlessness and lack of speech control exhibited on T.V., but 'you know', and 'er' and 'um' have been around for centuries, although I've never seen any recorded on a Greek or Turkish tomb.

The more you listen to yourself, the more you will learn to edit yourself. A tape recorder is a better asset than a 'best friend', however good his or her ear. Criticism of your speech is not easy to take. It's an intensely personal part of you, and yet without knowing it your voice may be responsible for people having a totally erroneous impression of your true personality.

Learn to count to five before you make a major statement and inhale and exhale as the yogi does, being aware of every breath. Whisper a speech that's important. Then say it a little louder, and then louder still, *thinking* about what you are saying in order to gain inflection.

An easy way to remember vital points in a speech is to have clues in the form of pictures and/or illustrations. A big business in America is 'teaching people to speak as well as they think'; one of their secret devices is the picture and/or illustration clue – not the written word, which can all too often 'freeze' the words about to come out of your mouth.

Thinking about the purpose of your message is the all-important factor in putting the point across well, but putting it across does not mean shouting it across. Words, like music, are not appreciated because of their decibels.

The all-important fact to remember is that the way we speak, the sound and pitch of the voice, is just as important as the way we look.

How to Succeed in Love and Business

ALL WORK and no play – well, life certainly would get tedious, wouldn't it? Every working woman should realize that being in love can play a tremendous part in helping her get ahead in business (and not for the obvious reason), just as an engrossing job can help her have a great emotional relationship with a man.

Helena Rubinstein once told me, 'Work is the only excitement that lasts.' It never seemed to cross her mind that in expressing that belief so fervently she was perhaps giving away the reason why she had a rather unsuccessful record as a wife.

Anyone who concentrates 100 per cent on their job is invariably not succeeding in life – or necessarily in the job either. Perspective gets out of hand. Decisions become too stereotyped if every waking hour is devoted to the business in hand. It's safe to say this can be a sure route to poor health, too. Remember, our emotional and physical life are one and the same. Without an emotional outlet, a release, the body can begin to rebel with sickness.

On the other hand, if the love in your life is all-important and your job is just something you do to pass the time when he's busy (or to earn enough to buy your bread and butter), it can be predicted that the relationship won't last. Suffocation will sniff the life out of it, leaving you bereft and empty.

The obvious answer is to be greedy, to want out of life all that it can offer – satisfying both one's need for an emotional life *and* one's aspirations and ambitions.

An interesting job can only be described that way if you set out to make it so, whether you're working for a company making nuts and bolts or sitting at an airline counter from nine to six. The more interest you put into it, the more the adjective 'interesting' can be applied to

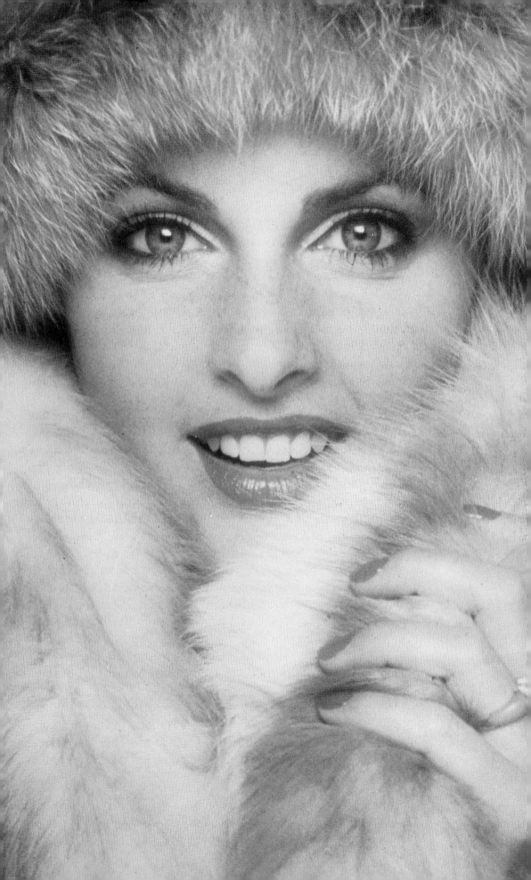

you, and, surprise, surprise, the object of your affections can become more *interested*, too.

If you feel you aren't scoring that well on either the emotional or the ambitious level, analyse how you cope with day-to-day situations. Are you uptight with newcomers at the office, those you think may affect your position or even those who have nothing apparently to do with your activities? Do you sulk when the person you care about phones to cancel a date unexpectedly, or take offence when your husband asks you mildly when dinner will be ready?

Analyse the reactions you have to life's many situations and see if you can't immediately comprehend why there are false starts in your life pattern. To help yourself, study someone you admire, who appears to move ahead steadily as you would like to do. Imitate that behaviour, little by little, so you can make intelligent comparisons between the way she or he copes and the way you would usually cope.

Start by being willing to listen and learn. You will find it amazingly easy if you set out to do that as an exercise in living. Once you appear to be receptive to others, even if you don't necessarily agree with them, you'll find coping *much, much easier*.

Ask questions and listen more carefully, too. Delay your reactions for a minute or two, and if you feel unhappy and want to cry, go somewhere to release that feeling and cry. Or yawn. All this helps you feel less stress, and strengthens your self-reliance. For it is your *attitude* that counts, that allows others to evaluate you and place you up or down on the success ladder.

Become aware that you can be your own best friend by paying attention to how you react to decisions and circumstances. When you feel 'uncomfortable' try to adjust your attitude until you feel 'comfortable'. Positive thinking is far more than a cliché – it is the tried and true way to success in love and business. You are beautiful . . . in more than one way and now you know how to prove it.

Index

357

ABOUT THE AUTHOR

Jane Carter started writing ten years ago. Before that, she went from being a production assistant for Film Australia to mustering sheep on her husband's property, raising five kids and helping to run their livestock trucking company. Moving in 2016 to Narrandera, she and her husband are following their dream and breeding Corriedale sheep. These last forty-odd years have seen her become passionate about the people she lives and works with, the men and women of rural Australia and their inspirational stories.

JANE CARTER

PRODIGAL DAUGHTER

First Published 2017
First Australian Paperback Edition 2017
ISBN 978 148924113 9

PRODIGAL DAUGHTER
© 2017 by Jane Carter
Australian Copyright 2017
New Zealand Copyright 2017

Published by
HQ Fiction
An imprint of Harlequin Enterprises (Australia) Pty Ltd.
Level 13, 201 Elizabeth St
SYDNEY NSW 2000
AUSTRALIA

® and TM (apart from those relating to FSC ®) are trademarks of Harlequin Enterprises Limited or its corporate affiliates. Trademarks indicated with ® are registered in Australia, New Zealand and in other countries.

Cataloguing-in-Publication details are available from the National Library of Australia www.librariesaustralia.nla.gov.au

Printed and bound in Australia by McPherson's Printing Group

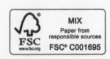

MIX
Paper from
responsible sources
FSC® C001695

For my mother

CHAPTER ONE

Gospel Oak, London, February

The pub was still crowded. Colliding with the wall of hot thick air, Diana stopped, weighing up her options. At least it was alive with human body-warmth and deafening noise. Pushing her way through padded bodies, she undid the buttons on her coat and loosened her scarf and let the sympathetic glances thrown her way float right over her head. A couple of Charlie's football cronies were arm wrestling over in one corner, encouraged by a few enthusiastic supporters. It looked more like a party than a wake. Good. It was what she had wanted. Was it time to get Bart, the publican, to stop the tab? She looked over towards the Suttons, Charlie's parents, who sat in a booth, talking quietly with a few friends. They were the only oldies left and they looked exhausted. It had been a horrible day. The Suttons were not a demonstrative couple but she watched Bill's arm slide round his wife's slim shoulders and give her a little squeeze.

'You should be pleased, it's a great send-off, Diana.' Sebastian handed her a half pint of Guinness.

She studied the clover leaf embellished in the creamy head. 'Charlie would have loved it. I know I should be pleased, I'm just wondering how I get them all to go home.' She put the glass back down on the small high table in front of her, untouched.

'They're all having a great time.' Sebastian grinned, then leant over and patted her hand. His hands were soft and milky white with the nails neatly buffed, and she wanted to pull her hand away. 'Turn off the tab, my dear.'

'That's what I thought.' She'd never felt so tired in her life.

'Don't worry about that consignment for the Japanese family. There's time, I can put them off. And you know the lad's paintings have just doubled in price.'

Diana looked blankly at the gallery owner who was also her agent. Sebastian could have been talking Japanese for all she knew. God, he was a heartless bastard. Money was what drove him. Since her pots had taken off and she'd become known in the art world she'd left most of the organising up to him. And paid him the fifteen per cent quite happily.

She also knew that however tired she was, turning around, walking out that door and going home was going to be hard. The numbness would help. Honestly, if someone pushed a pin into her right now, she wouldn't feel it.

Okay, she would do the walk and not think about it. It would only get worse, thinking about it. People were looking at her, 'one tough lady' they were saying. Well, she was tough enough to take the pitying looks.

It was walking out the door alone.

She'd just gone to say goodnight to the kids. She hadn't let them come to the pub; she hated the way people had looked at them this afternoon. She'd spent half an hour with Sienna before she'd dropped off to sleep. The kids were so lost. Milo and Saskia had gone to sleep immediately. But not Sienna. She'd just stared at her—her eyes wouldn't shut. As though if they did, her mother might disappear. Bridie would ring her if any of them woke.

She studied the bottles over the bar. This was her second funeral where she'd been personally involved. If anyone cared to ask, she could tell them that it didn't get any easier. But for this one, the wake was different—a real party. A hell of a send-off for one of the great partygoers. She was going to do it even if it killed her.

Although that wasn't an option, Diana took a deep breath. Then she smiled vaguely, careful not to make eye contact.

Why had she come back? Simple. For Charlie. *Breathe.*

She watched Janet Sutton get up slowly and come towards her. Usually tall and upright, her mother-in-law had shrivelled over the last few days. So had Bill, Charlie's father. He was one of those round-faced, silver-haired Englishmen with a belly laugh. Charlie was their only son, so Diana had been surprised they'd left the decisions this week to her. But she could see how they'd reached the end of their limit now. Having the wake here at the pub had been her idea, not theirs, but they'd come round. So many people had turned up. *Oh Charlie, why am I surprised?*

Janet put a hand on her shoulder. 'Why don't you go home, Diana? We can walk back with you.'

'The kids have just gone to sleep; Bridie's watching them like a hawk. I thought I'd stay a little longer. But thank you,

Janet. Why don't you go home.' She gave her a hug. Oh God, Charlie was her son.

'Ar—sen—al!' A few people burst into raucous song and she caught Bart's eye and made her way to the bar. 'I think that's it, Bart, if you want everyone to leave any time soon.'

'Don't you worry, Diana, I can keep the lid on this.' He grinned, polishing a few glasses with his towel.

She smiled. 'We've had some good times here, Bart, haven't we?' She felt her mouth tremble. *Not now.*

'We'll miss him, sure enough.'

Miss him. It was hard to know what that meant. It was so difficult to comprehend or understand the concept of death. Charlie was gone and she'd never see him again.

She should know, she'd faced it before when Cody died. Her baby sister, only six years old. That was what, twenty-five years ago? At least her family had been there to support one another, kind of … now it was just her children and Charlie's parents and they didn't know each other well enough to share the grief. There was no one to support her. Her family wasn't here. It was a long way from the farm in Australia to Gospel Oak, London. Too far. They'd offered, her mum had said, 'We can come, Diana, if you want us?'

'No,' she'd said. 'We'll be fine.'

There was at least one thing she could hang on to. Diana looked around. *Charlie, you'd have loved this. You really would.* She picked up her glass. Breathe. *Here's to you, Charlie! Here's mud in your eye.*

*   *   *

Two weeks later, Diana stood apart from the other mothers waiting for the end of school. It was interesting, the way the eyes didn't quite meet hers. The faces were solemn; no one was behaving naturally. Charlie and she had moved here three years ago, so they were hardly strangers but they weren't natives either. Probably being Australian didn't help. She would have loved someone to bounce over and say 'What a bugger,' and give her a hug. Pulling the coat around her and burying her face in the tartan scarf, she couldn't wait for the bell to ring. She missed Australians.

Children streamed past her, toting backpacks, coats and scarves. First off the block was Sienna, arm in arm with Polly, her best friend, and then Saskia trailing behind a group of classmates. Finally, there was Milo walking along in a dream, as usual. His face brightened when he heard her call and he picked up his pace as he changed direction.

'Hey, had a good day?' She hugged them and then they turned and were out the gate. 'Bye Polly.'

It was only a five-minute walk from the school to their house and the kids usually did it by themselves, but since Charlie had died, Diana had been walking them all to school and picking them up in the afternoon. There was an almost drizzle in the air, not enough to wet them.

They hadn't gone far when Saskia, her hand in Diana's, turned, her face alight, and asked, 'What would Daddy be doing now?'

Diana didn't hesitate. 'Today he's having afternoon tea with my grandfather Frank. They haven't met before, you know, because Frank died when I was only little and he wasn't alive when Daddy came over to visit.'

She'd started this game a couple of days ago—What would Daddy be doing now?—to divert them all from falling into a deep depression. The girls had been listlessly watching the telly and Milo had just been kicking a ball relentlessly against the wall beside him. Diana was ready to try anything.

So far Charlie had eaten dinner with his own grandparents and gone to kick a football with George Armstrong, the only Arsenal player she could think of who was dead. There were still a few to meet—her grandparents on her mother's side, for instance. If she ran out, she thought they could always have a few re-runs. Bobby Charlton might be a good one, though he was from the wrong club. She wasn't sure Charlie would have wanted to meet him.

'What is he eating?'

'I think they have special afternoon tea in Heaven. Daddy loved cinnamon donuts, didn't he? I think perhaps they'd be eating a huge plate of them, don't you think?'

'That sounds good. Does Grandfather Frank like donuts?'

'Actually he's your great-grandfather. He was a farmer in Australia and he did love them. Peg used to make them. She's your great-grandmother.'

'What was the farm in Australia called, Mummy?' Milo asked.

'Mog's Hill. I've told you before.'

'That's a funny name.' Sienna frowned. 'Who was Mog?'

Diana laughed. 'I don't know, but I think he found gold there.'

'Wow, did you find any gold when you were growing up?'

'No, I think it had all been found by my time. We were too busy looking after the sheep to worry about finding gold. Umm, actually Rosie and I did go prospecting once.' Diana stopped, wondering if she should continue. It was one of the few times she'd been smacked. 'I thought we should go look for some gold so Rosie and I went down to the creek with a shovel, a strainer and a bag, to hold all the gold. I thought it might be a good surprise if we came back rich. But I neglected to tell Mum where we were going. I got into some trouble that day.'

Diana looked down at her children. She could finally appreciate her parents' concern. 'Please don't go anywhere without telling me, will you?' She laughed, but caught her lip between her teeth. They were so infinitely precious, these children of hers, and this time they spent together … she well knew how quickly it could all be swept away. In a nanosecond their lives had changed completely.

Milo and Sienna were up ahead with Saskia trailing behind as usual. They were nearly home when the voice came from nowhere.

I'm not sure you're helping. They have no idea what dead means, you know.

She glanced around cautiously. *No, Charlie, you have the handle on that.*

The trouble was, as she looked at the figures tramping ahead, she wasn't sure she knew either. Not when Charlie was right there, talking in her head.

I'm not sure how to tell them the truth, Charlie.

Hey, that's what I used to say. Telling the truth is hard, isn't it? You used to go on and on about being honest with each other.

Never did me much good. You and I never saw eye to eye on the truth, did we?

My problem was always working out what was truth and what was fiction.

You just lied to get out of trouble. Remember that first interview I did for the art magazine?

She certainly remembered. She remembered how he hadn't turned up.

*   *   *

Charlie was finally walking in the door, four hours after he'd promised.

'Where have you been?' Diana stood in the doorway, watching him throw his coat on the hat stand.

'Sorry, I got caught up in a traffic jam, delivering those pictures round to that new gallery. How'd you get on?'

'Luckily, the journalist was an angel. Walked in the door and straight away took Sienna, who was screaming blue murder. She's had lots of experience with babies, apparently, and had her quietened down in a few minutes, thank God. I was going crazy.'

'Interview went well then?' Charlie turned on the television and sat down.

'It would have been better if you were here. The photographer pitched in and helped me move the pots around.'

'When does it get published?'

'Next month. "New Aussie Potter on the Block", or something like that. The photographer took some pictures of your sunset painting. I think he liked it.'

'Good for him.' Charlie got up and went into the kitchen and took a beer out of the fridge.

'Have you been drinking?'

'No.'

'I just thought you might have rung and let me know.'

'Bit hard when you're stuck in three miles of traffic.'

'I rang the pub and they said you weren't there.'

'Well, I wasn't, was I?'

* * *

Diana shook herself.

You never owned up to it, did you, Charlie? But I found out later you were in the pub all afternoon. I just wished you hadn't lied about it. You could have said you didn't want to be there, at the interview.

I could have. If I'd wanted to start World War Three.

Why were all these negative thoughts popping up out of the blue? Why was she so angry? *Where are all the funny, lovely memories of you, Charlie?*

They hurt too much.

* * *

Six weeks now and she hadn't slept again last night. Diana sat at her wheel but the shapeless lump of clay lay motionless. Out of the window, the tiled roofs stretched endlessly into the iron grey sky. April, and it was supposed to be spring, nearly summer, and there were floods and snow still in the north and murky, dark days. She walked down the stairs from her studio and pulled the sheets off the girls' beds. She was running out of time. The kids would be home soon.

What was wrong with her?

Blankly, she stared in the washing machine and the full load of sheets, freshly washed. Then she looked at the pile of sheets in her arms. Seriously, she'd just done the beds and now she was doing them all again. She banged down the lid and ran back up to dump the sheets back on the beds as the phone rang.

'Hi, Diana, just wondered if you'd forgotten something?' Her friend Lainie sounded smug.

'No.' Her mind raced through various options. 'Can't say ... Oh no, Sienna! Have you still got her?'

'Yes, my friend, don't worry, everything's under control. We were hardly going to chuck her out in the street. She's too nice. I had an interview at four but it was cancelled. The girls are okay, I was just wondering ...' A delicate pause.

Three hours late. How could she? 'It's fine. I'll be there.' She put the phone down, grabbed the keys and rushed out the door. She'd forgotten to check the fridge also. Never mind, Milo was on top of the stuff they were out of. Thank God for Milo.

The next morning it was raining again. Diana looked out the window as umbrellas pushed into the wind on their way up the hill. Everything was struggling—the hawthorns had their blossom whipped off before they'd come out. She was struggling. Where was her strength? She'd screamed independent for so long, it was her mantra, her flag, her cloak. Now look at her. Pathetic.

Charlie's paintings were stacked against the wall, his brushes still in jars of turps, one of his rags on the floor at her feet. They'd always fought over rags—he'd claimed hers were always so muddy he couldn't use them. They wouldn't be fighting over them again.

Diana now had no energy to fight and it was impossible to make a decision. Sienna asked her yesterday if she could go to the mall with Polly—by themselves. They were eight. And she'd ducked the confrontation and said she'd talk to Polly's mum.

You should have just said no.

Ha. Now you're the fired up authoritarian, Charlie. You wouldn't have said no, not in a million years. I said I'd talk to Polly's mother and I will.

Which she would now have to do.

She got up and walked to the window. The rain wouldn't stop. Sluggish she felt, and useless.

'Why can't I pot?' she railed.

But there was no answer.

It had never failed her before. It was her world away from reality. She made beautiful things, now they looked alien, like junk. If she brought up a hammer she could smash them all into pieces and start again. That was the beauty of clay. Who was the girl who wove all day and then undid it all at night? Ulysses … someone waiting for him? Diana couldn't remember. What did it matter?

Six weeks since Charlie died. He might be a voice in her head but he wasn't coming back, no matter how long she waited.

Australia was in drought, or so her parents said. The sun would have to be shining. Outside it was dark for nine in the morning, with more black clouds moving slowly in. What would she give to feel some sun on her face.

The kids were up. There were noises downstairs. Television, scraping of chairs, endless chatter. Milo didn't want to go to Zack's birthday party. She could hardly force him. Saskia on the other hand, desperately wanted to go to Farah's party but hadn't been asked. She was broken-hearted.

'Can I cook pancakes, Mummy?' The question floated up the stairs towards her.

'No, Sienna.' Not this morning.

'Why? I can make you breakfast in bed.'

'No, Sienna. I'm already up. But thank you.'

'Why? You like my breakfasts.'

Oh, but she could really do without the unholy mess that magically appeared with it.

'How much flour do I put in?'

'Sienna won't let me crack the eggs!'

'Don't Sassy. Put it down. Mummy, Milo's taken the maple syrup.'

'I'll be there in a minute,' she called down. Maybe they needed the diversion. She walked down the stairs to supervise the pancakes.

After breakfast she found the tickets. She'd pulled open the drawer of the hall table looking for stamps, and there were five train tickets to Scotland. She'd bought them ages ago for the Easter break and totally forgotten. Her fingers were shaking. No, they couldn't go. Not with Charlie, an empty seat beside them all the way to Scotland and back.

She wanted to go home and see her mother and her father and her sister, Rosie.

She ached to go home.

It was the first time she'd allowed herself to acknowledge it in ten years. What would her parents say if they just turned up, out of the blue?

Milo walked past her on his way upstairs. 'Mum, what's the Australian anthem, you know, like we sing "God Save The Queen"?'

Diana looked blankly at her son and then put the tickets back in the drawer.

He didn't know the Australian anthem.

*　　*　　*

It was only three days later that she met up with Sebastian in a local cafe. 'September—I can't do it.'

'Of course you can. That's what I'm here for.' Sebastian pushed over her coffee cup and passed her some sugar straws. 'September is five months away and we've got lots done already. Come on, you'll be back on track soon, this is an opportunity not to be missed.'

'Damn you, Sebastian, I tell you I can't. It's not working. I'm not working. I can't think, sleep or pot.' She paused. 'I'm thinking of going back to Australia.' There she'd said it out loud. She looked around—the coffee shop was almost empty. It was nearly three, she had to go and get the kids.

'Not a good idea, Diana. We've worked very hard to get you to this point. The children will be miserable. Anyway, you haven't been back for twenty years.'

'Ten.'

'Whatever, they'll be out of place and they don't know your family.'

And wasn't that the truth? 'Suppose something happens to me and they don't know my family, never met them? I'm feeling quite vulnerable. Just like that—poof,' she snapped her fingers, 'and it can happen.'

'Don't be maudlin. This invitation to exhibit at the Fulham Gallery is not to be sneezed at. I was very excited when they contacted me. It's the next step, my dear.'

'I won't do it unless they hang some of Charlie's paintings.' She looked at him.

Sebastian sighed heavily and lifted his cup. 'You ask a lot, my dear.' He examined her face. 'All right, you have some for me to look at? Our Charlie was fond of showing me pieces that always had "just a little bit more" to do before they were finished.' Another huff.

Diana closed her eyes, shutting out the piles of unfinished works leaning against the wall. 'I'm sure I can find ten, fifteen ... please, Sebastian?'

'For you, Diana, I'll do it. Now forget about going off to some far off country. How about a little car trip to Bibury if you need a bit of country air? That's an enchanting little place.'

'Honestly, Sebastian, I think I need a little more than a couple of hours' drive out of London to get my head back together,' she said.

'All right. You go off to Australia and come back nice and refreshed. Two weeks, three?'

'I don't know.' Diana sank miserably into her elbows. 'I've got to find the passports and book seats. Get the Suttons to look after the house. Pack. Ring my parents and tell them we're coming.'

Should she ask, or just tell them? Just tell them. She pushed the coffee cup to one side

'There you are,' said Sebastian, 'You have a plan already, that sounds more like you, Diana.'

So she did. And didn't it feel good? She stood. 'Sebastian, thanks for the coffee. You've been a great help. Trouble is, I have no idea what they'll say. It's been so long.'

*   *   *

'All packed?' Diana stood at the door. Milo was a tight ball on the bed, facing the wall. The room was unnaturally tidy. She could see the floor.

A muffled 'yes'.

She went to sit on the bed and reached out gently to touch him.

'You've done a wonderful job in here.' She felt bad for not coming sooner to help him. She'd been emptying the fridge. 'Have you remembered your charger?' Janet and Bill had bought him an iPhone.

'Yes. What shoes will I wear on the plane?'

'Trainers, I think. They'll be comfier than your new riding boots.'

'Why do I need riding boots? Am I going riding?'

'No. Everyone wears riding boots on a farm.' Saskia had refused to wear them. They weren't pink. So Diana had bought gumboots for the girls—pink gumboots.

'I call your father Tommo.' He turned to her restlessly. 'And your mother Stella?'

'Yep, that's what they want.' She bent over to kiss him. 'It's okay, you'll love them and they'll love you.' No answer. Diana pulled up the duvet and tucked him in.

The girls were sitting up in bed intent on yet another change of clothes for their Barbie dolls. She noticed not a huge effort had been made to clean up the room. Diana sighed and started to pick up the day's cast-offs.

'Right, turn out the light. Could you please do a little tidy-up in the morning? This is a mess, guys.'

'Are you sure I can only take one bear, Mummy?' Saskia looked up. 'I really want to take Horry.'

'He's too big—he'd need a whole seat to himself.'

'He could have mine. I could stay with Polly or Grandma.' Sienna didn't look as though she was joking.

'Listen, it's going to be great. Your grandparents are dying to meet you, and I want to show you the farm where I grew up. Come on, kids, a little more enthusiasm.'

Sienna gave an exaggerated sigh and turned off her light. Diana went to sit on her bed and held her tightly for a moment, breathing in the scent of the freshly washed hair. God, she hoped she was doing the right thing. Five years since she'd seen her mum, ten since she'd seen her dad and

Rosie. She would take the first steps and surely they would follow. They had sounded pleased. Would time have washed it all away? The past was a long time ago.

'Mummy, in the plane, we'll be awful close to Daddy, won't we? Will he ask us for tea?'

Diana held her breath, not sure whether to laugh or cry. 'I hope not, Sassy. But we can have a good think about him. It's a special feeling being up there above the clouds. You'll love it.'

Not sure she could physically do another thing, Diana turned off the downstairs lights. The stair light fell on her picture. The picture Charlie had painted for her, of her. Laughing, sprays of happiness—it was such a joyous picture. In his favourite acrylics. He'd done it soon after they returned from Australia and their terrible trip. He'd set it around Mog's Hill—well, his interpretation. There were a few sheep … she squinted. They could be sheep. It made her laugh, even now. Her dad would be horrified. But her Mum would love it. A Ned Kelly figure running down the hill behind her.

So, Charlie, you never told me who was that person in the body armour with a gun?

It's not that difficult to work out, Diana.

And now you never will. She sighed looking at the picture. He'd said that the last time she'd asked.

Just a couple more days and they'd be there. She swallowed the nugget of worry that was worming around in her throat. It had to be all right.

Slowly she walked into the bedroom. Moved the suitcase and crawled into the bed, gathering Charlie's pillow to her and rubbing her face into it, trying to catch the last lingering scent of Charlie. It probably wouldn't be there when she returned.

Charlie had given her back herself. He'd helped her to crawl out of the wombat hole she'd dug for herself—that she was not worthy of being loved. Not deserving, not since Cody had died.

Without Charlie, who was she?

CHAPTER TWO

Mog's Hill, Australia, April

Diana stood at the closed gate, her fingers fumbling with the stiff catch, just looking at the house. Simple white weatherboards topped with a grey corrugated-iron roof. Concrete steps painted green split the wide front verandah. The whole lot was overdue for a coat of paint. The white post-and-rail fence around the garden was netted to keep out the sheep. The wildlife too, mostly rabbits, wombats and the kangaroos. Not that her mother had ever declared it to have been very successful. The wombats went under, the kangaroos straight over the top and the rabbits ignored it altogether.

Charlie had been standing here with her the last time she'd seen it. 'Is this it?' he'd said.

'Yes.' She'd turned and punched him lightly on the arm. 'My home, my dad's and my grandparents'. Three generations of us Crawfords of Mog's Hill, and don't you forget it.'

But he'd just laughed at her, three generations meant nothing to an Englishman. And it had pretty well gone downhill from there.

She suddenly realised Milo had come up behind her. 'This is your job,' said Diana. 'The oldest child opens the gate.'

'Why?'

'No real reason. We've always done it that way.' She smiled at him. 'It was always my job. I'll show you.' Yanking at the chain didn't work. Gates at Mog's Hill were usually easily opened, it was one of her Dad's fetishes, swinging gates. Diana had to stand on the gate to free it. She ruffled Milo's hair as they walked back to the car.

Turning off the road at the entrance to Mog's Hill, the rumble over the ramp had silenced them all. Maybe feeling her tension, curious to be finally here.

Diana lifted her eyes, raking the familiar slopes and the soft, rounded hills around the house. Grey granite boulders, smoothed over the last forty thousand or so years and splotched with lichen, were scattered in unruly clumps over the ground. It was as though someone had painted a light green wash over the paddocks. There wasn't much grass, considering it was April. But despite all the talk of drought there must have been some rain recently. It was a reflex action, checking for grass; apparently you didn't lose that over the years. Diana had always thought she'd have made a good farmer if she'd ever been given the chance.

England, when you got out into the country, was all earthy and pungent. Here the light was brighter, the colours more intense and the smells clearer. She could almost taste the fresh, clean smell of Australia, and at last, there was sunshine on her face.

The late afternoon sun bathed the country in a soft glow, the best time to show off your sheep, her father had always said. The tall Lombardy poplars were turning into golden torches down by the creek. The willows had lost their leaves already.

Jeez. Ten years, where had they gone? Two dogs were barking, one of them jumping up and down on the spot with excitement. But more importantly, a figure waited on the verandah.

Driving through the gate Diana couldn't take her eyes off the figure.

'Milo, could you close the gate, please?' She pulled at the tops of her leather boots and nervously plucked at the soft wool of the grape-green pashmina draped around her shoulders.

'I did it, Mum.' Her son looked for reassurance.

'Thanks, darling. Good work.' The figure hadn't moved.

The garden, her mother's pride and joy, was hardly recognisable. That there had been so little rain over the last few years was finally impacting. Diana had liked to think of it green and lush, no matter what her parents said about the drought. This wasn't how she'd remembered it.

It was funny parking at the front, she'd normally have driven round to the back door, but her mother was out waiting for them here. Then they were all out of the car, clambering up the steps.

Her mother looked much the same. Slighter somehow. Still straight as a die and wearing a tweed skirt and a jumper in a soft mauve colour. Her mother had always liked lilac shades—they toned well with her fair skin and blonde hair. Her hair hadn't changed, short with blonde streaks and not a grey hair in sight. If she was nervous she was hiding it well. She'd always hidden things well.

'Hello, everyone … Milo, Sienna, Saskia.' Awkward hugs for the children. Her mother straightened. 'Diana.' There was nothing awkward about the bone-crushing hug she was receiving. Her mother's strength was always surprising. Diana had overtaken her in height by the time she was twelve and was, at the very least, a good six inches taller.

'Oh, Mum!' But she couldn't say any more as she squeezed the tears back in. The distinctive waft of Fidji, her mother's trademark scent, hadn't changed.

At last the interminable journey was over.

Stella patted her back stiffly. They pulled apart, and stood looking at each other before she managed a shaky, 'Thank heavens. Come on in. Did you have a good trip?'

Two cement pots, painted dark green and bursting with shocking pink chrysanthemums, flanked the steps. The screen door squeaked and banged shut behind them. It was almost dark in the front hall as she passed her parents' wedding portrait on the left, and that of her grandmother and grandfather on the right. Her eyes skipped the photo of Charlie and herself and stopped for a moment, examining the picture of the three of them—Rosie and herself with Cody in the middle, the light from the open door to the kitchen spilling on it.

Everyone trooped through into the kitchen. There was a roast sizzling in the oven and warmth from the Aga stove.

'How are the Suttons?' her mother asked.

'Bearing up, I guess.'

A plate heaped with fresh buttered scones lay on the well-scrubbed table. Three blue hard-plastic mugs were placed next to three, very familiar Willow-patterned china cups, with a small bowl of the shocking pink chrysanthemums in the centre, next to her great-grandmother's old silver teapot, rubbed down to the brass on the handle. For some reason that brought a lump to her throat.

She had to have some space.

'Out. Why don't you all go outside and I'll call you in a minute when tea's ready. Does that sound a good idea, Mum?' Diana didn't wait for an answer.

Milo would go. Milo was trying so hard to do the right thing. He'd been trying so hard for the last eight weeks, it was infuriating. Sienna would go if he went, but Diana would have to really work to get Saskia outside. Transferring Sassy's hand to Sienna's, she pushed the two of them towards the back door.

The back screen door jumped shut behind them. She watched them go down the back steps and stop on a patch of the dry brown grass. They stood there quietly, Sienna still holding Saskia's hand, Milo scuffing the dirt into little clouds with his new boots. Why wouldn't they go and do something?

'They've grown so much.'

Her mother sounded wistful. She shouldn't be all that surprised, it had been five years since her mother had come to England to visit, but they'd sent plenty of photos.

'Where's Dad?'

'Getting in some sheep he's thinking of selling tomorrow. The truck will be here in the morning. The meat market for sheep is good. They're off to the Middle East with a bit of luck.'

'How is Dad?'

'So, so.'

That wasn't very revealing. 'How are Rosie and Mal?'

'Fine. They'll drop by in the morning. They're dying to see the kids.'

Her sister and her husband lived not far away, in a cottage about half a kilometre down the road.

'And Granny? I couldn't believe it when you told me.' Diana leant against the faded laminex counter and reached over to take a piece of one of the scones that had crumbled off.

'It's been ghastly, really. We're trying to get her to move into a nursing home. Getting her to move and finding one for her to move to seem to be equally as difficult. She's so stubborn. Perhaps you'll be able to talk some sense into her. You and she always got on so well.' Her mother busied herself filling the teapot.

'Does she really have to go? Can't you get help? Isn't there somewhere local?'

'Judge for yourself,' Stella answered.

These conversations were familiar—getting nowhere with her mother. Diana took the mug and stopped her from adding the milk.

'Just black, thanks.'

'You used to have milk and two sugars.'

'I stopped.' About twenty years ago, when she couldn't afford milk and sugar. 'How long has Granny been—how long have you known?'

'I suppose we've known for three years. Dementia is not entirely unusual in a ninety year old, but the last six months it's really got a lot worse.' Stella poured herself a cup of hot tea, steam rising above the rim of the blue-patterned cup.

'I was in England, not Jupiter or Mars! Why didn't you tell me before?'

'We did tell you, or tried to. It was difficult to talk about it and you weren't here to see. It's been so gradual, and Rosie and I felt we could cope.' She paused. 'Then there was the accident and you had so much to deal with ... But when you said you were coming I had to tell you before you saw her. I knew it would be a shock.'

She made it sound so straightforward and simple, but it was hard to take in changes when you were half a world away. You didn't really want anything to change somehow, it was important that it all stayed the same.

'On the phone she always sounds so good.' Diana still couldn't believe it.

'I know. If you're talking about the past she can be very convincing.'

Diana felt ashamed. She should have rung more often. There'd been a flurry of calls after the accident; before that they were fairly sporadic, she had to admit. It had been so hard these last few weeks just trying to keep her and the kids together. It was as though they'd been living in bubble wrap. Nothing seemed real.

Her mother spooned homemade jam into a small dish. Diana couldn't resist a swipe and taste.

'Mmm, yum.' She sighed. 'Poor Granny, I can't wait to see her. I was hoping to stay for a few weeks. I want the kids to get some Australian sun, if nothing else. To breathe some fresh air and develop some roots. Get to know their grandparents.'

That, more than anything, had brought her back to Australia, for her children to get to know her parents. But they'd never know their great-grandmother now, not like Diana had known her. Her relationship with Peg had been so special. Someone she could always talk to.

'We'd like to get to know your children too,' said Stella. 'It's been almost six years since I came to London when Saskia was born.' She looked up and smiled rather wistfully at Diana. 'I am *so* glad you're here,' she added, as she poured lemon cordial into the mugs. 'Well, I think we're ready.'

Diana put down her cup, went down the back steps and joined her three children. Granny couldn't be as bad as her mother had described. Peg was such a strong person, always had been. She'd been brought up on tales of Granny and Grandfather Frank carving out Mog's Hill, how they'd turned it from a 'bush block' to a superb sheep farm.

'Come and look at the dogs,' said Diana. Taking Saskia's hand, she pulled her along, the other two trailing behind. The four of them went to stand in front of the dog's run. There was one young dog and one old one. The young dog was the one that had been jumping straight up and down on all fours, barking, when they'd arrived earlier. It was now straining on the chain towards them. Saskia retreated behind her mother, pulling at her hand and whimpering.

Milo looked as if he were trying to be brave. For heaven's sake, it was only a young dog. And it was on the chain. Yet they were all three apprehensive. Living in London there'd been no room for a dog. Her kids had had so little contact with animals. Growing up, she and Rosie's lives had been packed full of pet lambs and working dogs and there'd always been a cat somewhere. She'd always loved the sheep, not surprising when her father had such a passion for them. So she'd brought her kids home to touch a sheep, make friends with a dog.

And some space for all of them.

She knelt before the young dog, noted it was a male and put out her hand.

'Look, this is how you say hello to a dog—let him sniff you first.' The dog, he wasn't much older than a pup really, licked her fingers enthusiastically. Diana laughed and patted his head.

'See, he's really very friendly.' She turned to look at her children. 'Come on, Milo,' she urged. He made no effort to step forward. Diana sighed and stood up, dusting herself off.

'Come on then, we'll go inside and have some tea.'

*   *   *

The children sat quietly drinking their lemon cordial when Diana heard the motorbike coming. The engine stopped and then there was a clump of footsteps up the back steps.

'Hi, Dad.' Another hard hug, she wound her arms tightly round his neck and drank in his scent. 'I can smell sheep.' And they were both laughing. Her father was only a little taller than herself, but he seemed to have shrunk too, their eyes were level now. She pulled back to look at him. Same lean face, with the deep grooves running down to his mouth. His hair was salt-and-pepper grey now, his forehead reaching back further than it had, but the eyes were just as blue behind his glasses. The wide, welcoming smile on his weather-beaten face did wonders for her poor battered soul. The bands around her heart eased another notch. She was home.

'Well now, aren't you a sight for sore eyes?' He turned to the children. Obviously he thought better of approaching the two little girls, as they sat there, stiff and withdrawn. 'Hello, Milo.' He put out his hand to shake. Diana watched her son reach out his small hand, manfully, in return.

Tom leant back against the kitchen counter and accepted his tea from her mother with a buttered scone. In his thick socks, work-stained woollen jumper, blue-checked flannel-ette shirt and dusty jeans, he looked so good. Just the same. Diana saw him wink at the girls.

'I was just asking Mum if it would be all right if we stayed for a few weeks. Reacquaint these kids with their Australian heritage. Give me some time to work out what I want to do. I know it'll be a bit of a squash.' Diana looked from her father to her mother and caught the 'I told you so' that passed between them. It didn't surprise her; what did surprise her was how much it still hurt. 'Of course, if you think we'll be too much trouble ...'

'Of course not, Diana, you know you're always welcome here,' her father cut in.

Yes, he meant it. She looked at her mother.

'Diana, don't be ridiculous. We love having you all here.' Stella turned to the oven and poked at the meat. And with a short look at her husband, she added, 'Your father could do with some help.'

'Dad? Where's Mal? Why isn't he helping?'

'Mal is working down at Lost Valley now, for Patrick Morley.' said Tom. 'His contracting business is pretty well defunct. Anyway, I don't need Mal's help.' He frowned at Stella. 'I can do everything as I've always done here. Numbers

are down, but we've still had to feed right through summer.'
Her father was matter of fact.

Twenty years ago her parents had announced they were
leaving the farm to Rosie and Mal, that it wouldn't provide
enough of a livelihood if they divided it. So Diana had taken
the plane ticket offered to her and left, angry and bitter, in
her usual, hot-headed way. Upside was, they'd been right—
she had made it on her own and she had her potting. It was
interesting how one's view could change over the years.

'What's Rosie up to?'

Her younger sister by two years, Rosie had been considered the beautiful one, while Diana was known as the artistic Crawford. Their little sister, Cody, had been just six when
she'd died, not enough time to leave much of an imprint,
just an awful hole in all their lives. Cody had been such a
bright spark, she might have been the intelligent one.

'Rosie has a job in town, at the hospital,' Stella began.

'Hang on,' said Diana. 'I'll just move the kids to a telly.'
They looked so tired, sitting there like three little zom-
bies. 'They'll be right in here, won't they?' She shepherded
the children into the sitting room and handed Milo the
remote.

Her mother came to the door to watch. 'Since Philly
left she's put in a magnificent vegie garden, and is running
chooks and sells the eggs in town.'

'I remember she always loved chooks.' But Rosie and vegetables? Diana couldn't even imagine Rosie as a glorified
waitress at the hospital, washing up and mopping the wards.
They came back into the kitchen.

'And Phillipa?' Rosie and Mal's daughter, she'd surely be
nineteen by now.

'Phillipa is enrolled in college in Albury, doing her second year of Hospitality Management.'

Diana hadn't remembered that. 'What does she want to do?'

'It should get her a job running hotels.'

Diana was impressed. When she'd last seen Phillipa ten years ago, she was the same age her kids were now. Wasn't that incredible?

Diana suddenly felt very tired. She picked up the mugs, put them in the sink and then went back to look at the kids.

Everything was so upside-down since the accident. Usually Sienna and Milo would be arguing over which program they'd watch. Sometimes she found herself wishing for a bit of fighting spirit, or even just some whingeing from the kids.

'I think I'll go out for a while,' she said. 'Do you want to come?' They were sitting quietly, Saskia snuggled up to Sienna with her thumb in her mouth. None of them even looked her way. 'Okay, I won't be long.'

CHAPTER THREE

Stella watched Diana grab a jacket from the hall on her way out. There were dark circles under her eyes and she was thinner. She picked up the green shawl Diana had discarded on the back of the chair, squashing the soft fibres between her fingers.

Diana was home. How Stella had prayed for this day. Already there'd been so many wasted years. After Charlie's accident she'd thought surely they would come, and had asked Tom whether they should suggest it. That was after the funeral. Stella had wanted to go but it was too difficult—too much money, and they were hand-feeding the sheep. It was so constant, impossible to get away.

Diana had been hard to get through to these last couple of months, very vague. Living on the other side of the world hadn't helped, and so much time had passed. Where had it gone? Tom had said to let her sort herself out. Stella crushed the shawl to herself. Now she was home and those beautiful children, her grandchildren, were finally here. She moved into the sitting room.

Two pairs of eyes were trained on the television. Milo was hunched over his phone. Dark-haired like Peg, she thought, and so serious. No, he was Frank all over, definitely a Crawford. He hadn't smiled yet. None of them had.

Stella smiled at them. 'It must have been a long trip. Does anyone want to use the bathroom?'

The girls looked up at her standing there with Diana's shawl nervously wound through her fingers. Milo was still absorbed in his game.

'That's our mummy's pashmina.'

Sienna had spoken. She was blonde like Charlie, but there was something in the directness of her look, or the stubborn set of her chin, that reminded her of Diana.

'It's lovely, isn't it?' said Stella.

'Daddy bought that for Mummy.'

'We all bought it. We went to the markets, remember?' Milo looked up briefly. 'It's Australian wool. That is, we think it is. Mummy said it must be because it was so soft.'

'Daddy says it's the same colour as her eyes,' Saskia spoke up. She was like Rosie, with the same hair and eyes. So beautiful.

None of them had Diana's eyes. Her daughter's eyes were so unusual—a frosted light green, made more startling under those straight, black eyebrows. Nothing about Diana had been what she expected.

'It is, isn't it?'

A six-year-old Rosie smiled up at her, and Stella's heart melted.

'Would you like a biscuit?'

'No, thank you.'

Those high-pitched English voices. She sat in a chair. 'What are you watching?'

'We don't know.' After briefly scanning the unfamiliar cartoon figures on the screen, Stella realised neither did she. It didn't remotely look like *Postman Pat* or *Thomas the Tank Engine*, the English shows she remembered watching with Phillipa.

'ABC Kids is usually quite good. That's our Channel Two.' She gestured towards the phone Milo was fiddling with. 'I wonder if you'll get much reception in here, you may have to go outside.'

'It's an iPhone. Grandma and Grandad gave it to me.'

Surely he was too young to have a phone? Stella hoped he wasn't trying to ring the UK, but she couldn't say anything. The reception was appalling here. She fell silent, not making head nor tail of the flickering images on the television screen. The children must be feeling so strange when even the television shows were different. Poor babies. This was going to take some time. And time, thank heavens, appeared to be something they might be going to have. She could hardly believe it when Diana had rung and said they were coming.

Her prickly, defensive eldest daughter was finally home. She sighed. There were so many unresolved issues. She was determined to make it better. All she needed was time.

*　　*　　*

Diana drew a deep lungful of clean, crisp air. It was so beautiful. No doubt about it. The sky went up and out for miles. Not a single person or another house to be seen. How amazing was that? The sheer feeling of space was glorious, liberating. She walked with an easy stride, out the back, past the dogs. England had civilisation going back thousands of years, but out here it was the land that was ancient. The rock screes on the hillside shone gold in the late afternoon sun. The far off hills, covered in thick woolly scrub, had barely been touched by man. The paddocks of Mog's Hill stretched out to the base of the closest range. The sun would set shortly. It was a red, round circle surrounded by a few fluffy-pink clouds, striping the paddocks in gold and pink.

Happy now?

What do you think, Charlie? Look at this view. Sensational, isn't it?

I always preferred tiled roofs and a few smokestacks, myself.

Diana smiled, and wasn't that the truth.

Once upon a time this could have been mine, you know.

* * *

Diana lifted the suitcase onto the bed. She looked at her image in the mirror on the dressing table and pulled her hair back into its elastic. The flush of excitement beamed right back at her.

A change of plans. And she hadn't told anyone.

It was such a great feeling to have finished. Away for three years at Art School and now the rest of her life in front of her. She'd been ecstatic when she'd heard her uni tutors had negotiated a resident scholarship with a commune of potters in London for her. And until last week, that was what she was going to do. But now she'd changed her mind. She'd always have her potting, and it would always be part of her life, but home—Mog's Hill—was where she wanted to be, where she belonged, on the farm with her dad. She'd worked it all out. She was going to do a wool-classing course through TAFE and help with the sheep on the farm. It would be hard to get a job in some sheds but girls were doing it now. She could do it. Their shearing contractor would help. Her dad could concentrate more on the cropping. He'd be happy.

She walked down the hallway. Entering the sitting room she heard the pop of the champagne cork and everyone laughing. She'd thought it was for her. To celebrate her return, her good marks, a new beginning.

Everyone was in the sitting room, which was unusual, but then champagne wasn't a common occurrence. The scene was freeze-framed in her brain. Mal was there, his sleeves rolled up, sitting with Rosie on the sofa. Rosie wearing a new pink shirt. The two chintz-covered chairs patterned with large lilac roses, and her mother sitting with a broad smile on her face. Her dad was pouring champagne into the wide open glasses they used to have. She suddenly noticed Mal and Rosie were holding hands.

'To Mal and Rosie! Congratulations!'

Then they were all standing, clinking glasses. She hadn't known.

'And to Diana, the beginning of a future in potting. We've been told you have what it takes, or so your lecturers said.'

Her dad had looked at her proudly, but all she heard was that Mal and Rosie were engaged, and eventually would be given the farm. Not just yet, but Mal would be working with her father. To this day, Diana avoided champagne, the bubbles in her nose brought on that sick, empty nausea, because what followed had been the beginning of her night-mare. Her father handed her an envelope and when she'd opened it there was a return plane ticket to London. She was numb. All she could think of was that at last, her father had what he had always wanted. A son. Not that they said it. Oh no. They were so proud of her. This was such a great opportunity. She must be so happy.

But she wished someone had asked her what she wanted.

*　　*　　*

Diana wandered round the collection of sheds: the large machinery shed housing the tractors and a four-wheeler bike, a tool shed, a meat shed. She stopped suddenly. Sadly, she touched the ruins of her kiln, now a crumbling pile of bricks. No one would ever guess what it had been. She remembered poring over the plans of the do-it-yourself kit with her dad. It had taken them months to build.

Hearing soft footfalls behind her, she turned to see him now.

'I thought I'd find you here,' he said. 'We're so sorry about Charlie, Di. It was a terrible thing to have happened.'

Diana couldn't answer, the lump in her throat too large.

Her dad put his arm round her. 'Come, the tool shed is locked. I brought the key.'

He inserted the key into the door of the small corrugated-iron shed and waited for her to go inside. In the corner was a knee-high object, covered in an old wool bale. With a little cry, Diana skipped over and pulled off the dusty cover.

'My potting wheel! I can't believe it. It's still here! Dad!'

Tentatively, she reached out and felt the smooth surface of the kick wheel with loving fingers. She moved the treadle with her foot and watched the wheel start to turn. No fancy electric wheel this.

'Do you remember going to Albury to buy it at the auction?' said Diana. 'We'd seen it advertised in the paper.'

'I remember being nagged to death until I relented. You were always a determined minx,' her dad smiled.

'And when we got there we saw we needn't have taken the truck after all.' Diana laughed. 'You moaned about it all the way home.'

'I wasn't exactly told what to expect, was I?'

'Thank you, thank you so much.' All of a sudden she wanted to cry. What was the matter with her?

'Don't have to thank me for anything. It's yours.' His voice was gruff.

'I haven't been able to pot since the accident. I just couldn't do it or face anything. That was scaring me. And the kids are so quiet. It's breaking my heart. The only decision I've made is to come here. I hope you don't mind. Really,' she whispered.

Her father put his arms round her and held her. She took a breath.

'We're glad you're home, Diana. Everything will be okay now, don't you worry.'

Somehow the words didn't have the impact she'd hoped for. That's what she'd told herself in the plane coming home—*When I get home, everything will be all right.*

But she'd shut that out right now. 'How are those rams you bought a couple of years ago working out?' She picked a subject she always knew would light her father up. They turned to leave the shed and she waited while he closed the door behind them.

'Things have changed.' Tom chuckled. 'Now we're looking for meat on their bones. Lambs are worth good money
at the moment. I can't wait to show you. They're looking
quite good.' And that was high praise from her father.

'Can we have a look now?' They'd always passionately
shared this interest in the sheep.

'It's getting dark, we can see them tomorrow. There are a
few going tomorrow, we'll have a good look at them then.'

Tom kept talking as they made their way back to the
house. Diana needed a rest from being in charge. Just a
little time off. Strung so tight, she was afraid she'd shatter.
Her dad's words, however, they didn't ring true. How was it
going to be okay?

She had to come to terms somehow with the fact that her
Charlie was dead. Killed in a bloody car wreck. She had to
get away from the scent of him, that sick feeling it was all
a horrible mistake and he was just about to walk right back
in the door with that silly grin on his face. His voice hadn't
had a problem, coming all this way with her.

I didn't want to disappoint you, Diana.

*Charlie, Charlie. You wouldn't come with me before. You
said never, remember.*

She wanted her resilience back, to lose this feeling of
being in limbo. Like when she'd gone to England, shrugged
off the hurt, said she didn't care and made a career in potting. Couldn't she find the same strength again?

*　　*　　*

The next morning the truck arrived at 6 am to load the 160
lambs being sent to the market. The kids stayed motionless lumps under their duvets, despite Diana's half-hearted

attempts to wake them. They needed the sleep. Yawning, she'd pulled a sweater over her T-shirt, as she knew the morning would be chilly. Then she'd gone out with her dad, like they used to.

Watching the big truck slowly backing up, she hoped it wasn't going to bump the old wooden ramp which looked like it might fall over with the slightest provocation. The yards weren't as solid as they'd been twenty years ago. The wethers hadn't taken long to load, they'd flown on despite the so-called help they'd had from the new kelpie pup, whose name she'd discovered was Dave. Eventually she'd had to tie him up just to get him out of the way. Then they got in the ute to go check the sheep.

'Some things haven't changed. Dad, how long have you had this ute?' She gave the stiff door a second bang to close it.

'No need to change something that isn't broken. The old girl has given me good service.'

'You've sold the bikes. I couldn't see them in the shed—only a new, red quad bike.'

'I kept my old BSA Bantam. I'm going to do it up, restore it to its former glory one day.'

Diana smiled. Her dad had always loved his bikes. She looked over at the old dog in his usual place, standing guard at his shoulder. 'You're just an old bikey at heart, aren't you? And Sinbad's still going strong?'

'Mmm, maybe not as strong as he used to be, but the two of us should see each other out.'

'He certainly wasn't much use loading. He just sat in the corner with his tongue hanging out and giving the odd bark when he saw you.'

'We didn't have a problem loading, did we?' Tom asked mildly.

'No.' Diana laughed, shook her head and settled back, looking around her with interest. 'You must have had some rain recently.'

'Just enough to start the ploughing. I've been concentrating more on cropping lately. It's one way to afford to put a bit of fertilizer onto the land. Not a lot of money in the sheep, these days.'

'Pity, when you've got them looking so good.'

'They'll come back, always have.'

Oh Dad, you're just the same. You haven't changed.

CHAPTER FOUR

Two hours later they were back. Rosie and Mal were in the kitchen with Stella and Saskia.

'Di!' Rosie flew round the edge of the table to give her a hug.

'Oh Rosie!' Diana exclaimed, with a catch in her throat. Then they were laughing breathlessly. 'It's so good to see you!'

'I can't believe it!' they cried simultaneously. Everyone laughed.

Diana turned to hug Mal. He had to have put on ten kilos. Well, he could carry them; he was still a big, strong fellow. Was that a touch of grey in his dark hair? Rosie was just the same, like their mother, only her hair was still a tumble of light brown curls and her honey-hazel eyes were brimming with tears. Tears had always come easily to Rosie.

'Di! Your kids are so gorgeous. This Saskia is just *so* beautiful.' Retrieving her from Stella, Rosie settled Saskia comfortably back on her lap, kissing the top of her head. Having been her daughter's security blanket for the last three months, Diana couldn't help being a little astonished at the easy way she had transferred from her mother to Rosie.

'Rosie, Mal, it's so good to see you both. How are you?' Diana passed a mug of hot tea to her father who had come in behind her and then nursed her own, standing in front of the Aga, with its comforting warmth. The kitchen was always lovely in the morning with the sun streaming in. This was how she remembered it with the four of them together, the big room full of people and forever cups of tea. Her mother in charge, seated at the table with the teapot handy and within easy reach of the toaster.

'We had to see you before we started work,' said Rosie. 'Mal has a job at Lost Valley and I start at nine too, at the hospital. You'll have to come over for dinner, I'm dying to show you our renovation. Mum says you'll be here for a while.'

'Well, I'm pretty directionless at the moment. We needed a bolthole.'

Saskia had her eyes half closed, but reached out all the same to take the finger of vegemite toast her grandmother passed to her. Now, with the two of them together, Diana could see that Saskia was very like Rosie. Two peas in a pod.

'Careful, Saskia, you'll get vegemite all over your aunt.'

'Don't be such a grouch. We can wipe it off, can't we, poppet?' Rosie laughed and ruffled the top of her head. If Saskia had been a cat, she'd be purring.

'I'm so sorry about Charlie, Diana,' Mal said gruffly. 'We were all upset we couldn't get there for the funeral.'

'Not that we could have afforded it.' Rosie's muttered comment was perfectly audible. Followed by an awkward silence.

'We should have been there.' Her mother shot a look at her father.

'That's okay,' said Diana. 'I understood. It was pretty terrible. Seriously, I can't remember too much about it, only the fact I had an awful argument with Charlie's parents. I wanted him cremated and they wanted a burial.' The four faces just looked at her. Five if you included Saskia. She shouldn't be saying this in front of Saskia. She shrugged. 'I just couldn't face him being buried in the earth forever. He was such a free spirit, he would have hated it.' Her voice gave way.

'How are Bill and Janet?' Tom asked. He'd never met the Suttons but they'd spoken on the phone occasionally.

'They're fine. They understood when I told them I needed to come home. They've been wonderful, really. Luckily I had enough money in my bank account to get here. Probate won't be granted for another few months. Not that there's much. A bit of insurance, there'll be more if we sell the house. But my business is there and it's going pretty well. I have a lovely studio in the attic and all the equipment I need. I have to make decisions.' Not that she'd been making too many lately. Her head felt stuffed with mush most of the time.

'There's no need to make them today. Take your time,' said Tom.

'How was the flight over?' Mal asked.

'Long,' said Diana. 'No, it was good. The flight attendants were so kind, considering we stretched their patience to the limit.'

'You're not suggesting my beautiful grandchildren were difficult?' Her mother reached over to give Saskia a reassuring pat on the knee.

'Mmm. Everything was fine until *that* particular grandchild locked herself in the toilet.' Diana frowned at Saskia, who giggled. 'There were four attendants trying to explain to Saskia how to unlock the door, watched by a long queue of irate passengers. They were losing patience big time, as we'd all just had breakfast and it was about an hour to landing. It was getting ugly.'

Tom was chuckling. 'What happened?'

'Just as they were bringing in screwdrivers, the door clicks and out swans my daughter, looking fresh as a daisy and totally unfazed.' Diana looked round at her family and grinned. 'You can all laugh now but I tell you, it was touch and go. I was worried I might be lynched.'

'Get the wethers away this morning? How many did you send?' Mal was changing the subject. Diana watched him talking to her dad. Seeing him here in the kitchen was just like old times. He'd been around lots when they were growing up. He'd been her mate really; they'd go careering all over the farm on a pair of yellow Yamaha ag bikes. He'd dare her to jump the creek or a log, or she'd dare him. It had been good fun. The new quad bike looked practical and sedate. It wouldn't take much to get the kids on it, but was getting back on a motorbike the same as a bicycle, something you never forgot? She hoped so.

'Well, I'll see you at home.' Mal was addressing Rosie but he didn't look at her, and he sounded a bit short.

'I'll be a bit late home probably.' Rosie didn't sound too happy either.

'In that case I'll see you when I see you. Don't forget the mail.'

'Why don't you and Mal come over for tea tonight?' Stella said.

'That's a great idea. What do you think, Mal?'

'Sure, we'd love to.'

Mal was saying goodbye. Diana put her hands in her pockets and stayed leaning against the stove. He kissed her mother, but he didn't kiss Rosie—he barely acknowledged her on the way out after waving to Diana and Saskia.

'Oh,' Rosie sighed, 'I suppose I'd better go too.'

Diana watched her daughter transferred once again to her mother's lap.

'There you go, poppet. Say goodbye to the other two for me, won't you? I'll see you, Mum.' Rosie was pulling Diana by the hand. 'Come out with me and wave goodbye.'

Rather reluctantly, Diana left her warm position by the stove and followed her sister outside.

'Thank heavens you're home, Diana.' Rosie settled herself in her little Honda and fastened the seatbelt. She looked up at her sister. 'We badly need help convincing Dad he should retire. He's seventy, you know, and it's time for us to take over. Mum can't get him to even think about it.'

'What does he think he'll … they'll do?' Diana asked. She couldn't imagine her father moving anywhere else. He was the second generation of Crawfords on this farm. Mog's Hill was his life.

'That's the problem. He's got no hobbies, and holidays are something they used to do when we were kids. I don't think they've been anywhere for ages, and to make it worse none of his friends are retiring either. It's so infuriating.' Rosie started up the engine. 'See you tonight.'

Diana watched the dust rise behind the car as her sister drove off. Lord, Mal was forty now, the same age as her. He'd been married to Rosie for twenty years. She supposed he was ready to take over. A noisy flock of galahs wheeled and screeched above her, landing on the slender branches of a silver birch. They looked like fluffy pink and grey blossoms as they bobbed and swayed.

Diana leant against the big old gum tree in the garden and absently peeled off a strip of bark. It used to have a swing. Cody's swing. Damn, there were very few memories of Charlie here but plenty of Cody. Everywhere she turned there was Cody's smile, her freckled face, a question. She never stopped talking and asking questions. *Why is the sky blue, Di? I mean, how does it get to be blue?* No one had mentioned Cody this morning. Was that going to happen to Charlie? Twenty-five years on no one would talk about him?

She didn't turn around as she heard her mother come up behind her.

'You took the swing down,' Diana said.

'Rosie thought it was too dangerous for Philly. We had a little swing set for a while. Then we gave it away.'

'Rosie doesn't seem too happy.'

Her mother was carrying a red plastic bucket, which, at a guess, contained dish water. There were buckets all over the house—buckets for the showers, buckets for the toilets and buckets in the kitchen.

Her mother was carefully pouring the water around one of the straggly abelia bushes with its pinky white flowers and narrow bronzed leaves. Looking around, it was hardly a garden any more. The big gum tree was still going, but the silver birch covered with galahs was dead, and the beds had virtually disappeared. Suddenly the birds took off again, wheeling and squawking.

'Damn birds. They're always around when your dad is planting. They just follow the tractor, eating all the seeds. I'm surprised anything comes up.' Stella sighed. 'I guess Rosie and Mal are going through a rough patch at the moment. Mal is working for the new owner at Lost Valley—city money, and plenty of it. We tell him he's much better off there but he's frustrated, I think. What did Rosie want?'

'She thinks it's time for you and Dad to retire.' Diana stayed looking out into the distance, watching her sister's car make its way to the road.

Her mother gave a little shrug. 'I thought we'd be retired by now but your father doesn't want to. He can't think of a life away from here. Anyway, there's no money to set us up anywhere else. The drought has taken care of the little savings we'd been able to put aside, and we've got Peg to think about right now. We've got to get her into some kind of care … I can't bear the thought of a nursing home just yet and neither can she. So, I don't know. It's very difficult.'

'I don't get it. How come you can leave someone with dementia living alone in a house?'

'Your grandmother is very independent, Diana.'

'I thought I'd go and see her this morning. I might visit her by myself first, before I take the kids. Can I leave them with you?' She wanted to assess the situation. The news she'd heard only two days ago that her grandmother had dementia was a bit hard to assimilate.

'Of course you can. There are a few things she needs,' said Stella, 'and could you do a bit of shopping for me? I'll go and write you a list.'

Diana watched her mother carry the red bucket back into the house. She'd had fun explaining the water-saving strategy to the kids last night. The excess water from their showers was saved in buckets for the toilets. They were to put a quarter of a bucket in for number ones, and half a bucket for number twos. The kids were fascinated. Saskia had gone about four times before she'd gone to bed, which completely nullified the water saving.

'Why are we saving water?' her practical son had asked.

'Because we're in a drought. There hasn't been enough rain to fill the tanks. All the water for the house comes from the tank out the back. They used to pump it up from the big dam, but it's too low now.'

They'd all been waiting for Saskia to finish on the toilet, Milo and Sienna crowded into the bathroom with her.

'What happens when we run out of water?'

'We won't run out. A big tanker comes and fills up the tank when we get low.'

'Cool, will it come while we're here?'

'Probably.' At the rate they were all going to the toilet it would be sooner rather than later. Diana had flushed with the quarter bucket allotment and shepherded the three of them back to their bedrooms.

CHAPTER FIVE

It felt so strange driving back into town. So familiar, and at the same time Diana was noticing differences everywhere. The pretty church on the hill as you drove in hadn't changed, but now new trees boxed in neat brick paving lined the main street. Low growing roses, straggling with last of the season blooms, spilled over on the street corners. Half the shops were empty in the main street, but when you turned the corner there was a brand spanking new supermarket. Not a Woollies or a Coles, it had some other name. The town was nestled on the side of a hill. The steep, wide main street still had all the parked cars backed into the kerb, but Diana could see some new shops she hadn't seen before, including a trendy clothes shop Sienna would love. There was a fair sprinkling of people around for a Monday morning. The old two-storey bank building was now painted pink and was flanked by a row of riotous geraniums in flower pots.

Altogether, her home town had a much fresher look than ten years ago. Someone must have some money.

Slowly she pulled up outside her grandmother's house with the pretty leadlight windows. Granny had lived there for thirty years. For Diana, it had been a special place while she was growing up. Memories piled one on top of the other— when she was bullied by Tim Spelling and her grandmother threatened to go after him with a stockwhip; spinning dreams of potting before she'd ever remotely thought of telling her parents; her retreat, her refuge, when Cody died. Nothing but strong, unconditional love and support. Diana smiled, remembering apple cakes, plum jams, crab-apple jellies, marmalades, and then jars and jars of green tomato chutney when the last of the tomatoes were threatened by frosts. She'd loved the donuts best. Her grandmother never stopped cooking, and then giving it all away. *Granny, don't get old.*

Knocking at the back door elicited no response, and there was no key where there always used to be one, under the ceramic flowerpot. Diana reached for her phone.

'Mum, Granny's not answering the door.'

'She's probably taken her hearing aid out. There's a key at the neighbours—the one with the brick fence. The Mullens. I'm sure she's all right, Diana, don't worry.'

'I'll ring you right back.'

Moments later, Diana called her mother as she walked quickly back to Granny's house. 'Mum, they're not home.'

'All right.' Stella was quiet for a minute. 'Rosie's got a key. Go round to the hospital.'

Diana got back in the hire car and drove to the hospital. The red-brick building stood back from the road with a few

large pepper trees in front. Diana parked at the entrance
and raced inside. There was no one at the desk and it seemed
very quiet. Lord, where were all the people when you wanted
them? She strode down the corridor, glancing into rooms
that all seemed to be occupied by sleeping patients or visitors sitting in chairs—not anyone who looked remotely like
a staff member that she could see. Surely finding someone
on staff in a ten-room hospital shouldn't be that hard. Turning the corner she ran right into a solid mass of dark-green
woollen jumper and tweed sports coat.

'Oh, I'm so sorry! I'm looking for Rosie Burns.'

'Rosie. She should be here somewhere. Keep going down
to the end and turn right.' The voice was deep and amused.

'Thanks.' And she was off more quickly this time, half
running till she burst into the door marked 'Kitchen'.

'Rosie!' Diana exclaimed. 'Have you got a key to Granny's house?'

Rosie stood at the end of the laminated counter, loading
trays onto a large trolley. She looked up amazed. 'Diana.
What on earth's wrong?'

'I can't get into Granny's house. She won't answer the
door.'

'She's probably taken her hearing aid off. Calm down.'
Rosie disappeared out a door to her left and reappeared with
a large shoulder bag in hand. Diving into it, she took an
inordinately long time to find the key.

'This is what you need. Back door.' She passed it over
with a grin. 'We'll have to get you one cut. Or you can have
mine. Good luck!' But she was talking to a swinging door.

By the time Diana got back to the house, her hand was
shaking as she put the key into the back door and walked

in. It smelled stale. Old people smell. No one was in the kitchen, or the sitting room. With her hand on the knob of the bedroom door, she whispered, 'Granny.'

Her grandmother was lying on the bed, fully dressed, eyes closed. Diana approached her, terrified, putting out a hand to touch her shoulder.

The eyes flew open. 'Diana! What a lovely surprise! I haven't seen you for ages.'

Not for ten years, actually, Diana thought.

'Oh, I must have dropped off to sleep.' With a start of surprise she looked round the room. 'Goodness, it's hard to keep track of the time. How are you, darling?'

Her grandmother struggled to sit up. She swung her feet to the floor, looking around for something. Diana saw a walking stick leaning against a chair. She reached for it and handed it to her grandmother and tried to help her up.

'Don't. I'm perfectly able.'

Diana was reduced to uselessly watching as her grandmother put her stick to the floor and laboured to stand up.

Which she did, eventually.

'How are you feeling? It's so good to see you.' Diana couldn't resist giving her a gentle hug, felt the frailty of her shoulders and the papery skin of her arms, and noticed the lustreless white hair and her swollen ankles. She'd shrunk to a tiny old woman. Diana was shocked. All that was left of the feistiness she remembered was in her voice.

'What's that?'

'Where's your hearing aid, Granny? Did you take it out?'

'My what? Speak up! Oh yes, I'm sure it's somewhere. Those wretched people put it in places where I simply don't know ... Oh, there it is.' She shuffled slowly, painfully slowly, to the cabinet near the door, picked up the offending article and put it in her ear. They both winced at the sudden squeal and then she turned to Diana, beaming. 'That's better. Where have you been? I haven't seen you for ages,' she repeated.

'In England.' Diana was a little disconcerted. 'I've come back for a visit. I've brought the kids.'

'What kids? Do you have children? No one told me. But then no one tells me anything anymore.'

Diana followed her into the kitchen. The last time she'd seen Granny was ten years ago when she'd brought Charlie out to meet her family, just after they'd married. She'd never been able to get him to come again—it was not something he'd wanted to repeat. Her grandmother had thought he was wonderful. She was one of Diana's most favourite people in the world. This was breaking her heart. 'You remember Charlie, though?'

'That beautiful Englishman? Of course I remember. Had a sense of humour, very entertaining. Where is he?'

Diana left that right alone. 'I've brought some things for you. I've left them in the car. I'll just go and get them.'

When she returned to the house, Diana put the shopping down and looked round the empty kitchen, wondering where her grandmother had gone. She walked into the sitting room where Granny was sitting in what was a new armchair—or at least it was new to Diana. A fancy affair—very cushiony. Everything else was the same though: an arrangement of silk flowers on the tall bookshelf, beside two of her early plates. Diana gave a wry smile, remembering how pleased she'd been with them. Actually, examining them now, she realised they weren't all that bad. On another shelf, the French brass carriage clock that had belonged to her great-grandmother needed winding. Absently, Diana picked up the brass key and started winding it up. She set the correct time, five to twelve. She ran her finger along the row of books on the bottom shelf: H.V Morton's travel books.

It was Granny who had introduced Diana to a whole world outside of their country town. Peg had loved reading travel books, even though she hadn't done any travelling herself. She'd lived here in this house for … heavens, it must be thirty years since Grandfather Frank died. He was sixty-one when the cancer finally won out. Peg had moved in here, and her family had moved into the homestead on the farm.

'Where's your husband, Diana?' Peg asked suddenly.

'Umm, he died.' Diana swallowed.

'Oh darling, that's terrible, so young. Frank would have liked Charlie. Frank died way too early. I still miss him.'

'What would you like for lunch, Granny?' Diana asked, but her eyes were closed again and she hadn't heard the question.

Diana went back into the kitchen and was surprised by two women walking in the back door.

'We're from Meals on Wheels. You must be Diana.'

One of them was carrying a foam box, and picked up an empty one she obviously knew just where to find. She efficiently emptied the meal from the foil container onto a plate on a tray, along with pudding and a drink. The other woman squeezed out four pills from a Webster pack, adding them to the tray. Diana followed them in and watched them place the tray on her grandmother's lap.

'Here you are, dearie. Your granddaughter can have lunch with you. Isn't that nice? Been a while since you've seen her, I guess. Lovely fish today.'

And the two of them were gone.

Diana sat in the chair opposite her grandmother and watched her eat.

'I hate fish. Tastes like cardboard.'

'Have you thought of your next move, Granny? Where you'd like to go?'

'I'm not going anywhere, Diana.'

She couldn't help smiling. Her grandmother certainly hadn't misheard that question.

CHAPTER SIX

Diana drove home, and wandered into the kitchen with an armful of groceries. A picture of satisfaction, Saskia sat on the kitchen bench with a large spoon in her mouth, while Stella slid a tray of patty cakes into the oven.

'I thought I'd have a practice on the quad bike before I take the kids out,' said Diana. 'Milo will love it, Sienna too, when she gets over her sulk. I'm afraid she's missing Polly, her best friend.' She put the bags on the counter.

'Can I come?' Saskia asked.

'No, better wait till I get the hang of it, Sassy.' Diana grinned and wiped a bit of cake mixture off her nose.

'It seems quite easy for me,' said Stella. 'You should manage it all right. It's a key start and the gears are on the right, the throttle on the left, I think. Everything's on the handlebars, anyway. How was your grandmother?'

'It's been ten years since I've seen her. She's a lot older, but she's still got her sense of humour.' Diana felt defensive. Actually, it had just about broken her heart and been a little too hard to take in. 'I'll be back and we'll talk later. Thanks, Mum.'

As she ran down the back steps, Diana couldn't help thinking how everything had changed—her grandmother, Rosie and Mal were barely talking, and after they'd left this morning, her parents had had an argument, over cars of all things.

'I'm not having my grandchildren driving around in a car with no brakes,' Stella had announced baldly. Diana deduced she was referring to the family car.

'There'd be no need for them to drive around in a car with no brakes if you would just take it to Bruno's to have it serviced once in a while.'

Bruno's was the garage in town where they'd always had their mechanical work done. 'He's still going?' said Diana. 'He must be at least seventy by now.'

Her father didn't look pleased. 'His son Steven has taken over most of it, but Bruno is still "going", as you put it.'

Well that wasn't the most diplomatic thing she could have said.

'Before one has one's car serviced,' Stella continued, 'you usually have to come up with the money for filters and new brake pads and oil, and all the rest.' Her mother wasn't letting it go.

'Don't be ridiculous,' said Tom. 'You don't have to be driving round in a car that's not roadworthy. Take it to Bruno's today.'

'I'm not going in today. Diana's going to see your mother and do the shopping for me.'

'Well, take it in tomorrow, or whatever bloody day you are going in.' And her father had stormed out of the room. Her mother had avoided looking at her.

* * *

It was colder today. The wind had picked up and was quite chilly. Diana picked up her father's old crackly Driza-Bone and a woollen beanie, jamming it on her head on the way out.

Examining the bike, she could see that everything was pretty similar to the ag bike she used to ride. She got on and turned the key in the ignition. No problem, it started like a charm. With a little laugh she accelerated and was off. It had a different feel from the two-wheeler she used to ride. This was much more sedate. The kids were definitely going to love it. She set off for the creek, giving her shoulders a little shake, enjoying the rush, the sudden freedom.

She didn't recall her parents fighting like that. Perhaps it was selective memory and she'd just picked out the good bits to remember. Hell, she and Charlie had some beauties.

You were getting pretty short-tempered, if I remember correctly.

Hello, Charlie. That's nonsense. Someone had to keep you on the straight and narrow. You'd forget what day of the week it was when you were painting. I could never depend on you to remember to pick up the kids ... Tell me, why does thinking about you hurt so much?'

You always thought you were tough as, maybe you're not as tough as you think?

It hurt before with Cody, but I must have forgotten. You forget about the pain that comes with childbirth—maybe it's

the same? I supressed it all after Cody. Why can't I do the same
with you? I miss you. It hurts so much, Charlie.

There was a place along the creek that was Diana's favourite place on earth. Mog's Creek wound through the farm.
It was spring fed and in dry times it dried up into a chain
of holes, one of which had always been their picnic place.
Diana stopped the bike and looked down at the graceful
weeping willows leaning over the edge of the creek and the
enormous box trees grown tall with the water and shelter
from the wind.

You loved this place, Charlie.

Do you blame me? It was the only place I got to make love
to you.

I was too embarrassed to do it in the house with my parents
in the next bedroom.

Yes, they had made love there, stretched out on his coat
in the hot sunshine, long grass prickling the backs of her
bare legs.

Forget Charlie, forget Rosie's frustrations and her parents bickering. She turned the throttle round. The wind
was blowing straight into her face as she screamed down
the hillside towards the creek, her hair whipping her cheeks.
Her eyes were streaming from the wind rush. This was so
much fun. *Yes.*

'Wait for me, Di, wait for me.'

A whisper in the wind. Cody, or was it Charlie? Damn,
she was going too fast. Cody used to say it. 'Rosie, Di, wait
for me.' Charlie would say, 'Slow down, Di, slow down. Let
it rest, tomorrow will be okay. We'll do it tomorrow.'

Diana liked going fast. Getting it finished. But it was
Charlie that had been going too fast, Charlie that hadn't
waited for tomorrow. Damn him for walking out that door.

She opened her eyes. The bike had stopped, slewed sideways in a sandy ditch. She blinked. She'd nearly gone over the handlebars. Now she was bogged, she thought, as she roared the accelerator. In a drought. What a joke. Still shaking, she got off the bike and examined it. It had one wheel down and the other up. She was really stuck. What had she been thinking? It was too heavy to lift up. She'd never had that problem with the old Yamaha. Furious with herself, she started the long walk home.

CHAPTER SEVEN

Stella was worried. Diana had been gone for an hour and a half. Where was she? Where were Tom and Milo, for that matter? She glanced at the mobile phone sitting on the hallstand—it was supposed to be with Tom so she could contact him if there was an emergency, or vice versa. The girls were in the bath and she stood, hovering at the door of the bathroom, holding pyjamas and towels, when the back door slammed and she heard voices.

'Tom, is that you? Have you seen Diana?'

'No. Where is she?'

'She wanted to take the bike out for a run –'

'The bike? For Christ sakes, Stell, she hasn't ridden one for twenty years. Stay here, Milo.' He turned and struggled to put his boots back on. 'Why on earth did you let her go?'

Stella let her breath out slowly. Right, so it was her fault. You didn't tell Diana not to do something, it was like waving a red rag at a bull. You just hoped she knew what she was doing. Ever since she was tiny she'd been that way. And, she might add, usually aided and abetted by Tom.

'Girls, out of the bath, please. And how about you get in, Milo,' Stella called. But when she went into the bathroom the girls were out of the bath already, shivering on the mat, with Milo, white-faced, beside them.

Quickly she went down on her knees, threw towels around them and pulled them close. 'Hey.' She patted the girls down. 'Don't worry.'

'Where's Mummy?'

'Milo, she just went for a little ride on the bike. It's probably run out of petrol, that's all. Tom's gone to get her. She'll be back in a minute.'

'How does he know where she went?'

'It's okay, don't worry, Tommo knows where she would have gone.' And that was the truth. She would have gone to Mog's Creek, for sure.

*   *   *

The family sat round the table together. Her family. Her mother and father at either end, Mal beside her dad, then Rosie and the children. The table was set with two fat candles and the old silver, and another bowl of the bright pink chrysanthemums.

'So where's the bike now?'

Mal sounded amused. He was the only one. Her dad had given her a rocket. As for the kids, Diana didn't want to see that look on their faces ever again.

'Down nearly at the creek. There's an erosion gully I don't seem to remember being there before.'

'Just like old times, Diana.' Mal grinned at her.

'You were the one getting bogged mostly, I seem to remember.'

'Yes, you were good at pushing me off the track.'

'I don't remember that. Not remotely.' Diana raised her glass to him. 'It just helped make you a better rider.'

'I don't think the children need to hear how the two of you used to stack the bikes,' Rosie interrupted.

'Probably not. Would you kids like any more?' The three of them looked at each other.

'No, thank you.' Milo spoke up. 'Can we ring Grandpa and tell him we're here?'

'Of course.' Stella was up immediately. 'Is it a good time over there, Diana? I think it should be. Milo, come with me and I'll ring the number for you.'

Sienna and Saskia came over and wrapped their arms around her tightly.

'Don't worry,' said Diana, 'I won't do that again. Everything's okay, kids. Come on, say goodnight to everyone and we'll go and tell Grandma about the plane.' She got up and the three of them moved as one to the telephone in the hall.

It was almost half an hour later that she walked back into the dining room.

'Patrick told me today that you couldn't predict what the economy is going to do. Best to sit and wait it out.' Mal leant forward, pushing his plate aside.

'I just can't understand why wool won't go up when the dollar is so cheap against the American dollar. Nothing is certain anymore.'

'Who's Patrick?' Diana reached out and took a piece of crusty bread and buttered it.

'Patrick Morley, my boss,' said Mal. 'Honestly, Tom, why you stick with sheep is a mystery. If you had a few cows and a bull, you'd find that if sheep prices are down, cattle prices are usually up and you've covered your bets.' Mal was trying hard to hold back his frustration.

'Damn cows!' said Tom. 'I want them on the place like I'd want a hole in the head. If they're not kicking you for the hell of it, they're knocking down the fences and pugging up the dams.'

Her father wasn't giving in. Diana watched with interest Rosie's closed eyes and her mum's rolling ones. They'd heard this before. 'Farming's always seemed to me to be a bit of a gamble,' she offered.

'It all depends on your position. You can relax if you have everything covered and don't owe too much,' said Mal, as he passed the mutton casserole to Tom and reached for the mashed potatoes. 'I think farmers have been kicked in the guts for just a bit too long. If everything hangs on an inch of rain and you've lost badly the previous few years and you're hundreds of thousands in debt ...' He shrugged.

'That's why I like to stay with what I know and like.' Her father sounded grim. 'There's no one else to blame if you go under.'

'I hate the way these conversations degenerate so quickly,' said Rosie. 'We've heard it so many times before.' She turned to Diana. 'Did you know Philly did really well in her exams last year?'

'Mum was telling me about her course. She really likes it then?'

'It's the best hospitality course in the state, she told me last week.'

Stella frowned. 'I thought she said they had one of the best lecturers in the state, didn't she?'

Rosie tossed her curls back. 'More or less the same thing.'

Diana picked up her glass again and settled back in the chair. *Relax, settle*, she told herself, swirling the red wine around her glass. It was a beautiful Australian cab merlot. She squinted at the label on the bottle but she'd never heard of it.

'Well, at least we don't have to spend as much on fertilizer as we would if we had cattle on the place. You can't fatten cattle without it.'

Mal didn't answer.

'We'll never know, will we?' Rosie disappeared into the kitchen.

Rosie was always quick to point the accusing finger, and then equally as fast to duck for cover. Stella, as usual, was up and down and busy serving. Family, familiar—they must have come from the same Latin root. Which one came first, Diana wondered. She felt removed from the farming conversation, but what could she expect? There was a piece of her dying to be part of everything again. Once upon a time she used to have opinions. Her dad and Mal would listen to them, too.

Rosie was back with a tub of ice cream for the table. 'This must all be so boring compared to conversations in London!'

She sounded bitter. Everyone looked down or at the wall.

Diana was shocked out of her reverie. London.

No. She paled and the world went dizzy for a second.

There was a pause. 'Oh, I'm sorry, Diana. I didn't mean it like that.' Rosie went back into the kitchen.

Diana tried to rise and follow her but the room started to spin and she sat down again. The last two days had been huge—the drive from Sydney, stacking the bike, family politics … She was just so tired.

Mal frowned at her. 'Hey! You're probably better off just sitting for now.'

'I just wanted to tell her it was okay. Everyone doesn't have to go round treading on eggshells.'

'Rosie just speaks before she thinks sometimes,' Stella said.

And her mother was still sticking up for her. Diana swallowed the resentment and laughed. 'So do I. It must be a family failing. It's okay. I'm sorry, I can't … I just don't want to think about … London, right now.'

'Who'd like some ice cream?' said Tom.

'Not for me thanks, Dad.' Diana turned to Mal. 'So what's it like, working for this Patrick?'

'Okay, for a city bloke, I guess.'

'Oh, I think he's wonderful, Diana. Just wait till you meet him,' said Stella. 'We met him first in the bushfire we had about four years ago. I'm sure we told you. It took us all by surprise. It was the most horrible fiery day, anything could have happened. Temperature was over forty and the wind suddenly changed and Lost Valley was in trouble. Tom raced over to help Patrick save his home and the sheds.'

'We had to move pretty fast,' said Tom.

'And then I had to call Dad up on the CB to hightail it back here,' Stella went on. 'The smoke had thickened and was swirling round the house. I couldn't see more than a foot in front of my face. Patrick came back and helped us. He's been a good friend ever since.' She got up and stacked some plates. 'Coffee or tea anyone? Rosie, come and sit down.'

Rosie had reappeared and, rather unhappily, took her seat at the table.

'A little more red, Dad?' Diana held out her glass. 'Mal would like some more, too.' Mal laughed.

'Do you really think you need another?' her father asked.

She frowned. No one had said that to her for twenty years, and then she smiled ruefully at her dad. 'No, but it might help me get to sleep,' she said. 'Lost Valley is such a beautiful old place. It would have been a pity if it had burned down.'

'Patrick loves it. He's always tinkering with some idea or other. But then he's got plenty of money.' Tom poured some more wine into Diana's glass and went to fill up Mal's.

'Thanks Tom.'

'Don't you think that's enough, Mal?' Rosie echoed her father's comment.

'I think I should be able to manage a half a kilometre down the road without mishap,' he snapped.

'Yes, I didn't mean ... Oh, you are impossible.'

Diana's head started to pound. Nasty ones that did a zip round first.

'Can't you two let up for a while?' said Tom. 'Diana's not well.'

'Oh, that's right. Poor Diana! She's bogged the bike, had Mum and Dad worried out of their minds, but let's all consider Diana, shall we?'

Rosie got up and walked out. Mal took off after her, mumbling apologies.

Diana looked at her father. 'Jeez, I'm sorry, Dad.'

He shook his head and shrugged.

'No, I mean about the bike, I hope it's all right. If it needs fixing I can take it into Bruno.' She stood. 'I have to get the car back to him anyway. He can sort out getting it back to Sydney.'

'Don't worry about it, Diana. The main thing is you're all right. You're tired, you should go to bed.'

Diana weighed the truth in that statement and sighed gratefully. 'Okay. Goodnight, Dad, sleep tight.'

'Don't let the bed bugs bite.' Tom smiled, finishing off the rhyme they used to say to each other when Diana was a child.

CHAPTER EIGHT

When Diana woke the next morning Saskia was lying all over her. Damn, she was taking up most of the bed. Extricating herself, she carefully moved Saskia further over, lay back and examined the ceiling of her old room.

So you think you've done the right thing?

It's too early to tell but it has to be the right thing, Charlie, being in London was not good.

That's the bed your parents bought for us when we came over for 'the visit'.

It was our honeymoon. At least we didn't get another. So I guess it was.

It had all started okay. Charlie was on his best behaviour, then Rosie got spiteful and jealous and her parents became stiff and uncommunicative. And Charlie, well Charlie got all possessive. Diana had felt she was in the middle of a giant tug of war.

No wonder I didn't want to come back. The only person who liked me was your grandmother.

And that was the truth. *She remembers you, too. What a God awful mess it was.*

England seemed so empty without Charlie. England was Charlie. 'Time for bed, Di,' he'd say, when she'd forgotten the time and was up to her ears in clay. He'd stick his head round the door with a big grin on his face and refuse to leave till she'd packed up. Different matter when he'd been immersed in his painting. Strange, but she missed the annoying things almost as much as his endearing qualities.

Seven blurred weeks and she couldn't remember anything from one minute to the next. The four of them had been so lost. That evening, after she'd spoken to Sebastian, she'd waited till six o'clock, and then she'd picked the phone up and just told her mother they were coming home. Australia, Mum, Dad, Rosie and Mog's Hill. She'd needed it like a drowning man needed oxygen.

Diana considered her options now. Was she being selfish, dumping herself and the kids on her parents? Surely a few weeks in twenty years wasn't asking too much. No one seemed all that excited to see her. How happy were Rosie and Mal at the moment? Was there a problem? She must ask her mother. They looked as if they were going to jump down each other's throats, and her parents were no better. And Granny, that made her want to cry. What was wrong with everyone? She closed her eyes.

'Mummy.'

Diana groaned and opened her eyes again. A pair of honey-coloured eyes were trained on her with the intensity of laser beams.

* * *

After breakfast, Diana watched out the kitchen window as the red bike and Mal—with an ecstatic Milo on his lap— came into view, followed by her dad in the ute. The bike must have started all right. Mal and Milo were both wearing helmets. Funny, only wimps wore helmets twenty years ago.

'Thank heavens, they're here. It must be okay.' She went outside on to the verandah.

'Mummy, I've been steering.' Milo's eyes were shining and with a shy smile he looked up at his uncle. 'Thanks Mal.'

That had to be the happiest she'd seen him look for months.

Mal was undoing the buckle under his chin. 'It's okay, pal. Won't be long and you'll be doing it yourself.'

'Mummy, Mummy, the bike's all right!' Milo was running up the steps.

Diana laughed as he launched himself at her. 'Careful. I'm so glad everyone's got their priorities right. Where's the sympathy for your poor mother?'

'I don't suppose anyone told you, you don't lean in when turning a corner on these quad bikes.' Mal was amused.

'Well, better late than never. I'll know next time.'

'And next time you go out, you wear a helmet.'

Diana made a face at him and muttered, 'We never did before.'

'That was then, now you do.' Frowning, Mal turned back. 'No after effects? You're okay?'

'I'm fine. My pride is dented.'

They wandered back into the kitchen. Diana idly picked up an apple and bit into it.

Stella looked up. 'Who do you want to catch up with now you're home?'

'No one. It's so good to see you all and just be here. Making up for lost time.'

'What about Megan? Is she still down the coast?'

'She is. I should get down there, I suppose. The kids would love it. I wonder where Johann is?'

'Who was Johann?' said Stella. 'Oh, I remember, he was one of the boys in that flat you shared when you were at college.'

'He and Paul, Megan and I, we were going to conquer the world. Now Paul's dead, Johann wanders aimlessly round the world. Megan does random art things down the coast, and I'm a potter in London.'

'You're pretty successful though. You've achieved your aim.'

'I suppose.' Diana was thoughtful. 'What is success? I used to rate success pretty highly. I don't know what's really important anymore. I wanted to be a farmer. Do you think I would have made a good farmer, Mum?'

'Mummy, Mummy, we've found a sculpture!' Sienna's clear accented voice reached them before they saw the two little figures rushing out from the behind the sheds.

Diana exchanged a look with her mother. Puzzled, they went back out on to the verandah to two excited faces.

'Mummy, Mummy, Stella, come and look!' Sienna dragged Diana down the steps and behind the tool shed where she saw the 'sculpture'.

Collapsing with laughter Diana clutched Stella. 'What a hoot! It's a grader. You poor, over-cultured English babies!'

Before them up against the fence, in all its rusty-orange decayed glory, stood the Aveling Barford Grader. Her father had a passion for smooth, well-formed roads. This was just one in a long line of graders he'd bought over the years. God knows where it had come from. Diana circled the grand old machine, seeing for the first time its beautiful sculptured lines, the sweeping round discs above the blade.

'I do see what you mean though,' she said. 'It is magnificent.'

The grass was growing up through it. Obviously it hadn't been moved for a while. Milo tried to climb up into the cab but couldn't reach the bottom step.

Diana went to lift Milo up into the cab. 'Lord, it must be sixty years old, it's an antique. The kids would only have seen something like this in the sculpture parks we dragged them around in London,' she said, turning to her mother with a smile.

'It doesn't look like a grader,' Milo argued.

True, it had little in common with the modern, yellow variety. 'It's a very old one,' Diana explained. 'Tommo uses it for smoothing the roads. He loves to make the drive all even, with drains for the water to run off.'

'One of the advantages of the drought—there hasn't been enough rain to damage the roads lately,' her mother said drily. 'Tom does love that thing but he hasn't done any grading for a long while. He gets up in it every now and again just to turn the engine over.'

'You should get Tommo to show you his old bike. It's a beauty,' Diana told Milo.

Stella laughed 'Only if you've got a few hours to spare.'

A large truck with four tiers of hay was coming up the drive. They all went to watch it being unloaded.

CHAPTER NINE

The next week zipped past, introducing the children to the farm and trying to get them to be comfortable with her grandmother, which was a bit difficult as she never remembered who they were. Diana's main problem was avoiding heart-to-heart talks with her mother. She had no desire to open up and talk about herself. None whatsoever. Just thinking about Charlie was a no-go zone. She'd managed it before, pushed thoughts of home and her mother and father away when she'd gone to England, surely she could do the same in reverse. That was her plan anyway.

On the way into town, with Diana driving, Stella beside her and the two girls in the back, she saw the bare brown paddocks and the dusty gum trees beside the road. Either early winter frosts or the fact it had been some weeks since the last rain had dried everything off. The pale green fuzz she'd noticed on her arrival was fast disappearing. Slowly, the drought was making an impact.

'When do you think it's going to rain again?' said Diana. 'I don't know how you keep going. It's pretty depressing, isn't it? I mean you get, what, twenty millimetres the other day and the grass starts to grow and then it doesn't rain for weeks or months. I hadn't realised how awful it was.'

Her mother didn't answer.

'Why doesn't Dad want to come to town?'

'He never wants to come to town these days. I don't know, he's not very social at the moment, he doesn't seem to enjoy other people's company. Maybe it's because all any one talks about is the drought. At the moment I'm trying to get him to go to the Picnic Races. They're on in a couple of weeks. Patrick has invited us but he's saying no. Still, if anyone can talk him into going, it'll be Patrick.'

'How old is this Patrick?'

'In his fifties I guess, or late forties. He and your father get on really well. Patrick asks questions and then listens to the answer. It's very flattering, and quite unusual. You know, the older you get the less people really want to know what you think.'

'Mum, you're not old.' Diana laughed and gave her a little pat on the leg. 'I remember never being able to go to the Picnic Races because they were on a Friday.'

'They're on Saturdays now.' Stella sighed. 'We haven't been for years. Try to talk your father into it. We could all go.'

Diana dropped Stella and Saskia off at the shops and took Sienna to see Granny. Milo had disappeared with Tommo again, and she couldn't help feeling a little jolt of satisfaction—those two were getting along so well.

Sienna was the shyest of her children. It was only recently she'd removed her fingers from her mouth where they'd seemed permanently lodged. She hadn't just sucked her thumb, but at least three fingers at once. Of all the kids, she was getting on best with Peg, even though Peg never remembered who Sienna was. But Sienna sat quietly while they talked, and seemed to love to listen to Peg ramble on about the past.

After they arrived, Diana found the photo albums for Sienna to look at.

'What's this, Granny?'

It was an old photo, black and white, with an old truck and a youthful Granny and Grandpa standing beside it armed with sticks. Diana couldn't remember seeing it before. She lifted the album off the floor and placed it on Peg's lap. She and Sienna leant on the chair either side to see.

'Goodness, that was the truck that came to get the rabbits.'

'Rabbits?' Diana was stunned. Why would they need a truck for that? 'What rabbits?'

'When we were first married and went to Mog's Hill, there was a terrible plague of rabbits. There were rabbits everywhere. You'd look out and it seemed as if the hill was moving. Ugh! Frank employed an army of rabbiters—about thirty of them at one stage—and we got about twelve thousand one week.'

'Twelve thousand, that's impossible!'

'Tell that to the rabbits. We sold them to the local abattoir. Of course, they had to be skinned too. That was my job, to turn the skins inside out. We could get one pound for a pound of skins. Eight skins to a pound. Good money. Someone cut the head off and I helped pull the skins off and peg them out on some wire. Frank didn't trust them though, said you had to watch them.'

'Watch who?'

'The Rabbiters, of course. It wasn't in their best interest, was it, to get rid of them all? Leave a couple behind and hey presto, job continuity. Frank had to watch them, all right.'

Diana snuck a look at her daughter, and Sienna looked horrified. She turned the page quickly. Her grandfather was holding up a snake. It reached to the ground.

'He was a beauty, wasn't he?' Peg said with some relish. 'A king brown, quite unusual really, didn't find many of them.'

Diana wondered whether to close the book, find something her grandmother could reminisce about safely that wouldn't scare Sienna to death. She picked up another album. There were the pictures of herself and Rosie and Cody.

Well she'd asked for this one. The inevitable question.

'Who is that baby?' asked Sienna.

'That's me. That is Rosie and the baby is Cody.'

Diana was unprepared for the wave of sadness that swept over her when she looked at the round baby face. She and Rosie had adored Cody.

'Was Cody your sister too?'

She'd told the kids before about Cody. They'd obsessed about it at the time, but maybe Sienna had forgotten.

'How is Cody?' Peg asked suddenly.

Diana blinked. She never knew when she was going to come out with something random. 'Oh Granny, you remember, she died a long time ago, when she was six.' A look at Sienna's expression had her rising to her feet. 'I'm sorry, look at the time. We've got to go, Mum's waiting for us.'

They left, leaving Granny looking through the album on her lap, singing gently to herself.

*   *   *

On the drive back to the hospital, where they were to meet Stella and Saskia, Diana got sick of questions about Cody. How old? How big? Who did she like best? Where did she sleep? Why was she called Cody? It made her so sad.

'I've got no idea, ask Stella. That's enough questions. Look, here's where we can get some DVDs.'

'Why don't Tom and Stella have Foxtel?' Sienna asked, as they got out of the car.

'Oh Sienna.' Diana laughed. 'Here in rural Australia, they aren't quite as up to date as London in this stuff. Trust me, you can get some lovely films on DVD, and all the same shows,' she assured her.

'Mummy, why doesn't Granny know who I am?'

'Granny's very old and her memory's failing her, although she can remember what happened in the past as clear as day. I wish you could have known Granny as I knew her. She was such an amazing strong woman. She worked so hard mustering and helping Grandfather Frank with the sheep. I think she loved Mog's Hill as much as he did. I love her so much, Sienna, but she's getting old. We just have to be patient.'

'Okay.' Sienna slipped her hand in hers.

They left the store weighed down with seven DVDs—a full week's viewing in the white plastic bag.

Walking through the quiet hospital once again, without the sense of urgency she'd had last time, they pushed their way in through the door of the kitchen.

'Rosie!' Diana called.

She appeared round the corner , tucking her hair into the paper cap they had to wear in the kitchen.

'Hello, you two! Sit up here, Sienna, and I'll get you a biscuit. How was Granny?'

CHAPTER TEN

It had been just two weeks and, fingers crossed, they were settling in beautifully. The kids were so relaxed, a holiday was obviously what they'd needed—okay, what she'd needed. Diana grinned at her daughters, and shook the dice vigorously in her hands.

'One. Not good but not too bad. Your go, Sassy.'

Stella stuck her head round the door. 'Your father said to remind you he wanted you to come and look at the sheep.'

Diana looked up from the game of snakes and ladders she was playing with the girls. Her father had said this morning he thought more young lambs were ready to be drafted off their mothers. Then they'd send the next lot off to sale. 'Where is he?'

'He's up in the machinery shed. With Milo.'

Saskia threw a two. 'No!' she screamed.

'Down you go. Poor Sassy,' said Sienna with relish. 'Justice. I had to slide two rows on my last go.'

'Mum, you'll have to stand in for me. I'm nearly there, I only need a four.' Diana jumped up.

'But, Diana ...' Her mother relented as she looked at the entreating faces of her granddaughters. 'All right.' She sank to the floor. 'When is it my turn?'

Diana found Tom and Milo in the sheep yards. Tom was bent over, examining the wool on one of the mothers. He parted the wool downwards with his fingers, exposing the bright, white centre. 'Look at this wool, Milo, it's a good length, colour's good. Beautiful.' His excitement was infectious.

Diana laughed. She loved watching her dad with his sheep. Now here she was seeing her son experience the magic. She climbed over the fence into the yards. 'It's a real shame to be selling off these *beautiful* young merinos, just when you've got them so right.' She couldn't help teasing him.

'Times have changed. I can get good money now for these young'uns, it's been one of the benefits of getting them so big. I'm surprised they've done as well as they have, as the season has been pretty dry and not much feed. Diana, catch that one over there.'

She grabbed it under the chin with one hand, the other on its tail, and guided it over to the fence.

'You haven't lost your touch, Diana.' He chuckled. 'You've always been handy with the sheep. Now, this one's not so good, Milo. Look at the teeth—if they can't chew properly they'll never grow.'

Diana couldn't help but laugh as she watched Milo copying her father, peering into the sheep's mouth, seriously examining the bite and then scrunching the wool to feel its density.

Tom was concentrating on the sheep he'd nudged against the fence and was holding in place with his hip as he inspected its wool. 'Mmm, no, this one's a cull.' Then he let the sheep go. 'Milo, open that gate. I'll put him in the yard there.'

Diana found herself at the back of the mob just watching the two of them.

Your father never used to ask me to do things for him. Milo's not bad, though, is he?

Sorry Charlie, you were hopeless in the yards, always in the wrong spot. You never seemed to understand that sheep go away from you, not towards you.

He's not frightened of them, is he?

No, I'm so proud of him.

Was she creating these conversations with Charlie? Did they have these kinds of conversations, really? Or was it her imagination? Last night had been bad. She couldn't sleep. Charlie was in her head, asking what was it she wanted out of this trip home. There were no real answers. Or rather, so many it would have taken hours to sort them all out. She'd had to get up and make herself a cup of tea. Luckily Saskia hadn't woken.

'Thank you for taking the time to go and see Mum, it's so good for her,' Tom interrupted her reverie, as the sheep circled around them.

'You know I love her so much.'

'Two of a kind, you two. You know I see a lot of my mother in you, Diana, and frankly, I can't do it. See her like she is. So thank you.'

'I owe her plenty. She was always ready to listen to my problems in my teenage years.'

Diana looked at her father over the backs of the sheep, and then clapped her hands and whistled to get the sheep moving into the next yard.

* * *

'You've missed a call from the medical centre.' Stella looked up as Tom walked past her to the sink. He looked tired. 'Did you miss your appointment again?'

'Probably.' He stopped to fill a glass of water.

'Have you made another?'

'No, I haven't. I haven't got time. Stupid doctors, all they want to do is test after test. It's costing the country a fortune and for no bloody sense that I can work out.'

'Do you want me to make one for you?'

'No, I don't. I'm feeling okay, and it can all wait until Diana goes back. So just leave it.' Angry, he put the glass into the sink. 'And don't talk about it to the girls, either.'

Stella watched him go. What was he on about? His hands were shaking, it simply was not like Tom to act like this. It was probably pretty stressful, having everyone here, she guessed it might be taking its toll on him. She'd try to see he got some quiet time this afternoon. She looked at the clock. Damn, Rosie would be waiting. Stella had said ten minutes ago she'd meet her at the gate with Peg's washing, so she wouldn't have to come all the way up here.

Stella picked up the washing basket and slipped outside and into her little car. She felt a little guilty as she pulled up at Rosie's entrance. She hadn't seen much of her second daughter since Diana had come home.

'How're things?' Rosie was leaning against her car as Stella pulled up.

'Busy. I've got to get back to prepare lunch. They're big lunches these days, and Milo eats enough for four. I must admit I don't see a lot of Milo, he's Tom's little shadow.'

'Well, Dad must be enjoying that, I guess,' said Rosie. 'No worries. It fitted in perfectly as my shift starts at two. Could you do with some eggs?' She handed over two egg cartons as she took the basket of Peg's washing from Stella. 'Guess what, the hospital want more of my organic free range eggs—they love 'em. So I'm getting more chooks on the weekend.'

'Wonderful. You're so good with those chooks. When we had them, they used to look so smugly at me, as if to say "no eggs for you today". I never knew what I was doing wrong but I'd obviously insulted them.' Stella smiled. 'How are things with you? I'm sorry we haven't met up for our coffee recently. It's all been so hectic.'

'That's okay. I heard from Philly yesterday.'

'Oh, how's she doing?'

'Fine. I miss her so much but she'll be home at the end of this semester for the holidays. I'm dying for Diana to see her. Will they stay that long do you think?' Rosie asked. 'How's Dad doing with all the people in the house?'

Stella shook her head. 'I don't know what's the matter with him. He's not himself. He won't talk to me about it, he just blows up or stalks out of the room.'

'I wish you'd get him to talk to someone.'

'Ha, really, can you see that happening?'

'Granny is enjoying having Diana around, isn't she?' Rosie sounded a little wistful.

'Well, I think it's been good for Diana too. They've always had a special rapport. She was wound up so tight when she got back. I think she likes talking to Peg because she adored Charlie and they can just talk about the old days. And that's where Peg is happiest.'

'A few weeks here will be good for Diana. She can slow down a bit. She always goes at a hundred miles an hour.'

'Well, I'd like her to open up and start talking to me,' said Stella. 'I've tried everything I know, but Diana just clams up or changes the subject. She's not really coping. She gets up at two in the morning, wanders around the house and makes herself a cup of tea. I don't know who she thinks she's fooling.' She stopped and gazed at the empty road stretching out in front of her. 'I could never understand Diana's fascination with Charlie.' She glanced at Rosie. 'I shouldn't say that, should I? I did get a different side of him in England, but that honeymoon trip, when they came out here, he was so remotely polite. He seemed to think he was doing us some great favour, lending us Diana for a couple of weeks. It was difficult working him out.'

'Well, he's gone, and what's Diana going to do now?' said Rosie. 'That's what I'd like to know. She's not thinking of staying is she?'

'I wish she was. It would be the best—'

'I think that would be an idiotic move,' Rosie interrupted. 'She's a famous artist living in London. What on earth would she find good about living round here? Give me the opportunity and I'd be out of here like a flash.'

Stella looked at her daughter. 'Are you serious? I've never heard you say that before.'

'Never wanted to before.' she sighed. 'Mal gets me down sometimes. He's pretty frustrated at the moment. I wish you two would get a bit more definitive about what your plans might be?' She looked at her watch. 'Mum, I've got to go. Music Club auditions for the Soiree are tomorrow night—wish me luck. Don't pay any attention to my whinging. Love you.' And with a quick kiss and a hug she was off.

* * *

Lunch was nearly ready. Diana and the girls should be back from town any moment. Stella was humming to the radio and smiled. It was a long time since she'd cut sandwiches into little triangles.

Two sons-in-law she'd been allotted, but Mal and Charlie were very different men. She knew which one she liked best. Was she being unfair to Charlie? He certainly had charm. And he'd been so different in London. On her first and only trip to London, he'd shown her around one day, taken her to have her first pint of bitter at the 'local'. His parents, Janet and Bill Sutton, were good people, well meaning. Charlie was just … oh, damned if she knew.

Picking up a couple of Saskia's hair ribbons, she smiled and put them on the shelf beside the stove. She was so like Rosie. Stella couldn't help it, she just loved her to death. She was always saying such funny, bright things. Stella had gone to England for two weeks when Saskia was born. It would have been more fun if Tom had come too and if Diana hadn't been so exhausted. But at least she'd got to see Gospel Oak where they lived, where they shopped, just the little things that helped her see the kind of life Diana was leading.

They were really very good children. Sienna was just like Diana, stubborn as all get out. She didn't envy Diana the next few years while they were going head to head. On the other hand, it was poetic justice, wasn't it? With a little smile, she went over to the window.

She'd missed all their tiny, growing years. Photos just didn't do it, and the phone calls were fairly spaced apart. Longer and longer—the space apart, not the phone calls.

Tom had said not to worry, that they needed to live their own lives, but that didn't take away her need to be part of their lives. She could be happy with even just a little part. Being half a world away didn't help. There were simply a few things Tom and she didn't agree on. Not many, but more than there used to be.

In a marriage lasting forty-two years you'd think everything would be sorted. Were they just getting older and all the pressure of coping with all these dry years taking its toll, or was it depression, like Rosie said? Did she really want to know? She wished Tom would see someone. She couldn't imagine him going to Will Talbot, their doctor, and asking him something like that. He'd die first. Men were impossible when it came to their health.

And if it wasn't one child it was the other. Her youngest daughter was unhappy, restless. Or was it only Mal? And it's hard for a mother when her child leaves home. It changes everything. This was Phillipa's second year away and they were all missing her, but it must be really awful for Rosie. After being a mother full-on, you have to find another reason to be on this earth, another direction. If only she'd been able to have some more kids, it would have made such a difference for her. Rosie and Mal had even tried IVF around ten years ago, when Diana started having children, but the endometriosis flared right back up again. The IVF drugs had caused it, apparently. So it was just not meant to be, but it was very sad all the same. Rosie had wanted another child so much.

The weather report started on the radio and she turned it off. Damn the weather. The succession problem had to be resolved. The understanding was Tom would retire when he was seventy, but he was seventy now and he wasn't showing any signs of retiring. No wonder he was short-tempered all the time. Her husband and her son-in-law did not seem to be able to work together. Mal was a terrific stockman but he couldn't stand sheep, and Tom had never had cattle on the place. The thought of his flock dispersing just about broke his heart.

Stella put a tea towel over the sandwiches. But it was now Tom's turn to find another direction. Then there was the small matter of what they would have to live on. She'd suggested they move into Mal and Rosie's house, but that didn't solve the problem. What on earth were they going to do?

She walked over to the yards to get Tom and Milo for lunch, humming to herself. It was such a glorious day, with a blue, blue sky and not a cloud in sight. Clear and cool. A pair of Mountain Lorikeets swooped and chattered from tree to tree with flashes of blue and red. As long as it wasn't the white cockatoos, she didn't mind. They were so destructive, so raucous. She'd been known to get out Tom's gun and shoot at them on occasion, not that she'd ever hit many. They'd just fly around for a bit and then settle back down on the branches, swaying and chattering among themselves, as though nothing had happened.

She stood there watching for a little while. Tom was nearly finished drenching the mob of sheep in the yards. He was halfway down the last race. Despite the slight chill in the air, Tom was sweating. It was such back-breaking work, struggling with each sheep to put that wretched pipe down its throat. Using your knees and free arm to pull their head up for the second it takes.

The sheep weren't helping, not that Stella blamed them. She wouldn't much like that pipe thrust down her throat, either. Milo stood at the end of the race, opening the gate after Tom finished to let the sheep out. She used to do that. A hundred years ago, as a young bride. It had been so much fun. Then the girls took over. Then it was her turn again after they left home. *Tom is seventy years old. Hasn't he got any sense at all?* Surely he could see it was time to pack it in.

'Hey, lunch is ready.'

Later that afternoon Stella went to find Tom. He was in the office. There weren't many private spots in the house at the moment. She went in quietly. He was sitting at the desk with the accounts spread out before him. He was asleep with his head flung back on the chair, snoring slightly, and it was still an hour or so before dinner. She left him to it.

* * *

They were sitting round the table at dinner. Stella watched the children, Diana and Tom, picking their way through the lamb casserole, thick slices of bread and butter, and green peas.

'Granny talked the other day about the rabbit plague, just after they were married,' Diana said.

'Rabbits, I've forgotten all about them,' said Tom. 'Like they were, that is. Repressed it, more likely. That rabbit plague lasted for twenty years. I remember when all we ate was rabbit. Rabbit roasted, stewed and fricasseed. Put me off rabbit for life. Thank you, Stella, for never serving me rabbit.' He put out his hand to pat her arm. She smiled back.

'We fenced and poisoned and dug out and shot rabbits every spare minute we had. Everyone had a pack of hunting dogs, which we fed on rabbit. Lord, I remember the bastards were so thick when you drove them into a netting fence they just packed into each other. Then the rest could just run up over their backs and hop over the fence!' Tom shuddered.

'Why were there so many rabbits?' said Milo.

Stella smiled. She was learning Milo was never short of a question. He reminded her of Cody that way.

'Some fool brought some out from England. I think his name was Austin, the damn idiot. They just loved this country so much they went mad and bred up until they were totally out of control, because they didn't have any predators,' Tom said.

'What's a predator?'

'Something that eats it,' Diana answered. 'Everything has something to eat it, to keep the numbers down. I think it's called the food chain.'

'Who eats us?' Milo paused with his fork halfway to his mouth, as the thought suddenly struck him.

'Sharks eat us,' Sienna piped up.

'Oh come on, that's enough. Who wants pudding?' Diana stood, gathering the plates together.

One good thing was that Milo was coming out of his shell, and Tom was laughing. He didn't do that much these days.

CHAPTER ELEVEN

All of a sudden it was May and the days were getting shorter with brilliant blue skies. Nearly winter—but it was nothing like the English winter, where the sun had virtually disappeared by four in the afternoon, Diana thought, as she made her way to the meat house.

A sheep was hanging upside down on a curved wire hook outside the little shed. A large puddle of vermilion blood pooled underneath it on the concrete slab. There was nothing like the colour of real blood. The neck was severed and the head was still hanging by the skin.

Diana watched as her father cut the outside skin, down the belly from the top to the bottom. She observed how efficient he was. Quick, fast cuts from the razor sharp knife. The body was all loose and soft. She put her hand inside to separate the outside skin. Inside you could feel the warmth, the heat of the dead sheep.

She shivered. Charlie had been so cold.

The hospital where the policemen had taken her was a big place, enormous, with hundreds of people running every which way. They'd all been very kind to her, hadn't made her wait hardly at all before showing her into the cubicle where Charlie lay on the bed, his eyes closed. He was so still. Diana had picked up his hand but it was cold. She remembered rubbing it to try and make him warm again. Someone had to tell her he'd died. She'd thought he was asleep. His face, not a mark. There was nothing to show—

'Diana. What are you doing?'

Diana shook her head to lose the memory, the unwelcome images. 'Sorry.'

Punching, her father called it, but it was more a sliding, using the fingers and knuckles to separate the wool-covered outer skin from the skin that would keep the carcass in shape. It was important not to break through either of them. You had to slide between them. It was quite hard work, but she hadn't forgotten how to do it.

'Mum said you don't go to church anymore.'

Her father grunted. 'They are a mob of bloody hypocrites. I've lost my faith in a God that won't send rain to people who need it. I got sick of thanking him for disaster, every week, putting the little envelope in the plate. It was a waste of good money, I was thinking.'

'You and Mum used to make us go all the time. Every Sunday.'

The skin was off, and Diana carried it over to the fence where they always dried the skins, hanging it inside out to dry.

'You needed the instruction,' said Tom. 'Your mother liked to go. I don't think Rosie and Mal go much. Here hold this.'

Diana held the bucket steady as the guts spilled into it with a rush. So many slippery insides in a sheep, all quickly sliced away.

'What's the retirement plan, Dad? You must have some super stashed away.'

He lifted the bucket up. 'Bloody super. The little we had I cashed a couple of years ago and it's gone in feed bills. You tell me, Diana.'

'Rosie and Mal are champing at the bit. Impatient to take over.'

'Well, they might be—doesn't change the fact we've nothing to retire with. Now we've Mum to sort out, those retirement places cost a fortune. I'm not moving into town and that's that,' he said flatly. 'I've realised *we* could easily have another twenty years to go. It makes you want to hang on to what you've got for as long as possible. While I've still got two arms and legs in reasonable working order.' He looked up sharply. 'Hope you don't need money?'

'No, no, nothing like that. We're fine. It's just you lot that seem to be in a mess.'

'I'm sorry, Diana. Twenty years ago it all seemed so simple. There was going to be money for you, and there will be after Mum goes.'

Diana watched him empty the bucket into the pit. He looked strong but he was more stooped than he used to be. Crushed might be a better description. Not quite as quick in the yards either, she'd noticed.

'These last few years everything has fallen apart. Wool prices are bad, and the cost of fuel and fertilizer is sky-rocketing. Maybe it'd be better for Mal and Rosie to get out now, quit wanting to take over the farm. Maybe I'd be doing them a favour.'

Somehow she didn't think Rosie would agree. Diana used her weight to let down the sheep slowly, while her father took the carcass off the wire hanger and carried it over his shoulder into the meat house.

She followed him into the small room with its hanging meat hooks and the butchering block, a solid tree trunk that had been there forever. All openings were netted with wire gauze to protect from the flies, not that there were many around at this time of year. Steadying the hooks for her father, Diana couldn't help notice that it wasn't quite as easy for him as it used to be. She wished that he'd let her do more to help.

She sloshed water over the blood on the concrete. She didn't know where she stood in trying to talk her parents into leaving; they certainly didn't seem to be any closer to a solution than they'd ever been. She began to feel a bit sorry for Rosie. What an awful situation. Thank God she was out of it.

They walked back through the gathering gloom to the house, to light and warmth and family and the smell of dinner cooking.

* * *

'What do you think about putting the children in school while you're here?' Stella asked while serving out dinner.

'No, I don't want to go to school!' Sienna was quick off the mark.

'You'll make some friends and have fun. It's a good little school. Mummy, Rosie and Cody all went there, and I'm sure the Headmaster, Mr Lloyd, will let you in.'

'Why, have you asked him already?' Diana was amused. She'd witnessed her mother's not-so-subtle machinations before. She smelled a rat.

'I might have mentioned it. I saw him today in the supermarket. He said they had vacancies since the Collins left. Anyway, three more is not impossible, apparently.'

'What do you think, Milo?' Diana addressed her eldest, noticing the anxious look on his face.

'Do I have to, Mummy?'

'No. There's your answer, Mum. My children wouldn't know what hit them—a whole school with two teachers and thirty kids.' She loved her mother but sometimes she wished she was a little less meddling. Diana wasn't twenty anymore, and she'd finished needing someone to organise her, quite some time ago.

'Let's just leave it. There's plenty of time.'

CHAPTER TWELVE

Town was always busier on a Friday, when a lot of the city farmers came up for the weekend. The local cafe was almost full. Stella had managed to bag a table near the window and sat waiting for Diana and Rosie to join her. Tom was staying with the kids, so it was going to be just them. She waved to the Wallises as they loaded their ute with supplies. Maybe she'd chosen this table because it had been a while since she'd had her two daughters to show off.

Rosie walked in the door and looked around before coming over and plonking herself down.

'Hi Mum.'

'Hi yourself.' She leant over for a kiss.

'Have you ordered?'

'Yes, Fran's going to bring us cappuccinos, and I ordered Diana a long black. But she said she'd wait till we were all here.'

'I'm knackered.'

'Rosie!'

'Well, it's true. What does it mean anyway that's so terrible? I'm going to get a Diet Coke, Di will probably be ages.'

Diana arrived while Rosie was at the big double fridge. 'Hello. I've been doing Dad's list at Barkley's—except it's not called Barkley's anymore. I've got everything except the nails. Apparently there are no nails to be found until the next shipment from China. Hi Rosie, that looks good.' Diana eyed off the Coke.

'My memory's not that bad, I got you one too.' Rosie smiled at Diana and produced a second bottle.

'I seem to remember we used to share the same one.' Diana laughed, looking around. 'Hey, all the booths have gone. In London, they're putting them all back in.'

Stella sat back enjoying the sight of her two daughters sitting at the same table. They'd always been the best looking girls in town, and she wasn't prejudiced, was she? Rosie with her honey-coloured curls and Diana's unusual green eyes. Not that they were girls any more, she reminded herself. Her daughters were women with children of their own.

'How's Dad getting on at home?' Diana was asking.

'I think they were going to draft some sheep,' said Stella. 'I heard Milo telling the girls where they were to stand as he was opening the gate.'

'Nothing changes does it? The eldest is always the bossy one.' Rosie sighed.

'I might have been the bossy one, but you always got your own way.'

'Oh, I did not. Poor Dad, he'll probably still be there when we get home.'

'Have you heard from Phillipa?' Stella was pleased to see Rosie's face light up as she turned to her.

'Oh yes, she's off to a twenty-first in Wagga, wants to know if I can send her down my black dress.'

'I can't believe she's going to twenty-firsts already,' said Stella.

'One of the boys in her flat is twenty-one, I think it's his party. I'm just so thrilled she wants to wear a dress.'

'You're lucky, I can't get mine into anything else. And what's worse, they always have to be pink dresses. I even had to buy pink gumboots for them to wear here,' Diana grumbled.

'That time does pass, I can assure you.'

'Lovely to see you again, Diana,' Fran said, arriving at the table with their drinks.

'Thanks, Fran. This is a welcome change. Real coffee, I'm impressed.' Diana sniffed appreciatively.

'Yes,' she said. 'Change does actually occur here, slowly admittedly, but with all the new people in town there was a demand. I got the espresso machine last year and it's been very popular. Took me a while to get the hang of it, though.' Fran wiped her hands on her apron and looked anxious. 'Anything else I can get for you ladies?'

'What about some sandwiches or scones?' Stella asked the girls.

'Oh yes, some of your scones, Fran. That would be lovely,' Diana said.

'Coming right up,' she said as she walked away.

'Those are great boots, Di,' said Rosie, eyeing them off. 'Where did you get them?'

'Harvey Nichols. They're amazingly comfortable.'

'Actually, your whole outfit is wonderful,' Rosie sighed. 'It was the saddest day of my life when I stopped growing and realised I was never going to fit into your clothes again.'

'I bet.' Diana laughed at her. 'You used to always complain you had to wear my cast-offs. I can still hear those moans and groans.'

'That was before you came back in these wonderful outfits. I want those boots.'

'You always wanted what I had, right back to my first Barbie doll.'

'And do you blame me? Try having you for a sister.'

Stella felt it was time to change the topic. 'Did you get on to Megan?' she asked Diana.

'I've emailed her. I'm hoping we can go and see her.' Diana glanced around. 'Look at all these people in here. I hardly know anyone. But every person who's come in has smiled at you, Rosie.'

'It's hardly surprising, Di, I have lived here all my life. Tell me more about London and where you live, Gospel Oak? What's it like having an agent? Is he making pots of money for you while you visit Australia?'

'I'd like to think so. Sebastian is a good agent and I'm lucky to have him. I feel a bit guilty about not getting in touch, but I guess if there's a problem he'll contact me soon enough.'

'You've certainly been lucky, Diana, always,' Rosie said.

Stella felt uncomfortable with the way the conversation was going. 'You remember Megan, Rosie. Diana flatted with her in Sydney when she was in college. Did she ever marry?'

'No, she's the same old Megan. Doesn't ever change. She lives down the south coast now.'

'I auditioned for the Music Club's Soiree last week,' Rosie butted in. 'And I got in. It's going to be a Cole Porter night. Mum, they were wondering if you could do the costumes again.'

Making costumes or designing them for the local performances in town had become Stella's speciality. She loved doing it. 'Cole Porter—that's anywhere from the twenties to the forties. Has anyone narrowed it down?' Stella looked at Rosie's blank expression and laughed. 'Okay. I'll ask Helen.'

'So, all that *Young Talent Time* training finally paid off?' Diana teased.

'I was always much better than you at singing.' Rosie tossed her head.

'Says who? Mum, who was the better singer?'

'Honestly, when are you two going to grow up?'

'Never.' They said simultaneously.

'Jinx!' Rosie squealed. 'Got you!'

Diana opened her mouth and closed it again, glaring at her sister.

'Ha, now you can't talk till I say! Now I'm two up. I got you the last time too!' Rosie was jubilant.

'Girls, really! When was the last time?' Stella laughed disbelievingly at them.

'I'm not sure, when Di was fourteen maybe.'

Diana exploded. 'It was not—I got you the last time.' Then they both collapsed into laughter.

Diana insisted on paying when they'd finished. Stella watched her two daughters at the counter, still arguing over who'd got who, twenty-five years ago. She shook her head. And here she was thinking they were grown women with children of their own. Daughters. She was sad sometimes for Tom they'd only had girls, but not for herself. There was never a dull moment, that's for sure. All the same she couldn't help the pang as she saw the shadow of Cody standing beside them, reaching up to pull Diana's elbow, asking for a bag of mixed lollies like she always used to.

She'd lost a child and thought she'd never recover, but she had. Diana had lost a husband. If anyone could help her it was Stella. If Diana would only open up and start talking to her. Was there ever such a stubborn daughter?

CHAPTER THIRTEEN

The bickering voices rose above the TV commentary.

'Oh, oh,' Diana raced to the sitting room. 'Shh! Hey, quiet.'

Her father glared at the children and then at her. The kids had to be totally silent for the weather reports or her father lost it. She rolled her eyes and grabbed Milo and Sienna and shepherded them out to the kitchen.

'What is it about farmers and the weather?' Diana said to her mother. 'The kids don't understand the fanatical obsession farmers have for hearing these long and complicated weather reports. Why don't you get a computer and Dad could find out the forecasts whenever he wanted?' Diana felt restless. 'Would you two like to make biscuits?'

'Oh, no.' Stella frowned. 'Not just now, Diana. Can't they go outside?'

'Come on, let's go out.'

They didn't want to go. Milo shrugged her arm away and Sienna looked like she was going to burst into tears.

'I want to show you my first wheel.'

They relented, following her out the door as she led them towards the potting shed. They fell silent looking at the lumpy covered object with suspicion. Diana took off the dusty old wool bale. 'So, what do you think?'

'How old were you when you started to make pots?' Milo said.

'About thirteen. We had a fantastic teacher for art. We started making pots out of ropes.'

'Ropes?' said Sienna.

'Ropes of clay.' Diana laughed. 'I've shown you before. I got hooked, and badgered Dad till he bought me this.'

She could have kicked herself. She'd done it again. Reminding these two they didn't have a father to buy them a wheel. She had to be so careful. Diana went back inside leaving them looking at the wheel. At least it had got them out of the house.

'Why won't the kids go outside and play?' her mother asked.

'Well, outside isn't an option in London. Outside for my children means parks and walks and outings, not out the back door. They don't know what to do with themselves, the poor things. They just sit on the couch watching the television. I can understand it's driving you crazy. It's driving me crazy, too.'

'Diana, relax, it's okay. Let's have a cuppa. Put the kettle on.'

She stood stiffly, waiting for the kettle to boil.

'You're doing a wonderful job with those kids, you know. I don't know how you cope.'

'That's what Rosie said yesterday. It made me so mad.' Diana poured the water into the teacups with the tea bags. But her hand was trembling. 'I think I'll take this outside, check on the kids.'

She knew her mother wanted to talk but she just couldn't. She walked over to the yards away from everyone. Cope. What was coping? Wallowing in misery was not her style, neither was it an option. Her night time wanders were bad enough. Were you expected to tell a five year old, 'Sorry, Mummy has to have time out for a little cry right now'?

She had hoped coming home would ease the burden but they were still her kids, her responsibility. She sipped the hot tea, welcoming the burn, as she stared down the drive to the gate and the ribbon of grey that was the road. Such an empty, lonely road for the most part.

Moving in with her parents had its downside. Her family was in a right mess, and Diana couldn't see a solution. The thought of her dad finding a hobby to fill up his life was ridiculous. Maybe Mal could just hold off for a few more years. Maybe the problem was him. Was he going through a midlife crisis? Maybe that was her problem, too.

She felt a hot scalding behind her eyes. Tears? She hadn't had many of them since Charlie, since the accident. Angrily she wiped them away. More hot tears sliced out of her, along with the pain. God. Trouble was she didn't know who she was crying for—Charlie or herself. How pathetic.

Disgusted, she tipped out the rest of the tea. She heard running feet behind her. Milo went past flat out, followed by Sienna, both making weird noises. They were play-ing. Finally. She was so relieved. What strange games kids played—she really had no idea what they were doing. She and Rosie had played all the time, what did they use to play?

She'd better go and cover her wheel again—she bet the kids hadn't done it. With the old wool bale in her arms, she stood looking at her wheel. She couldn't pot. Was that what was really annoying her? That she couldn't sit still long enough without these horrible negative, swirling thoughts of Charlie disrupting her concentration? Before, she could disappear into her world of slippery clay, to the drone of the spinning wheel, and create pots, plates, dishes. It was so satisfying. Someone asked her once if she started out with a plan of what she wanted to make. She didn't like to say the clay had a life of its own and often she ended up with something quite different from what she intended.

She made anything that took her fancy, really. Last year she started creating little pairs of love birds, and they'd been a great success. She'd glazed them an incredible blue, using a barium glaze. It was a deadly poison, but all right if you didn't use it for anything that might hold water or food. They'd sold like wildfire.

Every minute she could afford, Diana was in her studio, lost in her own world. The rush it gave her was addictive. The money was not to be sneezed at either.

Hesitantly, she pushed the treadle foot up and down. It was stiff, it probably needed oil. Suddenly angry, she stood and threw the cover back on and walked out, not looking back.

*   *   *

The next morning Diana took Milo to the shearing shed.

He had been sitting on his bed, totally absorbed in the incomprehensible world of the wretched iPhone his other grandparents had bought for him for the trip out. What was so engrossing? It must be games as there was no reception in the house.

'Tommo's gone ploughing. Do you want to come and see the shearing shed?' she'd asked.

'Tommo isn't ploughing. He's sowing with the air seeder.'

He may as well have been talking a foreign language. What on earth was an air seeder? Trust her son to have the facts correct. She wasn't going to dispute it with him.

But at least he pocketed the damn phone and together they walked out the back and over the hill to where the shearing shed stood. Surrounded by the old wooden sheep yards it had been there a long time, built entirely of grey corrugated iron, with small glass-louvered windows. Steep wooden steps led up to a door with the paint peeling off. There was an open platform out one end of the shed, used to load the bales of wool onto the trucks. Diana opened the door and followed Milo in. She had always loved the shearing shed. It was the heart of the farm for her. Dim filtered light striped through the glass louvres and dust motes suspended in the air around them. The lovely smell of wool and sheep. Silence ... waiting to be filled with the noise and energy of men and sheep again. Inside, the uprights were solid tree trunks, the pens made from sawn Oregon.

'You know, this wood probably came out on an old sailing ship all the way from England,' Diana told Milo. 'They brought logs of Oregon and beautiful wrought-iron panelling as ballast to Australia, and loaded up with wool for the return trip.' She ran her fingers along the soft wooden surface, oiled over the years with lanolin from the sheep.

She went to stand in front of a shearing machine, the long silver arm dangling at an angle behind her. 'This is the board,' she said, pointing to the floor in front of her. 'The shearers pull out a sheep from the pen behind me, drag it out by its front legs and shear while holding it upside down.' She fingered the small triangular tin on the little shelf just behind the machine. 'The shearers keep their combs and cutters here, and oil for their hand pieces.'

Diana stopped, remembering standing at the doorway with her mother, hearing the buzz of the machines, and the chiacking between the shearers. Wool everywhere—fleeces on the floor, in the bins and bundled on the wool table. Everyone with a job to do. The frenetic energy. The farm came alive when the shearers moved in.

'It's dark in here.'

'When they're shearing, they usually open those roller doors at the end. That lets in the light and a bit of air. The generator has to be turned on before we can turn on the lights in here.'

Milo went over and pulled up the door at the back of the shed.

'After they're shorn, they push the sheep down the chute.'

Milo came back to examine the open chute. 'It's like a slippery dip.'

Diana smiled. 'Tommo used to throw me down there, too. Go on, off you go.'

Milo looked dubiously down the dark chute and sat tentatively at the top with his legs dangling. Diana couldn't resist and gave him a little push.

'Mum, yuk! There's poo down here! I can't get back up.'
But at last there was a smile on his face.

'Watch out, here I come.' Laughing, she followed him
down. 'Come on, we'll crawl out and I'll count you out, like
Stan does to the sheep.'

They walked back into the shed together, her arm round
him, feeling her son's knobbly backbone and the sharp, fine
shoulder blades under her fingers.

'Then they pick up the wool and throw it on this table.' A
couple of bundled fleeces lay on the old wooden wool table,
and a new press stood, metallic and shiny, next to the old
wooden Kurtz press.

Diana noticed the wool scraps littering the floor. Obviously no one had cleaned up after the last crutching. And
there was some old netting and broken fence posts piled in
a corner behind the shearing shed. This mess would never
have been left in her day. Never ever.

'Let's clean this up a bit,' she said. 'There's a broom over
there. You sweep, I'll pick up.'

Milo started to sweep, running in a straight line, the
broom in front of him. He ran from one end of the board
to the other, pushing the accumulated mess. Diana laughed
at his energy, picking up enthusiasm for the task. She really
was surprised at the state of the shed, it used to be so clean
you could eat off the floor.

She bent over, separating the stained and daggy pieces
from the woolly scraps on the floor.

'Yuk! Mummy, that's sheep poo.'

Diana looked up grinning. 'We learnt not to waste any of
the lovely stuff. Look over there on the old wool table. Feel

the softness.' She scrunched some fleece wool in her fingers, smelled it, and held it out to show him. 'Go on, smell it.'

Milo wrinkled his nose and she laughed at him. 'Let's pile everything up here. I'll get something to put it in later.'

Milo stopped suddenly. 'Sharks don't eat us, really. You said they don't. Lions and tigers eat us sometimes. But they like other things better, like deer and goats and things.'

'Yes, we only get into trouble when we're in their space, I suppose.'

'Is God a predator, then?'

Diana turned to look at him. 'No, no, Milo. Why do you ask?'

'Didn't he take Daddy?'

'No, it was an accident, a terrible stupid accident.' Diana knelt down, put her arms around her son, squeezing her eyes shut to stop the tears. Hugging him close. *Milo, oh Milo.*

'Didn't he want Daddy then?'

'Of course he does. That's where Daddy is right now—in heaven with God.'

But for the life of her, she couldn't explain why. Not to Milo, not to herself, either. She was so angry. So angry with Charlie. At the unnecessary loss, at the sheer waste.

She was so angry with herself.

'I like it here, Mummy.'

'Do you? Do you really?' Diana searched his round freckled face. 'So do I, Milo. So do I.'

CHAPTER FOURTEEN

Breakthrough! Her father had come to her while she was hanging out the washing, put his finger to his lips and pulled her along.

They stopped. Sienna was kneeling in front of the dog run, nearly, but not quite in reach of the young pup. It was sitting quietly, watching her intently. She put out a dry piece of dog food and pushed it slowly closer to the pup. The pup reached out and picked it up as if it was the greatest delicacy. Then he went back to waiting. Sure enough, Sienna pushed another towards it.

Diana nearly choked. Well, they weren't actually touching but it was the closest she'd seen any of the children to the dogs since they'd arrived. She smiled at Tom and gave him a thumbs up. They tiptoed back to the clothesline.

'Are you going to go to the races?'

'No. Bloody stupid idea. We haven't gone for years.'

'Oh. But you'll think about it, won't you?'

'No.' And he picked up the basket and clomped inside.

That wasn't a good start. Diana followed him in.

'Rosie wants you to go over for dinner tonight.' Stella was still washing up from breakfast.

'All of us?' Diana took an apple, scraped off the sticker and took a bite. 'I swear these apples are better than the English ones.'

'No, just you,' her mother continued. 'We thought you needed a catch up. Why don't you stay the night? The kids and I are getting into Scrabble.'

Diana chuckled. 'A sleepover. What fun.' She sat on the counter eating the apple. 'How does Sassy get around the spelling? She doesn't like coming last.'

'No problem. She gets three extra points for her words because she's three years younger.' Stella smiled.

'She's had a bad year this year. Joined the wrong group, and she's been bashing her head trying to get accepted.'

'She's got a wicked sense of humour, and she's bright. She'll work it out.'

'Why do you have to go through these battles your kids engage in? Why do I take it so personally?'

'I don't know. Can't answer that one. Only that it seems to be just as bad for you as it was for me.' Stella was drying the dishes and piling them on the counter.

'Mum, why does Dad hate the idea of going to the races so much?'

'He's always complaining that at parties he can't hear any one. Not that it would matter because all he would hear was drought talk.'

'He and Patrick are good mates, or so you say.' Diana put the apple core in the bin.

'Yes, he comes over with a bottle of whiskey, and he and your dad sit and talk about the state of the world. I think his latest idea is growing hops. Crazy, isn't it? He wants us to do it, too. Patrick's always asking us down to Sydney but we haven't ever been able to go.'

'Tell me, is this Patrick really very wealthy?' Diana grinned.

'Oh yes! He and his brother own pubs in Sydney.' Stella picked up the plates and handed them to Diana to put away. 'He has oodles of money for fencing, and has built state-of-the-art cattle yards. We don't have the money for that anymore, so here everything is running down. We can't stock like we used to, and so our income's reduced. The Powell's paddock came up for auction last month, a paddock your father has always hankered after because of its superb protection. But we were blown out of the water by the starting price. Didn't get a bid in.' Her mother sighed, picked up the bucket from the sink and carried it over to the back door. 'Lucky really, more debt we don't need.'

*   *   *

Diana readjusted her pashmina and paused at the door of the sitting room. It was dark already and the curtains were drawn. The standard lamp shed light on the newspaper her father was reading. Stella and the children were concentrating intently on the Scrabble letters on the floor, enjoying the warmth coming from the firebox with its glass door.

She remembered herself and Rosie, sitting in the same spot playing with her grandmother. Only it was her parents standing at the door ready to go out. The flickering from the open fire. Cody crying, in her Winnie-the-Pooh pyjamas, not wanting her mother to go.

She let out a breath. 'I'm meeting Rosie down at the ramp, to save her coming in.'

'Do you need a torch?' Her father lowered the newspaper.

'No there's a slip of a moon out already. I'll be fine.' Diana kissed him on his freshly shaved cheek.

She bent over Milo. 'What on earth is that word? Barph? That's not a word.'

'Yes it is.'

'Where's the dictionary?'

'No, Stella said if we could tell her what it meant it would be okay.'

'Well, what does it mean?'

'It's the stuff that comes out of the air seeder at the back when it's going along.'

Behind her she heard her father choke. She really would have to find out what an air seeder did. 'I give up!' said Diana. 'I cannot believe you are condoning cheating at Scrabble, Mum. You never let us,' she grumbled, kissing the girls.

'Your grandmother taught *you* how to cheat. Now it's my turn. I'm allowing the ingenious rule, and I'm enjoying myself immensely.'

'What's the ingenious rule?'

'Ingenious means clever, resourceful.'

'I know what ingenious means. I'm not all that sure my kids do.'

Her mother waved her away. 'Go on. Go!'

So she did. None of them looked up. For three children that had hardly left her side for the last three months, Diana wasn't sure whether to be thankful or a little bit hurt.

CHAPTER FIFTEEN

The little white Honda was pulling up just as Diana got down to the ramp.

'Good timing.'

'I hope you're not freezing. I've got the heater going. Do you want to turn the fan up?'

'It's the most beautiful night. I've been watching the stars come out. I swear there are millions more here than in London.'

'Ah, but in London you have all the nightlights, or should I say nightlife, to compensate. Trade me a few neon lights anytime.'

'You don't see much nightlife with three kids in the house. You're lucky if you make it to nine o'clock without falling asleep on the couch.'

'Well, I say enjoy the moment. Wait til you're staying up until they come home from a party, there's no sleep then.'

'Thank you for organising this, it is so good to have time for a real catch up.'

Rosie smiled. 'Just like old times.'

'Yeah.' Diana smiled across at her sister. 'Oh Rosie, I've missed you.'

'Me too, Di, me too.'

*   *   *

The house Rosie and Mal had bought when they first married was just half a kilometre away. It was a fibro, triple-fronted workman's cottage, and came with about one hundred and fifty acres, which was enough to run thirty odd cows, and a few chooks. Apparently Rosie ran chooks, now her mother didn't anymore.

'Wow!' Diana stopped just inside the front hall. The interior had gone through a transformation since she'd last seen it. All the front rooms had been amalgamated into an enormous open-plan family room, the kitchen at the back all gleaming black granite, with a computer corner, two dun leather couches, and the biggest plasma TV Diana had ever seen in her life, hanging on the wall.

'Rosie, this is amazing! When did all this happen?'

'About three years ago, after Mal started working for Patrick at Lost Valley. I have to say he pays well.'

Patrick again.

Diana sat on the comfortable leather sofa, where she could watch Rosie in the kitchen. 'He's asked Mum and Dad to go to the races.'

'So Mal was saying. None of us have been for years,' Rosie said, getting a bottle of wine out of the refrigerator.

'I was thinking if we all go, it would cheer everyone up a bit, wouldn't it? I'm guessing you and Mal are going. Mum and Dad seem to be sticking in their heels. What's happening there?'

Rosie handed a glass of white wine to Diana. 'My theory is, I think Dad's suffering from depression.' She sighed as she sat down, tucking her knees beneath her. 'I've been on to the Beyond Blue website and it's all there. I ticked the list— won't go out, won't talk. He isn't sleeping properly. What's worse, he's losing his temper all the time with Mum.'

'Can't Mum do anything?'

'She won't see it—and I mean, will *not*. She has her head in the sand. She has a foot in our camp and a foot in Dad's, trying to keep the balance.'

'Well, I talked to Dad the other day and there doesn't appear to be an imminent date of departure. He said they'd have nothing to live on.'

'Oh dear, I know. I've told Mal that until I'm blue in the face. We know damn well that Mog's Hill won't support two families, not at the moment anyway.' Rosie got up to consult the calendar on the fridge. 'To return to the subject at hand, when are the races … They're still two weeks away.'

Diana groaned. 'What about you two? Will you come?'

'I don't suppose Mal will have a problem getting the time off.' She grinned. The phone rang and Rosie reached over to answer it.

'Hi, Philly.' She smiled across at Diana and then frowned. 'Honestly! The money was supposed to last you to the end of term … Yes, I suppose so. How's everything apart from that? Fine. Diana's here for dinner … Yes, I'll give her your love. Bye, darling.'

Rosie brought the cordless phone over to the couch with her. 'That, as you might have guessed, was Phillipa. She's run out of money again. She lived on campus last year, but now she's moved into a flat with a few friends since February. Apparently they don't have enough to pay the electricity bill. You'd have thought they'd have put money away for the essentials.'

'All depends on what your priorities are.' Diana grinned. 'You must be pretty proud of her.'

'We are, oh yes. But I miss her.' Rosie's eyes filled with tears. 'She'll be back in July. It seems an eternity away. You must be so thrilled with your three. I adore Saskia, and Milo is so earnest and always asking questions. Mal says he's a hoot. I haven't got through to Sienna yet, though. I would have loved to have more kids,' she sighed. 'But it wasn't to be.'

Diana studied her wineglass, running her finger around the rim. She knew all about the IVF program Rosie had taken on after she'd had Milo. 'The kids are pretty good— amazing, considering they're in a strange country with their father dead eight weeks and living with people they don't know.'

'It might take a little while but kids are resilient, you know,' Rosie said.

'I don't think we were particularly resilient after Cody died. It took ages for me to get back to anything normal again.'

'You're right. It wasn't until Philly was born that I got back to normal again. We all adored her. She was our gift. Our atonement. But it does get better, Diana.'

'Yeah, I guess I know that.'

'Diana, I want to apologise. I was so jealous when you came back the last time. Swinging in with this up himself, English husband, who treated us like dirt—' Rosie stopped. 'I'm sorry, but that was how he seemed to us. No one paid any attention to me or Phillipa, you were the proverbial prodigal daughter. I'd been picking up the pieces, keeping everyone going, but there you were, taking all the limelight again. I shouldn't be saying this. But I know I behaved badly,' she whispered, her eyes bright.

Diana sat stunned. Then she got up and joined her sister on the couch and reached for her hand. 'Oh God, Rosie, if you only knew how scared I was. Charlie was terrified I'd want to stay in Australia. He wasn't rational. Mum and Dad were being impossible. I think they were hurt we got married so suddenly.'

'Of course they were. We all wanted to be included.'

Diana took her sister in her arms, felt the tears running down her cheeks as well. She wasn't sure how long they sat there. 'I'm so sorry.'

'No, I'm sorry Diana, really sorry.'

To hear that at last. To be able to let out just a little part of the pain. Share the hurt. Diana was so sick of being strong for everyone else.

'Good Lord, I'm turning into a watering pot. Where are the tissues?'

'In the kitchen, on the counter.'

Diana got up and went to find the tissues, and stopped at the picture of Cody sitting on a swing, smiling cheekily into the camera. 'Well, that's one thing I suppose, we've got lots of pictures of Cody. We never stopped taking pictures of her. I wonder what she'd be like, what she'd have done, if she'd had the chance? She'd be thirty-one now.' Her eyes smarted, she sniffed. Now she'd started, she might not stop.

'I know,' said Rosie. 'But you simply can't go down that road. The thing is, Di, we were so lucky to have her. Just be grateful for what time we had.'

'All very well for you to say, you weren't in charge that night.'

'Bloody hell, Diana, I was there too. Stop thinking you were the only person there that night. Between you and Mum, sometimes it's like I don't exist.'

Diana looked at Rosie. 'I'm sorry. Perhaps you're right.'

Carrying the box of tissues and the picture of Cody, Diana walked back to the couch. 'Being so far away, I put everyone in a sort of time capsule. You all stayed the same, Phillipa stayed nine, the farm was always green. It was the only way I could cope. I had to rely on myself.'

'You've always been tough, Di, and strong. I wish I had your strength.' Rosie pulled out a handful of tissues and blew her nose.

If she said that again, Diana just might hit her. 'Well, I needed it when I came home and found you two engaged.'

'You didn't love Mal, Diana. You might have thought he was going to wait around forever, but he wasn't.'

Diana looked at Rosie. She mightn't have wanted Mal to wait forever, but they might have said something to prepare her, just … something.

'No, I didn't love Mal. But I did love the farm,' she said slowly. 'That's what you took from me.'

'Well, it's all been for the best. Look what you ended up with—a career, three kids, a house in London.'

Diana looked at Rosie. Her sister hadn't just said that, had she? She'd forgotten to add 'dead husband'. Perhaps she'd best change the subject right there. 'Tell me about these vegetables. Since when did you start growing vegies?'

Rosie laughed. 'It was because of the chooks. I had all this manure and I read a book about growing organic vegetables, and so I tried some zucchinis. Well, you've never seen anything like it. We had zuchs for breakfast, lunch and dinner and still they kept coming. It all started from there and now I'm obsessed, particularly with this organic theory. Now the hospital want more eggs, and I've just bought more chickens to be able to give them a regular supply.'

Diana lifted her head to see Mal stop and hesitate before clearing his throat and coming in. He'd taken his coat off and was still dirt streaked and dusty and smelling of cows. Funny what a completely different smell it was to sheep. Her father smelled of sheep when he came in at night. They both looked filthy and tired. The two had that in common.

'Hello, Diana. Rosie.' Mal leafed through the mail on the benchtop. 'I presume you two are all right, I don't need to get the mop out.' He laughed. 'Don't suppose you'd like to go and cry outside. It might get the message and bring on some rain.'

'We've just been talking.' Rosie jumped up and threw herself at him, burying her face in his chest.

'So I gathered. Hey, I'm covered in muck.' Mal said, disentangling himself.

'What sort of a day did you have?' Diana asked.

'So, so. Feeding cattle is a never-ending task. We're thinking of sending some on agistment, up north. Tim's getting on to it, should get back to me tonight.' He was systematically opening the mail, reading it and screwing up the rubbish.

'Is that Tim Spelling from school, football god to all us mere mortals?' And bully, if Diana remembered correctly.

Mal nodded. 'He's got the local Stock and Station Agency in town.'

'Philly rang,' Rosie interrupted. 'Apparently she needs money to pay the electricity bill. She's sending us an email.'

'She's supposed to have enough to cover that,' said Mal. 'I'm getting a bit sick of this. When she comes back in July we're going to have to talk. She can have the money as an advance on next semester's money.'

'You can't do that. I don't want her to run short.'

'She can get a job then. Plenty of students work part-time.' He paused, scanning the letter in front of him. 'Apparently you haven't paid our electricity either.' He threw the over-due bill at her and turned in the direction of the bedrooms.

'Bloody hell.' Rosie went into the kitchen and started slic-ing a loaf of bread.

Diana was beginning to think this may not have been a good night to come. 'Mal looks tired.' Rosie didn't answer. 'Do you have the internet? Could I use your computer? I cannot understand why Mum and Dad don't get one. Actu-ally I think Mum secretly would like the challenge.'

Rosie laughed. 'Oh dear, did you bring it up? I bet I know how that was received. Of course, I think it's turned on.' She gestured vaguely in the direction of the computer. 'The internet is very slow, we can only get dial up. You're right. Mal is tired and so am I! Don't mind us. I work too, a fact he seems to conveniently overlook and I hate paying bills. It all comes back to his frustration that he can't take over Mog's Hill. He's forty-one soon. The other problem I can't see an answer to is the cattle versus sheep issue. It's a biggie. They've argued over it for years. Mal could see there was money in cattle but Dad wouldn't hear of it. There sure as hell hasn't been any money in sheep. Men, I'm so sick of them!'

Diana didn't look up as she went to sit down at the computer.

'Oh, I'm sorry. I don't know why I say these things.'

'Does Mal see how the farm is running down?' Diana asked. 'Gates need to be re-hung, fences are falling over, even just a general tidy-up. Dad doesn't seem to see the mess.'

'He's given up. Dad is impossible—he's so hard to help.'

The phone rang.

'Hi Tim … Yes he is. Mal, it's for you,' Rosie called.

Diana opened her email account. She got a shock to see so many. Her next door neighbour was wondering what to do with all her mail. Bills probably, though she wondered if there was any money. She emailed back the postal address at Mog's Hill.

She wasn't surprised to see one from Sebastian.

'Darling! I miss you terribly. I need more pots. Time to get back to the real world. September is scurrying along.'

Smiling to herself, she typed her reply that she needed a holiday and he should stop being such a slave driver. However difficult it was living at home with her parents she simply couldn't face going back at the moment. Too bad, she thought, scrolling down some more. Megan was asking her when she was bringing the kids down to meet her. It had been ages since they'd seen each other. It was always fascinating catching up with Meg's latest fad, whether it was painting, sculpture or her latest necklace creation. But Diana couldn't actually see how they were going to get down there either, there seemed to be so much happening at home.

Johann! She hadn't heard from him in years.

'Diana, so sorry to hear about Charlie. I am in England for a few months—or in and out, more likely. I'd love to see you again. Here's my number, Johann.'

'What's amazing?' Rosie walked up to look over her shoulder. She'd obviously voiced her surprise.

'Johann Pollack. Do you remember? We used to flat together—Johann, Paul, Megan and I, the four musketeers. Johann had put a notice up on the board at college for a room to let, and Megan and I both turned up at the same time.' Diana laughed. 'We decided to toss for it and both called out tails. We couldn't stop laughing and decided it was definitely a sign we would share the room. Luckily Johann made the decision to get a larger flat the next term.' Diana turned back to the computer. 'He's in England and says he wants to come and see me. That's so lovely of him; he was always a very thoughtful person. But I'm not going to be there.' She typed a quick reply and then exited the program.

'All the old boyfriends gathering around, I take it? Didn't take long.' Mal was back freshly showered, refilling her empty wineglass.

'Johann was never a boyfriend.'

'Just one of those platonic friends you used to claim, was he?'

'Yes.' Diana frowned at Mal. She couldn't believe he was standing there sounding ... jealous? 'Johann loved Paul actually.'

She watched curiously as Mal took meat out of the fridge and spices from the pantry, like he knew what he was doing and was going to start cooking.

'Paul died, didn't he?' Rosie said.

'Oh yes, nearly fifteen years ago now. I never got to go to his funeral. It was so sad.' Diana took a sip of her wine. 'Is Phillipa enjoying uni?'

'Oh, she loves it.' Rosie came and sat down next to her. She was obviously happy to let Mal take over the cooking. 'She's got Granny's car now, which makes getting home a little easier.'

'It was the best time the four of us had,' Diana said, a little wistfully. 'Did you miss not going away?'

'It's funny, but I didn't really. Mal was a deciding factor, I didn't want to go away.' Rosie raised her glass to clink with Diana's. 'But that was then. That's not to say I don't want to go now. I do, I'd give anything to go now. I'm a late starter, that's all.' Rosie grinned.

Diana snuck a look at Mal, studiously concentrating on cutting up onions. It didn't look like he thought much of that remark of Rosie's.

CHAPTER SIXTEEN

Empty plates and knives and forks were pushed to one side. Mal held the wine bottle over Rosie's glass and, at her nod, filled hers too.

'So when did you learn how to make a stir-fry, Mal?' said Diana. 'I can't remember you cooking.'

'Rosie was watching all these cooking shows and all the cooks were men. But suddenly there was Nigella Lawson and I was hooked.' There was the old Mal smile.

'Now I can't get him out of the kitchen, not that I'm complaining.' Rosie ducked as Mal threw a piece of onion at her. 'What about the races, Mal? Are we going?' she asked.

'Patrick's hired a marquee, booked a space and has organised someone to do the food. So yes.'

Rosie began gathering up plates and glasses. 'Ooh, I might have to buy a hat. Want to come shopping with me, Di?

'I don't like shopping, never have, and I don't want a hat, thanks.'

Mal got up. 'Who's for coffee?'

'Yes, please. What do you want, Diana?'

'Black, thanks.' She watched with astonishment as Mal went to the bench and started measuring coffee into a magnificent coffee machine.

Rosie dimpled. 'This is Mal's new passion. He can make you anything. Lattes, flat whites ... I'd love a cappuccino, thank you. His tiramisu is to die for, unfortunately he didn't have time to make it for you.'

'How do you get on with Patrick, Mal?' Diana asked as she stacked the placemats.

'He's all right. For a city bloke. Drives a hard bargain. He's got Irish blood, you know, got all the blarney as well. But Tim's not in his good books at the moment. Only half the mob of heifers we bought last month is in calf. Doesn't like being made a fool of, does our Patrick. Having said that, he goes along with most things. There's always a bottom line but I can usually get through to him, and the bills get paid. What more can you ask?'

Diana thought about that for a minute. If he was her boss, probably a bit more.

Mal served them their coffees. 'I'll let you ladies get back to the deluge. I'm bushed. See you in the morning, Diana. I'd appreciate you talking to Tom and Stella, maybe you can get them to retire. Rosie can't seem to move them.'

'That's not fair, Mal. If you'd just say you weren't going to sell all the sheep, maybe they'd change their minds,' Rosie spat back.

'It's got nothing to do with sheep or cattle, it's about money to live on.'

'Well, why don't they lease the place to you?' Diana asked.

'Because,' said Rosie, 'if you'd noticed, over the last ten years there's been a drought and no one's making a living off a farm, let alone able to lease and come out on top. We're all going deeper into debt. We couldn't run Mog's Hill unless Mal gave up his job.' Rosie turned on her. 'Why don't you lease it, if you've got so much money.' She stalked off out of the room.

Mal sighed. 'We own this house, and I could borrow half a million against it. But by the time I'd put in new cattle yards and re-fenced Mog's Hill and bought the cattle and paid the lease, there'd be no money for us to live on.'

Diana looked at Mal. 'Jeez, I'm sorry.'

'We're just tired of it all. Thing is, your father said he'd retire at seventy and he isn't showing any signs of it.'

'Have you talked to him properly?'

'He does not respond rationally to those sort of conversations at the moment, and hasn't for some months.'

Diana could easily believe it.

'Well, I'm for bed. Goodnight, Diana.' He stood up.

'Just before you go, Mal, what on earth is an air seeder?'

*   *   *

'I'm so glad Rosie and Diana are having some time to themselves,' said Stella.

'Mmm. Hope it doesn't bring on World War Three,' Tom grunted. He was already in bed.

Stella slipped on her nightie and jumped in beside him. 'Ohh, thank heavens for electric blankets,' she said blissfully, with her eyes closed.

'Your feet are freezing,' Tom complained.

'I remember way back, a long time ago, you used to warm them up for me.'

'Then I bought you an electric blanket. Stop wriggling and turn off the light.' He rolled over, away from her, she noticed.

'I had so much fun tonight, Tom. I loved it when the older two helped Saskia with her words. They get on well, don't they?'

'Mmm.'

'Do you think they'll stay?'

'Don't be crazy, Stella. What do you think Diana would do with herself here? Her world has changed. She'd never fit back in here again.'

'She could pot, and bring up her children, teach maybe,' Stella said wistfully.

'Dreamtime, Stella. Rosie and Diana in the same town! It's hard enough keeping the two of them apart as it is. Why have they got to be at each other's throats all the time? Beats me.'

'That's not fair, Tom, they have different ways of solving things, that's all. The eldest versus the middle child, the grass is always greener syndrome.' She turned over and pulled the doona up to her chin. 'She's still wandering around at night.'

'Who is?'

'Diana. And at last we are beginning to talk, at least about the kids. Rosie and I used to talk all the time about Philly and what she was up to. Today Diana told me that Saskia was having a hard time settling in to school this year. The fashionable group, you know, the one they all want to be part of, is ignoring her. Poor little mite.'

'Why doesn't she just leave them alone? Go off and do her own thing.'

'Oh, you don't understand, girls can be so bitchy.'

Tom grunted.

Her girls had experienced enough of it. 'Why do we all want what we can't have? I wouldn't be surprised if Diana wanted to come back here. I wish she would. And Rosie,' she sighed and turned off the light, 'I'm not sure what she wants anymore. Which is strange, as we've always been on the same page. Whereas I've felt Diana got on better with your mum. But all the same, I think she inherited that artistic talent from my side of the family.'

'More than likely. There's precious little of it on the Crawford side.'

'Does Milo remind you of your father? Little things ... he's so serious.'

'I guess he does. Taught him today we have crows not ravens in Australia.'

'Did you see some crows?' Stella winced at what that implied.

'They had a ewe down in the west paddock, picked out her eyes. Milo has to learn it's not all soft and woolly looking after sheep. The old ewes are a bit weak; I might have to increase their feed. I think a fox is nosing around. I saw one the other day.'

'Was Milo okay?' she asked softly. There were some grisly lessons to be learnt on a farm.

'Yes, he'll do.'

Tom's breathing was soon steady and regular. Stella couldn't sleep though. Her daughters were so different. They'd always wanted different things from life. Never having had a sister, she was sometimes at a loss to explain the ups and downs her daughters went through in their relationship. Bottom line though, she thought they'd always be there for each other. Well, she hoped so anyway.

Women nowadays had so many choices. Her mother-in-law had had no choice at all. She'd worked so hard, and she just seemed to pick up and do what had to be done. But all the same, Frank and Peg seemed to have had a great social life, from all accounts. There was time for going to church, and the races, and the dances every weekend. Of course, there was no television in those days.

She and Tom had been more isolated, although the cars were faster and the roads better. They had telly, of course, but the drink driving laws had had an impact, living thirty minutes out of town. You could hardly get a taxi to get you home. So that had put paid to drinking out. If only one of you drank it wasn't nearly as much fun. And there weren't so many community things, like dances, to go to any more.

All this talk of women's liberation was a farce in the country. Stella had always felt totally liberated, along with most of the wives she knew, while this younger generation were suddenly pressured to go out to work, and raise a family, and continue doing all the things on the farm.

So now they had to be superwomen. Have a job and help on the farm. Raise the kids, run, run, run. Drop them off, pick them up. Halleluiah, it made her tired even thinking of it. She yawned.

Tom had lost his temper again today. He had such a short fuse lately. Diana had been egging them on to get the internet, but the whole computer business, let alone the internet, was a world they knew nothing about. Diana had said that lots of farmers used computers. But not Tom. He was so stubborn.

'I don't need a computer, I have a pen and a piece of paper when I wish to send a letter and I have a telephone when I wish to communicate in person. I do not need a computer. I cannot see how I would be better off with one.'

'You could get weather reports and market reports,' Diana had suggested, and Tom had just raised one eyebrow—didn't he get them already ad nauseam on the radio and the TV? And that was that. Diana had rolled her eyes and walked out of the room. Tom had gone on and on about people living above their means, and how they should be satisfied with less. He got so worked up these days.

They never closed the curtains at night. It was very dark outside. Lots of stars. Stella loved moonshine with all the silvery light and shadows in the garden. There was no moon tonight though. Tom always liked to get up at the crack of dawn and it was beautiful watching the light creep over the sky, turning it from grey to pale pink, and then that delicate eggshell blue. Listening to the birds calling to each other. Lying in bed with the drumming of the rain on the tin roof was another of her favourite things. Unfortunately that was more of a dim memory these days.

She sighed and looked around the familiar room. She loved their bedroom, they'd painted it pale grey a couple of years ago, and she'd found some beautiful, washed-out grey silk for curtains that billowed and made a rustle if there was a breeze. The windows were always open, winter and summer—admittedly only a crack in the winter. The familiar noises of the night outside soothed her and she closed her eyes, thinking she must find the costumes she'd made for the girls. They should be in her chest if she remembered rightly. And she did have to talk to Diana about Peg. She'd hurt her leg and she had to remind her to buy Peg some support stockings. That could all be done tomorrow.

Sunday was Mother's Day. Her day for remembering Cody. Over the years it had just happened that she'd take the day for herself. Wrap the memories of Cody around her. Take them out, give them a shake before putting them away for another year. She'd walk up to the headstone on the top of Mog's Hill and sit there and talk to Cody. Tom and Rosie left her to do what she wanted. They'd usually go and spend time with Peg. With Diana and the children in the house, it would be different. Maybe it wasn't fair to be thinking about Cody when Diana needed a show of love from her children, when they needed to concentrate on the living. She could always do it another day, couldn't she?

CHAPTER SEVENTEEN

Diana walked in to her grandmother's house at around four.

'Granny!' she called, after letting herself in with her key.

Peg was watching the television. 'Diana! How lovely to see you. How are you darling?' She raised her soft powdery cheek for a kiss.

'Fine, just fine. How are you? How's your leg?'

She'd knocked a big piece of paper-like skin from her leg a couple of days before. The local health nurse had been coming every morning to keep an eye on it.

'My leg is doing very nicely. Doesn't hurt at all.'

'Good.' Or at least she hoped that was good. Maybe if it was numb that was a bad thing. It was so hard to judge if something was healing or not when you couldn't get a reasonable report from the patient. Yesterday, she hadn't even remembered what she'd done to her leg.

'I went to Rosie's last night for dinner,' said Diana.

'Did you have a nice dinner?'

'Mmm. Delicious food cooked by Mal. Did you know he liked cooking? Lots of homegrown veggies. We talked for hours.'

Diana pulled up a chair to face her grandmother, and sat and took her hands in her own. 'Do you remember Charlie, Granny, my husband Charlie?'

'Of course, dear. The Englishman.'

This was suddenly so important. Diana really wanted someone to remember Charlie, not the way Rosie remembered him.

Please remember.

'No, really, do you? I have to talk to someone. He came here with me, to see you. Actually, you came to the airport to meet us. Charlie wasn't all that tall, more medium size, blond hair, straight-ish, kept falling in his eyes, such beautiful blue eyes. Sienna's got his eyes.' Diana searched her grandmother's face.

'Of course I do, I think he's charming. Very like Frank, you know. They had that twinkle. I remember when I met Frank, he simply took my breath away.' She chuckled. 'Not that I let on to him any such thing.'

'Really, you remember? I want someone to remember him … Rosie was saying she didn't like him very much, but he wasn't like that—arrogant or stuck up. He wasn't. I can't bear that no one here knew him, loved him as I did. He was so funny, Granny, he was such a free spirit and he loved me so much. And I don't think I can bear it any more. It's not fair, it's just not fair.'

'Sometimes we have to accept God's will, dear, even though we can't make any sense of it.'

Diana knelt at her knee, put her face in her lap and cried again for the second time in twenty-four hours, Peg tsking and patting her head gently. Then the words, the thoughts she'd refused to think let alone utter, came tumbling out.

'What if it wasn't God's will, though? I feel so wretchedly guilty. I think it was all my fault, if only …'

'Hello, hello,' came a deep voice from the doorway. Diana looked up, startled.

An equally startled man stood at the open sitting room door. 'Sorry, the back door was open so I just came on in. You must be Diana, I've been shown your picture often enough. Will Talbot. I'm Peg's doctor.'

As he came closer, Diana scrambled to her feet. On her knees he'd appeared very tall.

'Hello, Peg, just thought I'd have a look at that leg. Is that all right?' He turned to Diana. 'You're here for a visit? How long?' Kneeling at Peg's feet, he pulled the white stocking slowly down her leg.

'I, er …'

'Diana was just telling me about her Charlie,' said Peg. 'Did you meet her Charlie, Will?'

'No, no, I didn't. When did he come out?'

Diana realised she was going to have to answer. She took a deep, shaky breath. 'Ten years ago. He only came out the once.'

A white handkerchief appeared in front of her face and she took it. She sat, blew her nose loudly, and straightened her shoulders, hands clasping the edge of the chair. 'Thank you, Dr Talbot.'

'Please, Will.' He looked over and smiled.

Diana did like the sound of his voice. And the look on his face was serious and concerned. But she had no desire to meet his eyes full on. She stared at the television.

'He was a lovely man, you know, her Charlie. An Englishman.' Peg said.

'How did you meet him?' he asked, as he carefully unwound the bandage.

'He used to come to the pub where I worked, in London. He'd sit at the bar there for hours, just talking. Eventually he said I'd have to take full responsibility for him becoming an alcoholic if I didn't go out with him. As a line it was pretty weak, but it worked.' Diana drew a shuddering breath.

'What does he do?'

'He's, um ... he was an artist. Painted landscapes.'

'So, modern, traditional ... what?'

'A bit in between. He loved crayon, it was so quick he used to say. But he did a bit of oil as well. He was always trying something new.'

'Did he sell them?'

'Oh yes, they were very good. There was a gallery in Hackney that used to take his stuff.' She paused. 'He died in a car accident.' Diana almost choked on the words.

'That must have been a terrible shock.'

'Dreadful. I can't describe how dreadful. Someone is there and then suddenly they're not. I can't quite accept that he's gone for good, forever. I feel he's going to walk back in, or at least ring me any minute and say "Hey, sorry I'm late". I think I'm going a bit crazy.'

If she concentrated very hard on the television she could hold it together. She was blabbing to a perfect stranger. He must think she was crazy too. No ifs about it.

Will Talbot didn't look up or stop his inspection of the nasty-looking wound on her grandmother's leg. 'That sounds perfectly natural to me. Acceptance is probably the first step you have to take, and the hardest.' He pointed to the two plates on the bookshelf. 'Are they yours?'

'Yes.' Diana shrugged. 'Very early Diana.'

'They're good though.'

Peg must have tired of being left out of the conversation. 'William, there's another thing I want to take up with you.'

'I think the leg's improving,' he said. 'It's not getting worse anyway, Peg. Hmm, Peg leg.'

'That's enough.' Peg was not to be diverted. 'Now, I want to get my driving license renewed. It's run out and I need a doctor's certificate. All you have to do is fill it out and sign something.'

Horrified, Diana looked at Will but he just calmly and gently rolled up the support stocking. 'Now you know I can't do that, Peg. Your license ran out a year or so ago, didn't it?'

'Goodness, has it been as long as that? I'm sure I was driving just recently. I was, wasn't I, Diana?'

'I don't know. I wasn't here, Granny.' Coward! Diana knew perfectly well her license had run out well over a year ago. That had filtered through, mostly from Peg herself, who had been incensed. Only now did Diana feel a prick of guilt as she remembered she'd taken her side at the time. What had she been thinking? Her grandmother shouldn't be driving.

'Surely it's better to let someone else drive you, Granny. Rosie's in town every day.'

'It's not the same as driving yourself. I've had my license since I was twenty. I remember the policeman gave it to me on the understanding I would never try reverse.'

Will Talbot burst out laughing. 'I hadn't heard that one before, Peg!'

'You gave your car to Phillipa, remember? She's taken it to university,' Diana said.

'I'd forgotten. Are you sure, Diana?'

'Well, Peg,' said Will, 'the last thing you want is a car right now. The price of petrol is sky high.'

'Oh, I suppose you're right. I'm a very good driver, though.' Peg didn't sound convinced.

'Of course you are, I've driven with you.' Will smiled and stood. 'I'm off now, back to the hospital. I think the leg is mending nicely.'

'If that's the case, could you give me a lift, Will?'

'Yes, of course.'

Once they were in the car, Diana turned to Will. 'I just don't know where I am with Peg. It's as though she has an on and off switch. It's very confusing. Will she get worse?'

'I can't help you there. Everyone goes at their own speed. I know she is a remarkable woman and it must be very hard for you.'

'Thank you Will, for listening to me talk about Charlie. I seem to be all over the place. One minute I feel like ranting, the next I'm in tears and then I want to kill him. And then I remember he's already dead. It's all so bloody difficult.'

'This is all part of the grieving process. Its early days, you know, very normal. If you feel you need an ear or a hand-kerchief, give me a ring.'

'Three months I've been living in a fog. People would say just to live from day to day. Getting through ten minutes was more like it.' Diana looked at the handkerchief crushed in her hand. 'Oh I forgot. I'll wash it and send it back with Rosie. Thanks so much.'

CHAPTER EIGHTEEN

The dogs were barking.

It was the middle of the night. Dogs shouldn't bark in the middle of the night. Diana heard the sheep then, baaing, calling to each other, and then she heard her father walking down the hall, past her bedroom door.

She got out of bed, pulled her socks on over her bare feet and a jacket over her pyjamas, covered Saskia and left the room. Tom was standing at the hall stand.

'What is it?' she whispered.

'A dog on the loose, maybe a fox.' He picked up his old .22 rifle, gathered a handful of brass bullets from the drawer and put them in his pocket. It was an old rifle with a long gleaming barrel and a polished wood stock; it had belonged to his father. It used to reside above the hall stand but Diana hadn't seen it since she'd been home, though the wooden pegs that had supported it were still there.

'Can I come?' She struggled into her boots at the back door.

'Sure. Can't sleep?' He handed her a big halogen spotlight.

'Not really.' Diana turned it on and off. 'Impressive. Now this is a light.' She grabbed a beanie and they went through the kitchen, and outside.

Her father hopped in the back of the ute while Diana got in the driver's seat and put the light carefully on the seat beside her. Before her there were myriads of stars in the black velvet void. The slip of a moon she'd seen the other night must have been the wane; there was no moon now. It was still. Cold too. She shivered in her jacket, pulling it up round her neck. She had to leave the window down to hear her father's instructions.

'Go through into the creek paddock.' Tom pointed.

At the gate Diana stopped and her father got out and opened it. She waited for him to hop in the back. He tapped on the roof when he was ready to go.

She saw the sheep first, mobbed and quiet, in the head-lights. She stopped the car and leant out the window with the spotlight, scanning it slowly over the sheep, their eyes gleaming like yellow jewels in the light. She picked out the two red eyes slightly over to the left and held the light steady.

The shot was almost instantaneous. A sharp crack in the night. The sheep didn't move. Wise under the circum-stances. People who didn't think sheep were clever should think again.

'Did you get him?' Diana asked.

There was a grunt from her father as he swung himself over the side of the ute. She watched him walk over the short grass, toe something on the ground and then pick up the carcass and carry it to the ute, where he threw it into the back.

'Move over.'

She shuffled over to the passenger side. 'Was it a fox?'

'Yep, a bitch if I'm not mistaken.'

'Good shot. You haven't lost your touch.'

Her father smiled. 'Not bad for an old fella. Dogs are the problem these days. Fellow down near the border lost thirty sheep in one night recently.'

'Dingoes?'

'No, not entirely—we've got a new breed these days. People go out with pig dogs to hunt dingoes and pigs, lose their dogs or leave them behind, and they've bred up into something quite menacing. They'd attack a grown man, no trouble.'

'How horrible.' Diana shivered.

Back at the house, Diana gestured to the wooden pegs where the rifle had rested before. 'You've moved the gun.'

'Mmm, they have to be locked away now. It seems to me the only people allowed out with guns these days are the criminals.'

Diana smothered a laugh. 'Good work, Dad.' She gave him a kiss on the cheek. 'Would you like a cup of tea?'

'Sure, I'll just put this away.' He walked quietly down the hall to his bedroom, nursing the rifle in his arms. When he returned, he sat at the kitchen table.

'You've been up nights, your mother tells me. Having trouble getting to sleep?'

'All these thoughts keep going round and round in my head and they won't let me alone.'

'You can't expect everything to come right all at once. I know you, Diana, you like to think once you've decided something, it's done. Not everything goes that way.'

'I know. You'd think I'd have got that through my thick skull by now.' Her elbows on the table, Diana leant forward and put her head in her hands. 'I know Mum wants me to talk to her but I can't, not about Charlie. The strangest thing was I could talk about him to a perfect stranger I met at Granny's today. Her doctor.'

'Will. He's a good bloke. I wouldn't worry too much. We know you need some time.'

They sat in silence, drinking their tea. Tom stood, giving her shoulder a squeeze on his way to the sink. 'Oh, Diana, it's Mother's Day on Sunday.'

'Good Lord, I'd totally forgotten. Mother's Day in England is in March.'

'Thing is, your mum likes to think about Cody on that day. Just wanted you to know, that's all.'

'What do you mean?' Diana asked.

'She usually takes off, spends the day by herself. Rosie and I go and see Mum.'

'Oh, what should we do?'

Tom looked uncomfortable. 'I don't know. Don't do anything. I reckon she'll tell us. Shouldn't have said anything.'

'Yes you should. I'd really like to do something for her. I don't get a lot of opportunity, being so far away. I'll put my mind to it.'

'Forget I said anything. Goodnight, Diana. Thanks for the tea. Sleep tight.'

* * *

'What are we doing today, Tommo?' Milo was attacking the four Weet-Bix in his bowl with gusto.

Tom regarded his grandson indulgently. 'We've got to feed the old ewes this morning. I've been thinking we should up their feed over the winter months, they're a bit weak.'

'Have we got enough to last?' Stella passed him another piece of toast.

'Should, if we get rain in the next couple of months.'

'Can we come too?' Saskia had finished her Coco Pops and reached up to put her bowl next to the sink, rather precariously. Stella absently raised her arm to push it further back.

'Sure, the more the merrier,' said Tom. 'Who wants to come?'

Diana walked in, a bit fuddled from her lack of sleep. 'Come where?' she yawned.

'Feeding this morning. Sure you don't want to go back to bed?' Stella couldn't help a smile.

'No, I'm better up, I think. I had horrible nightmares of being attacked by ferocious pig dog-dingo crosses, and when I woke up it was Saskia kicking me.' Diana groaned.

'Tea, darling?'

Diana nodded and Stella passed her a steaming cup of tea.

'Thanks, Mum.'

*   *   *

Stella sat in the front to drive, and after they'd loaded four bags of wheat and three children into the back of the ute, Diana and Tom clambered in with them.

Diana grinned at her father. 'We fill up the space pretty well.'

Tom smiled at her over the top of the children's heads. The sun was shining and the leaves in the gum trees trembled in the light breeze. Suddenly Diana felt a strong yearning to stay, not to go back to England. Could she?

'This is so much fun,' she said. 'I used to love doing this when we were kids.'

She watched as her father slit the stitching at the top of one of the bags and, bracing himself against the side of the ute, he lifted the bag upside down and a stream of golden wheat grains started to trickle out.

'Sienna, would you knock on the top of the roof to tell Stella to start moving.'

The ute lurched off to a slow start in a straight line down the paddock. Diana laughed and pointed at the sheep, scattered all over the paddock, as they started to call to each other and race towards the back of the ute.

'Look, see the one at the front,' said Tom. 'That old girl is always the first here. Sheep are very like humans, they have their own individual personalities. She'll have a quick nibble but she always thinks the new bit is better. See that one over there, she'll stay at the back and eat steadily until her pile is gone, and see that one over there, she'll circle around, trying to get into the mob where it's thickest. Whinging. Just like people, aren't they?' He smiled at Diana and gave the bag a shake. It was almost finished. 'Sienna, tell Stella to stop until I get the new bag started. Hold on, kids.'

And they were off again.

'You remember how I met Will Talbot the other day?' said Diana. 'He's an easy person to talk to. You wouldn't consider going to see him and asking him about your depression?'

'You've been talking to Rosie. I am not depressed.' He lifted up the last bag of wheat, braced himself and nodded to Sienna. 'There's nothing wrong with me a good wool cheque wouldn't fix.'

'Failing that, there's nothing that might make you a bit easier to live with?'

'Who me? I'm the most easy-going fella around.'

Diana couldn't help laugh. She watched her father, telling the kids about his sheep. He loved his sheep, he loved Mog's Hill. They were indistinguishable. She couldn't think of him anywhere else.

* * *

Her daughter's head appeared round Stella's bedroom door. 'Can I come in?'

She nodded.

'Dad says it's Mother's Day tomorrow. I'd like to cook lunch for you, bring Granny out, invite Rosie and Mal. We've done Mother's Day in the UK, it's definitely your turn.'

Stella examined Diana's reflection in the mirror. She appeared better than yesterday, not so exhausted.

'I'd rather not have any fuss.'

'Please, Mum, it's been years. Let me. Everyone can celebrate their own mothers. Dad, Rosie and I, and the kids. Does Philly come back?'

'No, not usually.'

'She might come up. I'll ring Rosie.'

Suddenly the mirror was empty. Diana had gone.

She should have said no. But Diana was right, it was a day to celebrate motherhood, not mourn children. It was just that it had become a day she'd carved out for herself. She didn't want to share it, or share her memories of Cody. Stella knelt on the floor and opened the camphor chest at the end of her bed. The chest had been her mother's. The camphor scent rose up sharply, the folded baby clothes, some dresses she'd made for Diana and Rosie. Cody had been more into jeans and shorts than skirts. Ah, there were the two costumes she'd made—one fairy princess and one Maid Marion. Picking them up and shaking them, she examined them critically and then laughed. Diana had wanted to be Robin Hood. They had compromised. Life had been a series of compromises with Diana.

There'd been a time when materials and fashion had been her life. A long time ago. A strange, unsubstantial kind of life, looking back on it, where fabrics and season colours and hot accessories were the most important things in her life, before food even. And strangest of all—it was so normal. Now she knew what was normal, everyday life and she wouldn't change it for the world.

Stella spread the gossamer fabric of the princess skirt and assessed the garment with a tilt of the head. She might have made a fashion designer. On the other hand, maybe not.

'What are you doing?' Tom put a hand on her shoulder. She hadn't noticed him coming in.

'Look, I've found these costumes. Do you think they'll fit the girls? They could wear them to lunch tomorrow.'

'Diana said something to you? Are you all right with it, love?'

'Sure, it will be good.' She smiled up at him and let him help her to her feet.

*   *   *

Diana rang Rosie.

'Mum will hate it, she does her own thing on Mother's Day, always has.'

'Well, she agreed. So how about it? What about Phillipa? Could she come up, do you think? I haven't seen her yet and she hasn't met the kids. You ring her, and I'll sort the food. Can you bring some beans?'

'I haven't got beans, Diana, how about some spinach?'

'As long as Mum likes it. Okay, see you tomorrow.'

Diana rang off. If she met any more negativity she'd scream. Surely Mother's Day was all about the living? They could bring Granny out and have everyone all together. Her kids and Granny hadn't exactly hit it off just yet—not really surprising when she never remembered they'd been born. It would happen. Just a little more time. This was a really good idea.

CHAPTER NINETEEN

Sunday morning, Diana was in the kitchen regarding the big piece of rump when Rosie arrived and handed over a bunch of spinach. She was well satisfied with her purchase she'd found at the butchers, just before he closed. Her mother would enjoy the rare pleasure of a different meat than lamb.

'So Phillipa's coming today.' Diana shook the water off the spinach leaves.

'Yes, I'm so excited. She said yes straight away. She might be a little late, depending what time she gets up. There was something on last night.'

'Oh those halcyon days.' Diana grinned, reminiscently.

'Mal just says he hopes she's not going to drive when she's over the limit,' Rosie said. 'But I'm with you. I'm glad she's having this time without responsibility, or having to answer to anyone. I want it for her.'

'There was no getting you to venture out of this town,' said Diana. 'And we tried, Rosie, all of us.'

'I know. So foolish I was, but my life was here. I had a good job and I had Mal. I knew I loved him long before he knew he loved me. There was no way I was going to leave him like you did.'

'Rosie, you know there was nothing between Mal and me. Just good mates, that's all we were.'

'You are good at seeing what you want to see, Diana, aren't you?'

Diana finished smothering the piece of beef with margarine, picked it up and put it gently in the pan. 'No, Rosie, I'm honest. You're the one who's built it up, way out of proportion.' She faced her sister. She had to finish this conversation, Rosie wasn't letting it go. 'There's absolutely no accounting for someone's heart. It's involved, taken, shackled, or it isn't. My guess is that Mal wasn't desperately in love with me.'

'How did you know you loved Charlie? It was very sudden.'

'Charlie and I needed each other. And we became parents so quickly.' Diana gave a little laugh. 'No time to think about it afterwards.'

Stella called out for Rosie. She shrugged and left Diana alone in the kitchen.

Charlie. Diana waited for the pain. She waited for the feeling of Charlie swirling around her. *Was it so bad, Charlie, to have married you so quickly?* She had wanted to love someone, wanted to belong to someone, and Charlie had wanted her. Lust and convenience—a good package. She'd been so lonely. He knew that, though. He'd thought he was getting this lonely person with no appendages, no family baggage. That was why he got such a shock when they came out to Australia. She did have a family, and they posed a threat—for him anyway, although Diana could never see it.

*   *   *

The airport departure lounge was packed to the rafters—men sitting on the floor using their backpacks as pillows; mothers, hot and tired and cranky, nursing children on their knees.

Diana looked up from rocking the stroller absently as her mother finally pushed through the crowd towards her. 'Another delay?'

'Half an hour at least before we start loading.'

'I'd suggest we go and get another coffee but the baby has just gone to sleep. I'm not moving.'

Stella laughed. 'Good idea. If there was only a seat here anywhere, I'd suggest you sleep, too.'

'How I could sleep in all this mayhem, I have no idea.'

'Just take the opportunity whenever it presents to rest yourself.'

'Thanks, Mum, for everything. I'm sorry I've been so useless.'

'Don't you dare, I've had a wonderful time.'

'If only Saskia had been easier.'

'I said stop now. I've loved every minute. Now when are you going to come home?'

'Home?' Diana looked blankly at her mother. Where had that come from? 'I have a home, Mum. You've just been staying in it.'

'Can't you talk Charlie into coming over for a few months, at least? I have a feeling he'd like Australia. He needs another go, don't you think?'

Diana rocked the stroller back and forward, trying not to lose her temper. 'We're pretty settled here, Mum. You know, I have a business, my pottery, Charlie's painting, and Milo's just started school. Moving is not on the agenda.'

'Just think about it.'

An announcement crackled above their heads and people started moving forward in a massive, slow-moving wave.

Her mother looked anxious. 'I've got to go.'

Diana didn't have the heart to tell her it was still going to be some considerable time before she could fall into her seat. And she had no idea when they were going to see one another again. 'Give my love to Dad and Rosie and Mal and Phillipa. Bye.'

They hugged and Diana turned and pushed her baby back down the never-ending hallway.

She found a tight parking space down the road from their house. She was so tired. She glanced over her shoulder at the sleeping baby in the car seat. Diana leant back. Maybe she could go to sleep now, too. There was a knock on the window and she opened it.

Charlie peered in at her. 'You've taken your time. It doesn't take that long to get to the airport and back.'

'The plane was late taking off, and we were talking.'

'That doesn't surprise me. You and your mother can certainly talk.'

Diana looked at him, puzzled. 'We've hardly touched base this visit. I've been trying to settle Saskia most of the time. You've seen more of her than I have.'

'Well, Milo and Sienna are driving me crazy. Having three kids was a terrible mistake. And add on top of it having to entertain your mother for ten days.'

'I had no idea it was such an effort,' Diana said stiffly. She got out of the car and went round to release Saskia.

'You haven't exactly been much fun lately,' said Charlie.

'I know. I'm sorry. I've just been so tired.' She picked up Saskia, who started to cry. 'Oh no, go to sleep, baby, hush hush.'

'Well, we're both tired. I haven't had much sleep either. I'm off to the pub. The lads are getting together to finish off that darts comp we started last week. The kids are in front of the telly.'

Diana watched him lope off down the road. She wasn't going to tell him about the conversation she'd just had with her mother. She'd hoped so badly for some recognition of what she and Charlie had achieved. Just a 'Well done, Diana. What a beautiful family'. No, all she'd got was, 'When are you coming home?'

Well, she wouldn't be repeating that to Charlie.

And she couldn't see a move to Australia any time soon.

*   *   *

She'd been wrong about that. Here she was in Australia and it was Mother's Day. And it was up to her now to make the decision. *To move or not to move …*

CHAPTER TWENTY

Stella wandered into the kitchen. 'My curiosity's got the better of me. Is there anything I can do? How long has that
meat been in the oven?' she asked suspiciously.

Diana shook off the memory of that trip to London. 'Oh,
no you don't, Mum, you are off duty. Go and sit down.
Have the girls finished doing your nails?'

'Yes, thank you for that idea.' Stella held up her hands to
show a rainbow of different colours on her nails. 'And the
massage was lovely, but I haven't seen them for ages.'

'Neither have I.' Diana frowned. 'Where on earth are
they?' She went to the back door and called. 'Sienna, Saskia,
Milo, where are you?'

No answer. Nothing moving round the sheds, no chatter.
Just perfect quiet.

'I think you'd better go and look for them,' said Stella,
frowning. 'They may have wandered away.'

'Don't be ridiculous, Mum. They're not going to get lost.' But Diana was moving down the steps. 'Milo, where are you?'

Three figures came round the shed. Diana blinked. 'What on earth have you been doing?' They were covered in mud from their knees down and up to their elbows.

'Mum, can we have a tray?' asked Milo.

'A tray?'

'We found some mud behind the tank and we've been making pots for you and Stella. Like you showed us, with ropes, but one I made just broke and I need a tray to put it on.'

'Mummy, look at mine.' Saskia started to run and nearly dropped whatever she was holding, and then slowed down to a steadier pace.

Diana started laughing. 'Give my children some mud and they know what to do with it.'

She was astonished when Stella ran past her. 'Where is it, where's the mud? Milo, go and find Tom. He's inside. No, don't, you're too dirty. Rosie,' she called, 'find your father.'

Stella walked quickly to the big water tank up the hill at the back of the house. Diana, still mystified, caught up with her. 'What's wrong?'

'Mud! They've turned on the tap at the back of the tank. All the water will run out. Or there's a leak somewhere. I hope the tank isn't leaking.'

'Oh, I hadn't thought of that. I'm sure the kids wouldn't turn on a tap to make mud pots.' Diana couldn't help feeling a little defensive.

'Oh my God.' Stella stood horrified at the huge pond surrounded by muddy edges where the children had been playing.

Tom came up behind her. 'Bloody hell. Bloody kids, what have they done?'

Diana rounded on him. 'My children haven't done anything.'

'They certainly have. They think water's free round here. It isn't. It bloody costs a fortune. I can't believe this. They need a whacking, well and truly. Milo, what did you think you were doing? Of all the stupid irresponsible things ...'

'Don't you dare talk to my kids like that.'

'I'll go and get a shovel.' He turned and stomped back down towards the machinery shed.

'Milo, did you turn on the tap?' Diana asked. 'Sienna, Saskia, what happened?'

'No, Mum, we just came up here and found it,' said Milo.

'I'm sure it wasn't their fault,' Stella said, staring at the pond. 'It's just that this is the last thing we need right now. Damn the water.'

Diana looked after her father. That was so unfair, to blame the kids.

CHAPTER TWENTY-ONE

'So it was a pipe joiner?' Stella asked.

'Yes.' Tom was exhausted and not very forthcoming. He and Mal had worked for the last two hours, digging, searching for the leak and draining the water away before they could fix the leaky pipe. Her husband was white-faced and looking old and tired. It was so worrying. He wasn't himself at all.

Stella had had to go pick up Peg, as Diana and Rosie were cooking. Now Diana was annoyed because she felt the children had been blamed, unfairly as it turned out. They'd had to wait to eat and the meat was overdone. Phillipa hadn't turned up after all and Rosie was upset. What a day. All Stella wanted was to walk away from it all and go to Cody's grave and spend some time with her. But if she left everything where it stood this afternoon it could easily implode. It was like standing on a knife edge.

Damn them all.

She made a decision. 'I'm sorry, I've had enough. I'm going for a walk. Thank you for lunch.'

If she hadn't been at the point of exploding, she would have found the stunned faces amusing. As it was she could hardly raise a smile, her face felt all stiff with making an effort. No more, she was out of here.

Stella grabbed a coat and pulled on her boots. Not the bike, not in the mood she was in. She walked down round the back of the shed and took the path through to the pine paddock. They'd called it the pine paddock after the row of pine trees Frank had planted as a wind break. The trees were old and gnarled, and thin on top after all these years, but they were solid still. And they were the way to Cody. A flock of cockatoos flew up and squawked in annoyance until Stella had passed and they indignantly regained their positions.

Just walk. Don't think. Tom, it was Tom she was mad with. Why did he have to go off at the children like that? He was always going off at everyone, her too. All the kids did was play in the mud. She blew out a breath.

Four generations had been at her table today. It wasn't the greatest mix. Peg was querulous and demanding; the children, quiet and nervous. Sienna had worn the Maid Marion dress and Saskia the fairy princess costume, but all that had done was make Stella feel like crying every time she'd looked at them, remembering her girls at that age. Rosie was upset because of Philly's no-show. Tom and Mal were tired from all that digging. To top it off, Diana had been so determined to cook a lovely meal, and she didn't like it when things didn't pan out.

Cody, help me.

*   *   *

Bed was very enticing that night. Stella was in it before Tom, for once. He hadn't apologised and she was so fed up. It was as though he didn't think before he said these things. She knew Tom had been exhausted and worried, but it didn't mean he could go off and yell abuse at everyone. Damn him.

The bed dipped, and she felt Tom's body slide under the covers. She was so angry, her whole body was stiff. She reached over and turned off the light. Outside the wind had come up. Rain, rain, rain, if only it would rain.

'I've spoken to Diana.' Tom's voice came out of the dark. 'I said it wasn't the children, just that I didn't need anything else to go wrong at the moment.'

Stella didn't reply.

'Sorry, Stell, Mother's Day and all. It wasn't too hot, and most of it my fault.' His hand slid over and touched her hip. 'Come and give me a hug. I just want to tell you you're the best mother, grandmother and daughter-in-law I've ever known.'

She rolled over into his arms.

'And I couldn't do this fathering thing without you.'

Stella wasn't sure whether to laugh or cry. 'Sometimes, Tom Crawford, you are impossible.' She buried her head in his chest and felt his strong arms tighten around her.

'I know, Stell, I know.'

*   *   *

Diana lay in bed and carefully pulled the covers up over Saskia and herself. If she turned over again she'd probably wake Sassy, and she didn't want to talk to any one right now.

Except Charlie. Oh she missed Charlie.

Things don't always go as planned, Diana.

I just wanted Mum to have a good day, thank her. It was a total disaster.

Just be thankful you've always got tomorrow. It's more than I've got.

Quietly she edged over to her side of the bed and got out. She crept down to the kitchen to make a cup of tea. What a mistake, she should have never ... no, that wasn't right, she should have come back. It was a mistake, though, to think about staying. She could never live with her parents. Today had shown her that.

She'd never seen her father go off quite like that at the kids before. They were devastated. Then her mother disappearing up the hill to sit by Cody's grave gave her the creeps. Diana was so glad she hadn't buried Charlie. His ashes were still in London but there was something about knowing he hadn't been permanently covered up. Cradling the warm cup in her hands, she walked around the kitchen, restless. She looked out the window into the darkness. Why couldn't she sleep? She'd never had trouble sleeping before Charlie died.

Because she'd always been able to escape to her wheel, that's why. And pot until morning, if she felt like it. Charlie had never got mad with her. He'd had to put up with a lot.

She rinsed out the cup and went back to bed.

*   *   *

Stella came in from the garden the next day with her empty buckets to find Diana reading the local newspaper.

'I can't believe it,' she said. 'Your father has suggested we all go to the picnic races. He thinks it would be good for you to get out and see some people.'

'Me?' Diana looked up. 'He is such a fraud. He's the one who needs to go. I've been poking and prodding him for days. What's changed his mind?'

'Atonement. He's sorry about yesterday.' Not that he'd said it. What he'd said last night was as far as she'd got in the way of an apology. What went on in Tom's mind these days was a total mystery to her. 'But I don't intend to give him any room to change his mind. I've rung Patrick to let him know we're coming.'

'So we're invited to his tent? Who else will be there?'

'He has a brother, Sean, and his wife Marnie. From what Rosie tells me there'll be a lot of locals.'

'What do we need to take?' Diana asked. 'Rosie and Mal are coming too.'

'Patrick told me not to worry about food.'

'We should still take some things for the kids, so they don't disgrace themselves. Or us, more to the point'.

'Good thinking.' Stella laughed. 'Sean has a couple of kids too. I think they're much the same age as yours. I can't wait to show my grandchildren off to everyone. Now, what have you got to wear?'

'Not a lot. I'll think about it. So how does this Patrick really get along with Dad?'

'They do a lot of talking. I think Patrick uses your father as a sounding board. I'm not sure he wants to go with the hops project, though.'

'Hops? What hops?'

'Patrick wants to grow hops and wants your father to join him.'

'Dad grow hops? I've never heard of anyone growing hops around here. How ridiculous.'

'Mal's thoughts exactly.'

This was just what Diana needed, Stella thought. She couldn't fool her, as if she didn't know how Diana was hurting. Dark, shadowed eyes meant sleepless nights, and there'd been another cup of tea at two this morning. Fresh air and sunshine was all well and good, but now she needed people.

CHAPTER TWENTY-TWO

'Milo, where are you?' Diana walked into the kitchen followed by her girls.

It had seemed to take hours for her and the kids to get ready. Diana bent down and brushed a mark off her short black skirt, and gave a quick satisfied look over her Harvey Nic boots. The white silky top she had borrowed from her mother was a little tighter than she would have liked, but definitely more dressy than anything she had with her. No hat, no sir. Rosie was wearing one of those feathery fascinators but Diana wasn't going down that road. 'Milo!'

'We're here.' Her father came in the back door with one of Milo's boots in one hand and the polish in the other. 'Can't have a grandson of mine going out with dirty boots, now can we?'

Milo limped in behind him, the other boot still on his foot.

They were going out to the farm where the races were held a little early, to help set up. Diana thought the children would enjoy being part of it all.

'Could you help me with this?' Stella held out a necklace.

'Turn around. I remember that, you've had it forever.'

'It was my mother's. One day it will be yours.'

Diana flushed. That was the first time her mother had ever promised her anything.

'It's lovely.' The necklace was yellow topaz stones set in silver, and lay flat, circling her mother's neck. Diana touched the smooth surface softly. 'Thank you, but it looks great on you.'

She and her mother exchanged a smile. It was odd. She was touching base with her mother after all these years. Perhaps it was for the first time—she'd been more inclined to exchange confidences and take problems to her grandmother in her teenage years. If only she'd stop trying to talk about Charlie.

'You don't think this is too tight?' Diana loosened the pashmina to show her mother the top.

'It looks a good deal better on you than it does on me.' Stella laughed. 'Do the children have their coats? It might get cold later. I've got the slices in the esky and drinks for the children. Tom, could you put the eskies in the ute. I think we're ready.'

With Milo hopping to put his boot on, they filed out the back door. They took two cars—Stella and Diana went with the two girls, and Milo and Tom followed in the ute.

'I'd forgotten it was such a long way in from the road.' Diana smiled as her first glimpse of the racecourse came into view. 'It reminds me of the county fairs in England.'

In the middle of the paddock, a race track had been defined by a double post-and-rail fence with a mown strip in between. The far side was lined festively with a row of white tents with blue roofs.

'Mum, Sassy's squashing me. Tell her to stop.'

'Hey Sassy, we're nearly there, hold it will you?' Diana half turned around, but all she could see was Sienna's scowl and an innocent Saskia face.

'There are so many more cars than I remember.' Stella was leaning forward to inspect the crawling queue before them. 'It's ages since we've been.'

It didn't look as though they were going to get anywhere fast. 'Tell me more about this Patrick,' said Diana.

'He's an interesting man,' said Stella. 'I think he likes to come to his farm and tune out, get away from city pressures. Luckily for us, he was around that weekend of the bushfire.' Stella gave a little shiver.

'Oh yes, you were telling me the other day. That was only a year after you came to stay, when Saskia was born.' Diana made a wry face. 'I wish I'd been a nicer person when you came to stay that time. I was so cranky and tired. I left you to Charlie's company mostly. We didn't do any of the things I had planned.'

'Not surprising, when you'd just given birth and had two other littlies running around.' Stella reached over to touch her knee. 'I didn't want to do things, just be with you and see where you lived and get to know Charlie a bit better. And get to know my grandchildren,' she added, with a smile at the girls in the back seat.

And want to know when we were coming home. That still rankled.

After parking the cars, they unloaded the eskies and trooped past the horse stalls, made of treated pine poles draped with hessian and decorated with eucalyptus branches. Some horses stood quietly in their shady stalls, seemingly asleep, while others snorted and looked around, their eyes wild. There were already a few bookies, set up under the trees with their chalk boards and leather bags. Further over was a hodgepodge of old-fashioned green tents, camper chairs and fold-up tables that people had brought themselves.

'Where are we going?' Milo asked, his eyes wide with excitement. He and Sienna were following Diana along, carrying an esky between them. They paused outside a timber pavilion that housed the bar and the jockey's rooms.

Diana asked for directions from a red-headed young man in a smart jacket with Official on his tag.

He pointed. 'Lot 37 is over there, third tent along.'

Fashion was quite dressy, Diana noticed, as she walked along. Girls stumbling along on high heels, wore shiny tight cocktail dresses with fascinators perched on top of their heads. The day was quite chilly and they'd probably freeze to death.

Oh dear, Diana bit her lip. She was feeling her age.

The tent the official had pointed out was obviously brand new, with white walls and a blue roof. It was empty except for a man and woman unloading glasses onto a trestle table covered in a white cloth. The man looked around. He was dark-haired with blue eyes and a slightly hooked nose. Diana smiled hesitantly. This must be Patrick. She held out her hand.

'Are you Patrick? I'm Diana Crawford.'

He looked confused.

'Ah welcome, Diana, you're early,' came a voice from behind.

She whipped round. The man behind her held out his hand. His eyes were very blue.

'I'm Patrick, and that's my brother Sean,' he said with a lopsided grin. 'And I recognise you from the photo in the front hall. Stella and Tom are with you?'

There was no mistaking his heritage. Patrick spoke with a full Irish lilt. 'I think they've been held up along the way, chatting.' For some reason she felt nervous. 'This is Milo and Sienna.'

'I must introduce them to my nephews. Sam, Alex, come over. Tom's grandchildren are here.'

Two boys skidded to a halt at the group and were introduced. The children eyed each other up and down. Sam appeared to be the oldest but both he and Alex were like peas in a pod with the Morley blue eyes and dark curly hair.

Patrick squatted down. 'My nephews haven't been here before either, so take a look around and get your bearings and then go and explore. I'd stay away from the horses.'

Diana opened the esky. 'Just help yourselves.'

They clustered like bees round the esky and each grabbed a drink. Then the four were off like a shot.

Without the children, the tent seemed suddenly cavernous. Diana was conscious of Patrick standing beside her. He had a quizzical look in those blue eyes. He was sizing her up, no doubt about it. She turned to Sean and tried to concentrate.

'Delighted to meet you, Diana. I don't often get taken for my brother, I'm flattered.' Sean's grin was all cheeky younger brother but he'd lost his accent somewhere along the way. The Morley brothers wore identical, crisp cream chinos and striped open-necked shirts and riding boots. It might be all RM Williams but they still looked different from the locals. Maybe it was because they weren't wearing ties. Diana looked around; everyone over the age of fifty-five was wearing a tie—that hadn't changed.

A young woman threw her bag and hat over a chair. 'I haven't been to a picnic races before. Everyone looks so happy. This is going to be so much fun.'

'Marnie, let me introduce you to Diana, Tom's daughter,' Patrick said.

Sean's wife was friendly, with her younger son's smile. Two more men arrived, carrying boxes and more eskies. There were more eskies than people.

Patrick was still looking at her intently. 'It's good to meet the famous Crawford sister at last,' he said.

Diana smiled. 'I wouldn't go that far. But it's good to meet you. My parents talk about you constantly.'

'And that would be very complimentary, I hope?'

'Yes.'

Patrick laughed and winked at her. 'It's all the whiskey I give them. I've made very sure of my welcome.'

Marnie handed him a bottle. 'I need space for the dips and breads. Let's open the Prosecco, Patrick.'

The tent filled up with neighbours of Tom and Stella, people Diana hadn't seen for twenty years. Patrick was a good host. He certainly seemed to know everyone's name, as just about everyone in the district flitted in and out of the tent. But it was a strange twist in the dynamics of country life—city money entertaining the country people. Still, something had to have changed in the last twenty years.

'I was sorry to hear of your loss.' Patrick was beside her, offering a refill.

'Thank you.'

'Stella and Tom were very happy you decided to come home.'

Diana looked at him and then away. 'We're just here for a couple of weeks.'

'I think they're hoping it will be longer.'

Diana watched as he made his way around the tent. He was very up-to-date with her situation. Then she remembered Mal was working for him too. No wonder he knew her family history. She wished Charlie was here. Suddenly there was a sharp pain twisting inside her. She could imagine him over there, head bent, talking to Marnie; he would have loved Marnie. She wanted him to be there so much she felt faint.

'Hey, are you okay?' Patrick was beside her again.

She couldn't speak. Just shook her head. He took her elbow and led her gently out of the tent to the fence onto the track, away from the crowds.

All Diana could manage was a deep breath.

'It's such a beautiful day for the races,' said Patrick. 'When do they start, I wonder? There's no horses down at the barrier. I guess it will be a while yet.' He rattled on comfortably, not waiting for an answer. 'I think I can see your children.'

She nodded. For the life of her she couldn't say anything for the ache inside. She scanned the crowds for her kids. 'Whereabouts?' she managed.

He pointed to where they were all standing next to a ditch, looking at something. 'They're over there. Piece of luck for my nephews. They don't know anyone else here. They certainly seemed to take to each other quickly.'

Diana held on to the rail tightly. 'Thank you. I thought there for a minute I was going to lose it.'

'No problem. It must be a very hard time for you.'

'It's just, I suddenly thought of Charlie, wished I could have brought him. He would love all this. He never saw Australia like this, our party side. He loved parties.'

'Hello, darling,' said Stella as she approached. 'Everything all right? Is the first race about to start?'

When Diana turned back, Patrick was gone.

CHAPTER TWENTY-THREE

Milo, Sam and Alex came into the tent—hot, dirty and dishevelled—to get themselves another soft drink.

'How are you boys getting on?' Diana asked.

'Great, Mum, we think we've found a snake.'

'In the middle of winter?' She regarded them sceptically. Sam looked a little sheepish. 'I think they might be having you on, Milo.'

'We saw something move, didn't we?'

'Well, don't touch it,' Diana called after them. 'Are you coming to watch the race? It's on in ten minutes.'

They all stopped and looked back. 'We'll be back, Mum. Can we put a bet on it?'

'No.' Diana laughed. 'I can, or Tommo, if you see a horse you like. They're all going round the parade ring now. Come on, let's go and look.'

She joined her father at the railing, the two girls beside him. The boys all climbed on the fence to get a better look at the beautiful horses, walking round and round the enclosure before the first race.

Sienna pulled Diana's arm to get her attention. 'They all wear such pretty shirts.'

'The jockeys all wear the horse owner's colours,' Diana pointed out to her children.

'We used to have our own colours,' said Tom. 'Black with red diamonds, I think. Wonder where on earth they've got to?'

'When did we have a horse? Must have been before I was born,' Diana said.

'You forget your grandfather was right into race horses. Always had one or two floating about.'

'The field is not huge,' she commented to her father.

'I think they're lucky to get five or six for each race. It used to be horses you brought out of your own paddocks, but they all come properly trained these days.'

The first race was being announced on the crackly loudspeaker.

'Come on, we'll line up behind Mal's bookie.' Diana looked at Milo. 'Which horse do you like?'

'The black one over there, number four.' Milo pointed.

'He's got a good eye, that son of yours.' Mal grinned and turned around as they all lined up behind him.

Diana scanned the page of the first race. 'Number four belongs to Patrick Morley.'

'Aye, he owns a string of them, trains them in Canberra. Loves his horses, does Patrick,' Tom said.

'Ah, speak of the devil, here's Patrick now. He's the expert,' said Mal. 'Who do you think is going to win?' He saluted Patrick as he joined the group.

'Hello, Mal. Which horse do you think is going to win, Milo?'

'Number four.'

'I'll go with that one too, then.' Patrick smiled. 'Let's go and stand at the finishing line to watch.'

They finished placing their bets and threaded their way through the crowd to the edge of the track, holding the girls' hands to keep everyone together. Milo raced after Sam, and Mal was caught up with someone wanting to talk.

Diana was being pressed closer to Patrick by the crowd at her back. She was distracted by his nearness.

'I think number four will win this time, Mummy.' Milo was back, squeezing in front of her.

'I think they're having trouble getting our horse in the barrier,' Saskia said from her observation post high on Tom's shoulders.

'Don't worry, Sassy, sometimes the last one in the barrier is the first one out,' Tom reassured her.

'They're off!' she squealed over Tom's head.

'Anything could be happening over there, it's such a muddle. I can't see what's going on,' Mal said.

The loudspeaker cackled and the caller went into race mode, drowning out any reasonable attempt at conversation. The horses came thundering up the straight beside them and number four flashed past on the outside to win.

'Go, Monty, go boy, go,' Patrick was shouting.

'We won, we won! Mum, we won the money.'

'And here's the ticket.' The euphoria of winning was infectious. Laughing, Diana kissed the ticket, gave Milo a hug and then straightened to meet Patrick's eyes full on. Her stomach went on a spiral. This was ridiculous. She tried to take a step back.

'Give it to me,' he said, 'and I'll take Milo over to collect our winnings. Good choice, Milo.'

Diana dragged her eyes from Patrick's wide smile to Milo's excited face and handed him the ticket. Then she watched the two walk off together.

*   *   *

'This is beautiful.' Stella reached for a piece of the flat bread and dipped it into the dish of purple beetroot in front of her. 'I've only eaten beetroot in a salad or on a hamburger before. What else is in it?'

'Some vinegar and yoghurt probably,' Rosie replied absently as she watched Mal and Diana on the other side of the tent, deep in conversation with Sean and his wife.

'What's this one?' Stella pointed to a pale green mash beside it.

'Baba Ganoush.'

'What's that? It's absolutely delicious.' She dipped her bread again.

'Eggplant. Honestly, Mum, where have you been living?' Rosie frowned at her.

'Obviously not in the right places. I've never seen anything like this before.'

Stella settled back and regarded the scene in front of her with some satisfaction. She put out her hand and touched Rosie lightly on her arm. 'I hope you're trying to help Diana through this time. It's been pretty rough. I know it's difficult to understand just what she's thinking sometimes; she always puts on a good front but she must be hurting so badly.'

They both watched the conversation happening across the tent. Mal was bending down, talking earnestly with Diana. Funny how things turned out. Diana and Mal had been really good friends a long time ago. A very long time ago.

'Mmm,' Rosie said, frowning. 'It's my observation that she's always been particularly good at landing on her feet.' She sighed. 'Yes, I know, Mum. I wouldn't wish what she'd gone through on anybody. It must be terrible. It's just that she always has someone to pick up the pieces.'

'That's what families are for. I wouldn't like to be standing in her shoes, all the same.'

'You're right. I wouldn't, either.'

Patrick joined the group. 'Hmm, Patrick, that's interesting,' Stella observed.

Down the end of the table, Tom put his head back and laughed. A deep belly laugh. It had been so long since she'd seen her husband laugh like that.

She saw Rosie join the group over the other side and surreptitiously give Diana a quick hug. They smiled at each other. Stella blinked away the sudden moisture. They were good girls, her daughters. Rosie might come up with the occasional cutting comment, but she was soft as butter underneath.

She settled back happily with Saskia on her lap. Sienna was standing beside Tom with an arm draped around his neck. The children were so much more comfortable with them. At last here they were surrounded by their family, so different from last Sunday.

Surely they'd stay.

More food kept appearing: platters of wonderful little pastries, dolmades and lovely plump olives in a shiny, citrusy marinade, heaped in dishes. Mouth-watering, all of it.

Working out what was going on with her eldest daughter was not easy, despite Rosie's assertions. Diana used to be transparent, but now … Stella wasn't so sure. There was a lot she wasn't saying about Charlie, about England. Patrick was just sitting back not saying much, but he seemed to be quite focused on Diana. Was she aware of his interest?

'It's good to sit down.' Tom drew up a spare deck chair and sat himself next to Stella.

'What do you think is happening over there?'

Tom sat back and closed his eyes. 'Speculation never did us much good before. She ran off from Mal when he was besotted, and turned up with Charlie, who I'd never pick for her in a million years.'

'I can't help thinking, wouldn't it be a good thing …'

'Stop it, now, Stella. She's not ready. You know there's something not right.'

'She just might be needing a good reason to stay. There's a good reason, right there, in front of us.'

'Let it be, Stell, let it be.'

CHAPTER TWENTY-FOUR

Diana heaved the second can of drench into the back of the ute, with a little grunt of satisfaction. She was pleased with her plan to leave Tom visiting Granny, who he hadn't seen since Mother's Day, and had gone to pick up the drench alone. She'd managed to pay for it with her credit card. It was turning out to be quite a battle to pay for things without her dad finding out. At least he wouldn't know until she'd gone back to England.

That made her frown. Strange, she hadn't thought about England and her life there for a couple of days. Gospel Oak felt like it was a million miles away. The plan to move London, together with Charlie, out of her head just might be working.

A large black Toyota pulled up next to her. The window slid silently down and Patrick leaned out. 'Hello, Diana. Feel like a drink?'

She looked at him curiously. Two weeks had passed since the races. 'I'm with Dad. He's visiting Granny.'

'Would he like to come, too? How about we meet at the club when you're ready?'

'I'll have to ask him. I think he'll want to go home. But thanks.'

'Well, if you can manage it, just give me a ring. I can meet you at the club.'

Diana nodded and watched Patrick get out and walk into the Spelling Stock and Station Office.

Tom did want to go home but he insisted dropping Diana off at the club.

'Patrick can bring you back, it's hardly out of his way,' he said. 'And don't you worry about the kids. They'll be okay. You need some time off.'

So that left Diana walking slowly into the club by herself. She should have put up more resistance, but her curiosity was killing her. She looked round but she couldn't see Patrick. There was actually only one club in town now; the RSL and the golf club had combined their resources and moved into the bowling club premises. There were quite a few people sitting quietly having a drink after work. Two men sat at the bar, and a couple of women were playing the pokies.

This hadn't been Diana's watering hole when she was young. She remembered drinking down at the bottom pub. Couldn't be any more different, either, from the Horse's Head, where she'd worked when she first arrived in London. Wood had been the predominant feature there. They'd gone for a wood finish here, too, but it was fake. Lots of timber-grained laminex for the panelling and the tables, plastic chairs and a garish carpet on the floor. Honour boards, with their gilt lettering, lined the walls. They dated back to the 1920s. Diana liked the large plate-glass windows that looked out over the bowling greens, always brown at this time of year. So there was lots of light and space, and it was warm inside. She sat at one of the empty tables.

In London, the bar where she'd worked had been made of old, dark oak. She'd loved to run her fingers over the raised grain. It could easily have been a couple of hundred years old, and then there was the lovely, malty smell of the place. The hunting prints on the walls. Spindly wooden chairs tucked into small wooden tables. Dark booths upholstered in green leather. The only windows were the tiny, multi-paned bow windows at the front. But the best thing had been the sense of family, of belonging, the good-hearted repartee with the regulars. The pub was their home and she'd been welcomed into it. But God, she'd missed her family so much at the start.

She'd met Charlie while pulling pints at the Horse's Head. He used to come in and sit for hours, just watching her. Chatting her up. *Go away, Charlie.*

A frisson of awareness. Diana looked up to find Patrick heading towards her. It was a little unnerving, as she hadn't noticed him coming in.

'Hello, Diana. Where's Tom?'

'He wouldn't stay.'

Patrick nodded. 'What would you like to drink?'

'A beer would be lovely. I don't know my local beers anymore, you choose.' She watched him go up to the bar and then noticed that she wasn't the only one watching him, either. The three other women were also looking. He was good to look at, she had to admit.

Patrick returned with two midis of a pale lager, a good inch of head on top, and placed one on the table in front of her.

Diana dipped her finger in the froth and sucked it. 'Mmm, different. I guess you know your beers backwards. What's this one?'

'One of the new craft beers. What do you think?'

'A bit sweet and syrupy.'

Patrick laughed. 'I'll get you another.'

'No, no, I want to finish it. It's different. You're interested in these new craft beers?'

'Yes, a bit of a passion at the moment. It's why I want to grow hops and then I can make my own.'

'Ah, so that's the reason for the hops.'

Diana studied his face, like she'd study a subject before attempting a sculpture. The bone structure was defined. Not perfect—his nose was slightly hooked to the left and the jaw too square. Strong, yes, but it was more than that. She was aware of the scent of power emanating from him. Funny, how you could tell. But then he had a nicely shaped mouth that liked smiling. The blue eyes lazily roved over her in return, unsettling her. She held his gaze steadily. Unfortunately the hairs prickling on her arm were another matter. She hoped he hadn't noticed.

'Are you wanting a meal?' a young waitress asked.

Patrick waited, so it was obviously up to her to decide.

'Thank you. That would be lovely.' Diana nodded and then picked her phone out of her bag. 'I'd better ring Mum.'

The girl was soon back with menu folders. 'Our new chef started this week and I recommend the lamb shanks. They're delicious.'

*   *   *

Dinner was excellent, and Diana made Patrick laugh recounting the story about Saskia locking herself in the toilet on the plane.

'I can assure you it wasn't very funny at the time.' Diana looked down, rather astonished, at her empty plate, and leant back in her chair. 'How did you find Lost Valley, do you mind me asking?'

'No, I like the way you say what you think. You're very direct.'

Her directness often got her into trouble. 'So why does an Irish pub owner buy a farm in the Australian bush?'

He grinned. 'I'm not Irish, I'm Australian.'

'Sorry. You've got an Irish accent.'

Patrick threw back his head and laughed. 'It's a long story.'

'I'd like to hear it.'

'My grandparents emigrated from Ireland when my father was still a child.'

'Where were they from?'

'Galway. Days of the ten-pound ticket immigration. They were keen to get out of Europe after the war. I went back there for a couple of years after school, and for some reason the accent simply stuck. It's a curse, maybe from my ancestors.'

'I don't know about that. I like it.'

The waitress returned to the table then, with two cups of coffee. She picked up their plates and was off again.

'Okay,' Diana said. 'So why pubs?'

He shrugged. 'My dad owned a pub, down in the Rocks in Sydney. I worked pubs in Ireland, then came back to work with my dad. I grew up with them. They're great places, or can be.'

'I know what you mean, I worked in a pub in London. My extended pub family kind of saved me when I first went over to England. I don't know where I would have been without them.'

Patrick smiled that gentle smile again. There was no doubt about it, he made her very comfortable.

'You know, I think everyone should have a stint working behind the bar.'

'Why?' Patrick asked.

'First of all, you get to see what drunks really look like.' She bit her lip, wondering if she should have said that. But Patrick only laughed.

'But the best thing,' Diana went on, 'is that you're there to listen. You're the dumping ground for people's dreams, their failures, their passions.' She glanced at Patrick uncertainly and was reassured by what she saw. 'It's important, somehow. And what gets said stays behind the bar.'

'I know exactly what you mean.'

She decided to change the subject. 'So then what?'

'When my dad died, Sean and I took over. It was a plus for me that Australians love their liquor. But a pub doesn't leave you much time for a personal life. Eventually I arrived at a time in my life where I needed,' he paused, 'something else. It all started with the horses. I bought into a couple and found they spent more time off the track than on it. I thought it would be good to have somewhere to spell them, so I looked around for some land. When I found Lost Valley, it was perfect. So here I am.'

He added sugar and stirred it round. He had a strong square hand with blunt fingers—they didn't look like city hands. Faces and hands always fascinated Diana.

'Now it's your turn,' said Patrick. 'How come you ended up in London?'

'I was lucky, when I finished college, I won a kind of a resident scholarship with a potting commune in London, run by five wonderful potters.' She was well aware how lucky she'd been. 'And one day, with their encouragement, I took some of my pots to the gallery with theirs. The gallery owner was standing behind me watching me unpack, and he asked me how much I wanted for one of my pots, then doubled the price. He didn't even blink. A few days later he'd sold them all. That was my first sale, and that man, Sebastian, became my agent. It went from there.'

Patrick smiled at her. 'That must have been an exciting day for you.'

'Mmm.' She shrugged. He could tone down the smile—it made her shivery. 'Lucky, I guess, very lucky.' She paused, and then couldn't resist. 'Is there a Mrs Patrick?'

'Not a present one. I was married before, to Vanessa.'

'Right. Any children?'

He shook his head. 'So what are you going to do, Diana? Are you planning to stay? I have a feeling it would go down well with your family.'

'I can't imagine why,' she said. 'I haven't been the best daughter to them. Actually, I was pretty bad, when I think about it. I kind of exiled myself from my family, pushed them away, thinking I'd be stronger if I weaned myself, you know?'

'We all have to wean ourselves at some stage.'

'Do you miss Ireland?'

'You know, there's definitely a connection. I think I may have inherited some farming genes along with my accent.' He was laughing.

'I could have been a farmer, if things had turned out differently. Isn't it weird? A throw of the dice.' She traced the rim of the small cup with one finger. 'Your grandparents were very brave coming to a new country. I've lived in England for the last twenty years but I'm still considered a foreigner. You get very sick of the convict jokes.'

'You haven't answered my question,' said Patrick. 'Do you think you'll stay here?'

She looked at him. 'There's no simple answer. I feel like I'm split down the middle. Charlie's parents want me back there, or at least they want the children. They have been very kind—kinder than I deserve really. They didn't want Charlie marrying me in the first place, but we got on better as time went on. After the kids ...' She trailed off. She must ring her in-laws; she would when she got back tonight. It was daytime there now.

'We live in Gospel Oak, a great community with lots of different people. There's a sixties' housing estate across the road and millionaire mansions around the corner.' She grimaced. 'The kids are at a good school, and we found this great house. It's in a row of Victorian brick terraces, you know, with a string of gardens behind them. We ...' She hesitated. 'I have a beautiful studio at the top of the house, with a tiny glimpse of Hampstead Heath between all the chimney pots. It takes me just two minutes to get to the bottom of the Heath. Now that is a beautiful open space.' Diana looked up to find he had that look in his eye again

It unnerved her. 'Downside, you're never without people around you. I used to run on Hampstead Heath, but all the people ...' She shrugged. 'The problem is you're never alone in London, are you?'

'You needed to be alone?'

'In my studio I was alone, with my clay and my wheel and my kiln.' She was talking too much. She looked away from him and laughed. 'Not that I ever got away from the kids. Now that Saskia is at school though, there is more time. You must enjoy the peace and quiet at Lost Valley.'

Patrick put down his coffee cup, pushing his chair back. 'That's for sure. I'm sorry. I'm enjoying this, but I think it's time to go. I don't want your parents to worry.'

'Oh! I had no idea of the time.' Diana flushed.

*   *   *

It was silent in the car. The easy conversation had subsided into an uneasy quiet. Diana watched the dials with their bright white lights, then moved her gaze to Patrick's hands, resting competently on the wheel. He switched on the radio. Music filled the car. She knew that song so well.

'No, turn it off please.'

Patrick swiftly turned it off. 'Sorry.'

'No.' Diana shook her head. 'It's me. I used to play it in my studio all the time when I was at my wheel. Charlie used to ... he used to sing it, and say it was written for me, only me.' Help. She took a deep breath. '"She". Do you know it? From the movie *Notting Hill*. You know at the end, where they're looking at each other?'

'Of course I know it. It had me in tears, too.'

Diana didn't answer.

Then he broke the silence. 'There's something I haven't told you.'

Diana turned to look at him and waited for him to continue.

'We—Vanessa and I—did have a child. He lived to twenty-seven weeks, but he was stillborn. Rory, we named him Rory.'

No, you've lost a child, not a child. Nothing could be as bad as that. Diana was silent. Words stuck in her throat. What could she say? How could you bear losing a child?

Her parents had. Cody. Sharp as a tack. So beautiful.

'That's just awful,' she said finally. 'Rory is a lovely name.'

'I got to hold him. He was still warm, and so perfect. It was just such a shock. We didn't expect—I guess no one expects that to happen.'

'No, you don't. Giving birth is all about life.'

'You know the worst thing was filling out the form, the registration, that was tough.' His fingers flexed on the steering wheel. 'So … It gets better, that's all.'

'Thank you.' Diana was quiet for a moment. 'You probably think I'm mad, but could I hold your hand, just for a moment?'

Patrick stretched out his left hand and Diana tentatively took it in both of hers. She ignored the tingle that ran through her. Instead, she concentrated on its strength, tracing the blunt fingers, the well-shaped nails, the warmth. She squeezed gently at first, and then harder, before raising it to her cheek and brushing her lips along the back. She sighed and closed her eyes. It would want to get a whole lot better.

You know, you could say you were sorry. She waited. It didn't happen. It wasn't going to happen. *Damn you, Charlie.*

The car had stopped and she was sitting there, still holding Patrick's hand. They were at the gate. She opened her eyes. Patrick was watching her but said nothing.

Embarrassed, she released his hand. 'Thank you. Thank you for dinner. I'm so sorry about Rory. Don't come any further, you'll wake everyone up.'

Patrick reached into the compartment under the radio and took out a card. 'I'm off to Sydney in the morning. Ring me if you need anything.'

Diana stood just inside the door, listening to him drive off. How weird was that? He probably thought she was a crazy woman. Realistically, how could she refute it?

The house was so quiet. Everyone must be asleep. They certainly had gone to bed early. She looked at the clock. It was only nine thirty. Diana got into bed, carefully moving Saskia to her side, and she turned right over and slammed into her again. Diana lay there, eyes wide open.

Time for a tea.

Quietly she got out of bed and wandered into the kitchen. She stood watching the kettle boil. They say you should never do that.

That was so weird in the car just now, holding Patrick's hand and talking to Charlie in her head. Could she fall for someone else just months after Charlie died?

Stella came into the kitchen. 'Hello, did you have a good night? Patrick's nice, isn't he?'

'Yes, thanks.'

'Nice' didn't describe Patrick. He was charming, sensitive and thoughtful. Diana smiled. Her hand still tingled. She went to reach for another mug. 'Do you want a cup of tea?'

'Yes, please,' said Stella. 'Charlie would want you to be happy, you know.'

She wanted to talk again. If only she'd let it rest for a while, until Diana was ready.

'Have you thought any more about putting the children in school?' said Stella.

'Are you getting sick of them?'

'No, of course not.' She went to get the milk out of the fridge. 'We, um, just thought ...'

'I'm sorry, I'm not ready to make a decision yet. There's no point in them going to school if we're going back soon.'

'Of course, take your time.'

'You know I appreciate so much being here,' said Diana. 'It's hard for you and Dad, I know that. Just, thank you. Goodnight, Mum.'

'Goodnight, Diana. Sleep well.'

She left her mum to finish her tea.

CHAPTER TWENTY-FIVE

'A picnic?' There were three blank looks from the couch.

It was time to move the bodies from in front of the television. Diana had bought some sausages yesterday and asked her mother to make dough for puftaloons. Which had resulted in a blank look from her mother, too.

'I haven't made them for so long, I don't know if I can remember how.'

But Diana had worked it out, and the mixture was in the back of the ute, along with a saucepan, an old plough disc, sausages and a loaf of bread, newspaper, matches, fruit juice poppers, and some marshmallows she'd bought yesterday. Her mother had come out with a litre of oil, which she'd forgotten, just as they were setting off.

'For heaven's sake, be careful with the hot oil,' said Stella. 'Will you be all right starting the fire? Put it out carefully, won't you?'

Diana grinned and, along with her hatted, coated and booted children squashed into the front of the ute, set off.

As for starting a fire, for heaven's sake, she and Rosie had done this hundreds of times. To be totally honest, didn't she need some time alone with her kids? It was amazing how good they'd been.

Diana glanced over. The three faces weren't exactly alight with excitement. She started to sing. Milo and Saskia joined in. Teddy Bears, picnics and woods.

'It's called "woods" in England, isn't it, Mummy? Here it's called "bush".' Milo, ever a fund of information.

'Sure is.' She stopped at a gate and without prompting, Milo got out to open it.

'Where are we going?' Saskia was renowned for not taking anything in.

'We're going down to the creek, to my favourite place on earth, Saskia, for a picnic.'

'What are we going to eat?' Sienna sounded doubtful.

'Sausages and puftaloons.'

'What are puftaloons?' asked Milo as he got back in the car.

'They are little pieces of heaven, but you'll have to wait to try them yourselves and see what you think.' Diana smiled, she could hardly contain her excitement.

They were wending their way, slowly this time, down the same hillside where she'd come off the bike. It was such a beautiful day, sunny, no wind rustling the pointed narrow leaves of the sharp-scented eucalypts. Oh how she'd missed the soft, grey-green of the gum trees.

They had come as close as they could get in the ute. The rest of the way they had to clamber down, loaded up with implements and food, Diana helping Saskia, sliding down the last bit. It was worth it. Just the look on the kids' faces made her smile. The creek did a sharp turn but the ground beside it was flat, covered in a soft grass, some blackberry bushes and ferns. Large granite boulders littered the creek bed, which was largely dry now with just a few pools and wet, springy patches. The trees here were huge, white box, that showered the ground with creamy white, fluffy blossoms in spring. It was pure magic. Birds were singing, and Diana pointed to a little grey wallaby as it hopped slowly out of sight. The three were speechless. It was their first wallaby.

'A kangaroo!' Milo was squeaking in excitement.

'No. That, my children, is a wallaby. Kangaroos are bigger. Okay, first things first. We need wood.' The three kids stood and looked around them but didn't move. 'I mean we all go and get some wood to make a fire,' she repeated patiently.

'A real fire, Mummy?' Sienna looked as though she was going to give her a lecture on lighting fires.

'Yes,' Diana replied firmly. 'A real fire.'

They gathered the wood, then she set about showing her children how to build a fire. The kids stood silently as she piled the wood and scrunched-up paper. Luckily she'd brought enough paper, and the fire soon started and was burning brightly. Next they had to hunt for stones to put the plough disc on.

Diana heard a shout from the other side of the creek. A man and horse were standing there, and she had to look twice before she registered who it was.

'Mal!' Diana waved and shouted. 'Come on over. There's a gate over there.'

There was a gate in the boundary fence in case sheep got caught down here during floods. It probably hadn't been used for years.

Mal led his horse carefully over the creek, which had pitifully little water in it. It really was just a series of puddles. He tied the reins to a low branch so his horse could feed on the short pick.

'Well, well, you on a horse, I never thought I'd see the day,' Diana teased him.

'Just because your dad was mad about bikes and you didn't know anything about horses, doesn't mean I didn't.' He squatted down before their fire, poking around it with a stick. 'This is going well. I saw the smoke.'

'See, I remember how to light a fire. How's Rosie? I haven't seen her since the races.'

Milo came up carrying a heavy stone, much too big for their purposes, and dropped it at their feet. 'That's a big one, Milo. Look who's here.'

Milo's face lit up and he stuck out his hand. Mal shook hands and then turned to Sienna and Saskia with a smile. 'You're all working hard.'

'We saw a wallaby.' Saskia was clearly dying to get in first to tell him.

'We're getting stones to put the disc on so we can cook sausages.' Sienna still sounded doubtful. She held out her offering—two small stones. 'Look, Mummy, what about these?'

'Fantastic but we need some more.' Something clicked. 'My parents didn't send you to check on us, did they?' Diana asked Mal.

'No, of course not. Well, they did tell me where you'd gone when I rang a little while ago.' He stayed staring down at the fire.

'Would you like to join us, share a sausage?'

He looked up then and Diana was surprised to see an almost shy look cross his face. A flash of a memory of how the old Mal looked, way back when. She grinned at him and his face lit up.

'If you've got enough.'

'Oh, we have more than enough.' Diana waved airily towards the basket on the ground. 'There's tons, much more than we need. So explain why you're riding around on a horse?'

'The boss loves his horses. He likes me to exercise them every now and again.'

'So he has stock horses on Lost Valley, as well as racehorses?'

'Yes, a few Aussie stock horses, but they're mostly race-horses. There are about ten here, and the others are in Canberra. He's got, I don't know, four or five in training, I think.'

'It's funny, isn't it, how horses disappeared from the scene while we were growing up and now they're back.'

'They were around because they were useful, now they're for pleasure.'

Diana and Mal both pushed two large rocks up either side of the fire to rest the plough disc on. Then she roped Mal into getting more wood, bigger bits than they had managed to find. The fire was really catching on now.

The children were all introduced to the horse, whose name was Satan. For some reason, the enormous black horse didn't frighten them as much as the dogs had.

'I've picked him some more grass.' Sienna held out her offerings and laughed as the horse blew most of it away. Mal showed her how to offer him grass with it lying on the flat of her palm. She laughed again as he nibbled delicately at her hand.

'It tickles.'

'Come on, Sienna, help me get drinks for everyone,' said Diana. 'I think the fire needs to quieten down before we put the sausages on it.'

* * *

Providing lunch for two was a very different agenda from lunch for six. Stella got two cup-a-soups out of the pantry and put some toast on and wondered vaguely if it was enough. It looked a bit sparse. She was waiting for Tom to come in and worrying whether the others would be all right. The weather was perfect. She'd had no idea how sick you could get of blue skies. But cloudless blue it was today. Again.

It's all the other things that could go wrong. The ute could break down, and all she could do was pray they'd be careful with the fire.

That night when Diana was at Rosie's, Stella had got the children to ring their other grandparents. They obviously had a good connection with them. Sienna talked for ages. She was the most like Charlie in looks—she had his eyes. Stella sighed, she didn't know why they got off on the wrong foot with Charlie, but there was no denying they had. They were all so uncomfortable with him. She thought it was because there was no 'wearing in' time. No time to get used to the idea of Diana being married to an Englishman and all that entailed. All she could think was that this strange man was taking their daughter away, forever.

A Londoner, he'd called himself. He'd never been on a farm before. All of a sudden they were married and he was there, Diana's husband. Mal had been so different. Stella stopped buttering for a moment. They had known Mal forever. He'd spent more time on their farm when he was growing up than at home. Not that she blamed him—he was an only child living with his grandparents. They'd died soon after he and Rosie had got married but they didn't leave Mal much, mostly a big pile of debts. When everything was sold up there was just enough for them to put a deposit down on those acres and the little cottage. They'd done an amazing job with that, though.

Tom should be finished the planting soon. Then they just had to wait for some more rain. The thirty points they had a few weeks ago was enough to wet the soil, get things going, but they needed follow-up rain, badly. Like they'd needed rain badly these last ten years.

Tom came in filthy, reddened eyes and covered in dust. He went to wash up and came and sat down at the table. Stella didn't think he was terribly impressed by the spread before him either and he got up to get the jam out of the refrigerator.

'Fancy Diana asking for puftaloons,' she said. 'Remember we used to cook them on picnics when the girls were little?'

By the look on his face he was obviously thinking puftaloons would be good right now.

'Well, I'm finished the planting. Tractor's back in the shed,' he said. 'That's it, now we need rain. Is this all?' He looked at the food on the table. 'I'm quite hungry.'

That was a surprise. He hadn't been hungry lately. He'd hardly been eating anything.

'There's a tin of baked beans in the pantry. I'll get it.'

'I think I'll give Milo some lessons on the bike when they get back. He's ten, plenty old enough.'

'You'd better ask Diana first.'

He smiled at her. 'It's good having them here, isn't it?'

She smiled back. 'Yes.' She was afraid to say how much she loved having them. 'I'm glad Diana's taken them out on a picnic. I'm so worried about her, you know she won't talk about Charlie at all to me. It's not good for her, is it?'

'It wouldn't be normal if you weren't worried about some-one or something,' said Tom. 'She'll talk when she's ready. Thing is, Stell, how about we go down and join them? At the creek. I've finished for the day, there's no reason we couldn't go, is there?'

Stella jumped up. 'Great idea. Oh, I don't know, should we invade their space? Do you think Diana wants to be alone with the kids? They've got plenty of food.'

'It's a great day out there. Couldn't get a better one. Come on, we'll go on the bike.'

Stella swallowed her surprise. Tom hadn't suggested something like this for ages. But she wasn't going to demur. 'I'll just find a hat.'

* * *

'So how do you like the arty world, Diana? Charlie would have fitted right in with it, wouldn't he?'

Mal was turning the sausages over.

'Yeah, I guess. I think he enjoyed it more than I did. It's very different to here. Just looking around makes me sad though, it's so beautiful. I've missed all this.' Diana waved her arm around. 'I wanted to be a farmer. You never know where life is going to lead you.'

'But you've done so well, been very successful, from all reports. You wouldn't have done that here.'

Diana was about to answer when they heard shouts from above.

'Hi, there, any one home?'

They looked up. Two bodies were scrambling down the steep bank.

'Tom, Stella!' The children yelled in delight and rushed over to greet them.

'How did you get here?' Diana asked.

'We came on the bike.' Stella laughed. 'Tom finished early so we thought, that is, can we—'

'Of course,' said Diana. 'That's wonderful. Look who's here? Mal found us, too.'

'Um, I could have been responsible for that.' Stella looked a little guilty. Diana laughed and gave her a hug.

This was something they should have done before. Everyone relaxed, and the kids were being normal. Diana felt so happy. Mal was throwing stones into the water with Milo to see who could make the biggest splash, and Stella and the girls were looking for fairies—a game she remembered from long ago, with Rosie and Cody. She turned to the sausages.

'Help! They're burning.'

The sausages were only a little charred and they ate them in a slice of bread. No sauce—the sauce had been forgotten, but no one minded.

Diana filled the saucepan with the oil to cook the puftaloons. 'Just you wait, kids! These will be fantastic. Mum, thank God you're here to show me how to do it.'

'Oh no, you'll do a much better job than me.' Stella shook her head.

'Hey, give it to me, I haven't forgotten.' Mal reached for the dish that held the dough and dropped three spoonfuls into the hot oil.

'Wow,' said Milo. The children were fascinated. They all watched the little puftaloons magically expand and begin to colour as they rolled slowly in the oil.

'I didn't bring any sugar. Oh, I know.' Diana went to the basket and found the packet of marshmallows. 'Look what I've got.' She was jubilant and sent the kids looking for sharp sticks. Milo came back and showed her the stick he'd found

'Perfect,' said Diana and handed him a marshmallow. 'Right, now put the marshmallow on the end and hold it over the fire. Not right in. Just a little closer, that's right.'

They all agreed that melted marshmallows on top of puftaloons, served on a plate of folded newspaper, were just the best thing that any of them had ever tasted.

After lunch, just Diana and Stella were left sitting beside the dying fire. Tom had taken Milo back with him on the bike and Mal had left soon after. Diana sat propped against a tree trunk and Stella was sitting on a rock where she could keep an eye on the two girls who were playing near the water.

'This has been so good for them, Mum, thank you.'

'The picnic, or us joining you? I hope you didn't mind.'

'Absolutely both. Look at them.' Diana looked in the direction of the girls, heads together, engrossed in some game.

'What do you think about Patrick?'

'Mmm. He said he'd been married before but that was a while ago. Does he bring a lot of women down to Lost Valley?'

'Not that I've noticed. He seems to keep the farm a private place, I think. Sean and Marnie and the kids seem to come a lot.'

Diana yawned.

'If you want to close your eyes for a moment, I can watch the girls.'

'No, I'm fine, really, I think I'm finally beginning to relax a bit.'

There was silence for a minute or two.

'I got to know Charlie so much better in London, when I came over,' said Stella. 'He was a fun person, wasn't he? It was tragic to lose him so suddenly. But the hurt, missing him like you must be, it gets better. You mightn't believe me, but it does.'

Diana looked down where the girls were, fighting the tears. Why now? What could she say? *Well, actually, Mum, he wasn't that much fun that night. And what if it wasn't an accident that killed Charlie?* That would go down a treat.

They got back to the house without saying any more to each other. A little white Honda was parked at the back steps.

'Rosie's here,' Stella said.

Saskia was out first, having sat on Stella's lap on the way home. 'Hello, Rosie,' she said. 'We've just been on a picnic.'

'So I've been hearing.' Rosie turned furious eyes on Diana as she got out of the ute. 'I hope you've all had a lovely time. It's been ages since we've all been on a picnic. In fact I can't remember when the last one was. And Mal was there, too. What a treat for you all.'

'Your father and I crashed it, and Mal, well, I asked him to check on Diana … If we only knew you were here … It just evolved, Rosie.' Stella looked worriedly at Rosie as she came round the back of the ute. 'Sorry, darling.'

'Things don't change, do they?' Rosie stormed off, got in her car and drove away.

CHAPTER TWENTY-SIX

It had been over twenty years since Diana had been to a clearing sale and it looked exactly as it had when she was a child. The same red sign was fixed to the gate: Auction.

Forty or fifty cars were parked in straggly lines over the paddock; there must be over a hundred people here. Mal had brought her and the children. He wanted to look at a couple of tractors. Rosie and her mother planned to come over later.

To Diana's eyes, the rows and rows of heaped items for sale looked a little more decrepit and a little more useless. Maybe that was because they were the same items she remembered from her childhood. They sure looked the same. Cleverly, each lot held maybe one piece you might conceivably want, lumped together with at least ten you would never, ever have any use for. Milo had set off and thoroughly inspected every single lot and was now playing on the tractors with Sienna and Saskia. There were kids everywhere—running around underfoot, in strollers and prams, and strapped to tummies. If there was any worry about the population numbers in Australia, Diana smiled to herself, all anyone need do was come to a clearing sale to be reassured.

Wandering over to the tent, where lukewarm coffee in foam cups could be bought for one dollar and a glad-wrapped ham sandwich for just two dollars more, Diana was surprised to hear her name.

'Diana Crawford!'

A tall, elderly man with a great silver mane of hair emerged through the crowd. He was dressed in an old green corduroy jacket and sported a silk paisley scarf wound around his neck. He was balancing two cups of coffee and two sandwiches in his hands.

'Mr Herschel!' Diana cried.

Her old art teacher was smiling widely at her, and the fact that he had his arms full was the only thing stopping her from throwing her arms round him. 'It's so good to see you!'

'It's been too many years, Diana. When did you get back?'

'A month or so.'

He hesitated. 'I am so sorry for your loss.'

When Diana looked blankly at him, he nodded, 'Rosie told me.'

Just then, a tiny round woman with white hair pulled into a bun on the top of her head, popped up beside Mr Herschel and rescued one of the coffees from him.

'You haven't met my wife Una. This is Diana Crawford, one of my best students.'

Una positively beamed at her and offered her hand. 'Of course. I've heard you're now a very famous potter.'

'Oh no.' Diana shook her head. 'But I am a potter, and that is largely thanks to Mr Herschel.'

In the distance, Diana caught sight of Patrick. He was talking to Mal. Mal hadn't said anything about him coming. Not that she'd asked. The conversation in the car this morning had been pretty mundane. Rosie had not been happy about the picnic and Diana couldn't really blame her. She'd have felt the same way.

'I'm sorry.' She'd missed Una's last comment.

'Have you anything you've got your eye on?' Una repeated patiently.

'Um, no, I've just come to have a look. These are incredible affairs, aren't they?'

'We wouldn't miss them for the world,' said Una. 'I am a collector of just about anything. Sid didn't know that when we married, but they say "for better or worse".' She smiled mischievously at her husband.

'Diana, I was hoping to see you,' said Mr Herschel. 'Have you brought any of your work with you? Would you come to the school to show the children, give some tips and talk to the art class?'

'You are not still teaching!' Diana couldn't help her amazement. It was rude, she knew.

Mr Herschel laughed at her. 'Goodness, no. But I know the art teacher, very well. I could organise it.'

'Mummy, Mummy!' Milo ran up and tried to pull her by the hand. 'Mummy, I've found something for Stella. Can I buy it, please?'

Diana grimaced. 'Oh no, Milo, we don't need any of this junk.'

'It's not junk, Mummy. It's really beautiful. Please, come quickly.'

'I'm sorry, I must go. I'd be happy to come to the art class, Mr Herschel. I have a couple of things. Ring me. So nice to meet you, Una,' she added over her shoulder, as she was literally pulled away by a very determined Milo.

The lot was indistinguishable from all the others. A pile of junk: two faded old Arnott's Biscuit tins with the signature rosella on the lid; three Fowlers preserving jars without lids; a handful of mismatched cutlery and a double-sided toaster with a very frayed cord. And then she saw it. A large white enamel pitcher with a wide lip, chipped, and with a rusty stain down one side.

'See, Mummy, Stella would love it. She can water her plants with it.' Milo looked anxiously up at her 'Can I buy it for her?'

Diana felt weak. 'You've got to buy the whole lot with it, Milo.' It was such a lovely thought. Milo had an uncanny ability to hit on the perfect present. He would have worked out Stella could use it for watering the garden, as she spent a huge amount of time recycling water out of the wash tub and the kitchen sink onto the garden. Diana bit her lip and looked around. The small crowd surrounding the auctioneer was still a long way off. It would probably be some hours. Now what was she going to do?

'Hello, Diana.' Patrick had come up behind them. 'Hello, Milo.'

Milo ignored him. He hadn't taken his eyes from Diana and she knew he wouldn't until she'd given him an answer.

'Say hello, Milo. All right, you can buy it for Stella. But it will be ages before the auctioneer gets to this lot.' She turned to Patrick. 'Hi. I didn't know you were coming.' Or why she felt so pleased to see him.

He was wearing a sleeveless vest, jeans and boots—all spotless. City farmer fashionista. He looked good though.

'I wanted Mal to have a look at a tractor.'

'Have you heard the news?' Mal was striding up to them. He looked shocked, horrified even. 'Pete Summers is dead.'

The Summers were friends of Diana's parents. Pete was much the same age as her father. They had four boys, and Alan had been the closest in age to her.

'Has he been ill?' Diana asked.

'No,' Mal said. 'It was a shooting accident.' He paused. 'He didn't come in last night and Shelley went out looking for him, found him near a fence. The gun must have gone off when he was getting through the fence, they think.'

'A bit odd,' said Patrick. 'Usually you put the safety catch on when you're climbing through a fence.'

'I know. Not the sort of thing you forget to do, is it?'

Diana remembered Mal had been a good friend of Alan Summers when they were growing up. 'How are the boys, and Shelley? She must be devastated. Does Mum know?'

'I'm not sure,' said Mal. 'Diana, I'm going to have to go. Alan rang me and asked me to come over. I'm sorry, Patrick, I'll have to leave. Diana, could you gather the kids?' He turned to go, not waiting for answers, making his way through the lines of sale items, shoulders hunched and hands in his pockets.

'Mum?' said Milo. 'I can't go yet!' His stubborn little face was set in a look Diana knew only too well.

'We have to go, sweetheart. Mal has to leave right now.'

'Why don't you stay and I'll take you all home,' Patrick interrupted. 'There'll be nothing much for you to do about all this. Your parents might want to go with Mal when they hear.'

Diana thought that might be all too probable. She wished she had a car.

'Mum, please can we stay?'

She looked at Milo, weighing up her chances of getting him to leave. They weren't good. 'Thank you, Patrick, if you're sure?'

'Certainly, it won't be a problem.'

'I'll go tell Mal.' It would be better if Mal didn't have to worry about them. 'Are you coming, Milo?' Again, a stubborn shake of the head. He was staying put.

Diana hurried after Mal.

The news had shot around the sale like wildfire. It seemed everyone knew within minutes. Not long after Mal had left, other cars were winding their way slowly towards the gate, trailed by puffs of dust. Faces were saddened and shocked. Everyone knew and liked Pete Summers.

'Did you know him?' Diana asked Patrick as they stood beside Milo, who wasn't moving from his intended purchase.

'Yes, I met him at the saleyards, drafting and counting out. He used to help Tim Spelling.'

'He was such a quiet, nice man. I don't remember him ever saying anything horrible about anyone. He adored his boys, used to go and watch them play football. My father used to enjoy going with him; he didn't have any sons to watch.'

By this time, Sienna had heard Milo was buying the enamel pitcher and she wanted to buy something for Stella, too. Diana rolled her eyes but had to go to inspect all the piles again. Sienna pounced on a faded bunch of artificial flowers.

'Stella would really love these, Mummy, wouldn't she? We could put them in one of Milo's jars.'

'But you've got to buy all the other things too,' Diana remonstrated, looking at the broken picture frames and the sad bunch of flowers she was sure her mother would hate. There'd never been artificial flowers in the house, ever.

'We could put pictures of us in the frames for her and she could hang them in the hall too.'

'Oh dear. I don't think Patrick will have room for us and all this, too.' One last throw of the dice.

'No, Patrick has a really big car, Mummy.'

'No problem, Diana, there's plenty of room.' Patrick had come up behind them. She had a feeling he was enjoying this.

'I wish you would stop saying there's no problem. What am I going to do with all this?'

'I'm not sure, but I certainly wouldn't be game to tell them no. They're a determined lot, aren't they?' Patrick was smiling. He hunkered down to talk to Sienna. 'I think Stella will like those very much, Sienna.' He was rewarded with one of her rare smiles.

'Stella doesn't have many flowers at the moment,' she told him shyly, 'because of the drought.'

All Diana needed was Saskia wanting a pile too. She didn't take long. Her offering was a little more obscure. A pile of broken toys that included an under-stuffed, spotted dog lacking an eye.

'No, Saskia.'

'But Mummy, he doesn't have a home!' Saskia's eyes filled with tears and she buried her face in Diana's stomach.

Oh brother! 'Don't say anything!' she glowered at Patrick, who was trying not to laugh.

Saskia's pile came up first and then Sienna's and then Milo's. Diana had had to go and register at the official tent and come back with her number to bid. She had to admit they certainly hadn't broken the bank. By the time they had got to their lots, the crowd had thinned considerably and she felt Tim was just grateful someone would relieve him of the goods. It came to about seventeen dollars altogether.

CHAPTER TWENTY-SEVEN

Pete Summers dead! Stella couldn't believe it. Just last week, or was it the week before, she'd seen them both in the supermarket. Shelley would be devastated. What a terrible way to find ... No, she didn't want to think about it. Mal was coming to pick her up on his way over. She'd taken a casserole from the freezer and found a tin of peaches, and luckily she had just finished icing a chocolate slice. They were sitting on the table in a bag ready to take with her. Pete! He was one of the gentlest men she had ever met. It was too terrible for words. Those poor boys!

Tom had thought about coming but he'd changed his mind. He thought it would be better if she went and stayed with Shelley. He'd gone back out again. He was shocked. Stella felt quite shaken, herself.

She must leave something out for Diana. There were some sausages and chops; that would do them. They were really enjoying meat. Did they ever eat meat in London, she wondered.

Stella watched the road from the front verandah. She shuddered. It was all coming back—twenty-five years ago seemed like yesterday.

She remembered so vividly the shock of not being able to wake Cody up that morning. The little chest rising and falling; she was flushed and hot to touch but she wouldn't wake up. Yelling for Tom, Stella had grabbed a blanket and wrapped it around her child, meeting a tousled Tom in the hall.

'Something's wrong with Cody. Quick, you hold her while I get dressed.' Tom followed her into their bedroom and laid the horribly limp body on the bed while he pulled on jeans and a shirt and jumper.

'What's happened to her?'

'Diana ... Diana!' Fifteen-year-old Diana appeared mystified at the doorway, yawning. 'Did you notice anything last night when you put her to bed?'

She seemed shocked. 'No,' she said slowly. 'Maybe she was a bit quiet, but I gave her Panadol like you said and she went straight to sleep. Not a peep.'

'Ring the hospital and tell them we're coming in straight away.' It was as though everyone was moving in slow motion. This couldn't be happening. Cody had been perfectly well yesterday. Stella hadn't been at all worried to go with Tom last night, leaving Diana in charge. Okay, maybe Cody was looking as though she was coming down with something, so she'd told Diana to give her some Panadol if she thought she needed it.

'What else happened? Something else must have happened!' She was yelling at Diana. Where was her other shoe?

'Shh, Stella, not now. Diana and Rosie, you stay here. We'll ring you from the hospital and keep you up to date.'

The frantic drive to town. The road was mostly dirt then but it didn't slow them down any.

And then watching her daughter die. No parent should ever have to do that. The silent scream building up inside her. Nothing to be done. No answers. Nothing could have been done. An out-of-the-blue, massive bacterial infection. Meningitis. Words, no action, just words that didn't mean anything.

Why wouldn't someone do something?

But there was nothing anyone could do, was there? So many times she'd gone over that scene in her head. So many times.

Seeing Mal's white four-wheel drive turn off the road and bump over the ramp galvanised her into action, and she walked back to the kitchen for the bag of food.

Once she was in the car and they were on their way, Stella asked, 'How did you hear?' He was driving just a little too fast, she felt.

'Alan rang me at the auction.'

'Did he say how his mother was?'

'Pretty bad, apparently she found him.'

'How horrible.' The thought of it made Stella feel quite sick.

'She's pretty cut up.'

'You don't think, Mal, do you, that he ... that it wasn't an accident?' Stella couldn't help but ask the question.

'I don't know Stella, I don't know. It's the sort of thing you don't want to know, do you, for everyone's sakes. Go gently with Shelley, won't you? Don't even think it, is the best way to go.' Mal looked over at her. He was so sad. He was a very thoughtful person.

'Rosie didn't want to come?'

'Best if she doesn't. Alan and the other boys will be there. It hasn't been much of a female household—they don't really know how to cope with women. None of them are married. I think they'll want to have a few beers. Shelley would like you to come, though. Pity Tom didn't want to.' They drove on down the dirt road, gravel scattering under the wheels as they cornered on the way to the Summer's farm.

'I don't know why Tom wouldn't come. He was one of his good friends. There's no accounting for how Tom is going to react these days'.

'Don't suppose he's given any more thought to handing over?' Mal concentrated on the road ahead, changing down for the next corner. 'I'm not sure how much longer I can wait, Stella. I'm going to have to go and do something else. Find a good job. Rosie's very restless too. Patrick doesn't want a cattle man; he's talking now about putting in hops. What do I know about growing hops? Nothing. I'm wasted there, I think. I need to know something concrete, soon, cause I'll have to look for another job if not.'

Stella didn't know what to answer. She could talk to Tom again, go round in circles again, try for an answer but get nowhere. 'I'll try, Mal, I'll try.'

They had arrived at the farm. Alan was at the door. Shelley was inside, sitting on the lounge, ashen-faced. Stella went to make some tea.

So many men in the room, not knowing what to do. The Summers were all tall, strapping boys. But they looked stunned. Strange, the aftermath of death. Everyone was quiet, no idea what to say or how to make anything better. The phone would ring, one of the neighbours would answer it and write names on a pad near the phone. Stella sat down next to Shelley and gave her a cup of tea.

'He didn't come in last night,' Shelley whispered. 'He's usually in by dark. Sometimes, when the days are short like this, he's a bit later, but by six he wasn't in and I took the car, and a torch, and I was shining it around and ... Oh God.'

Stella took the cup quickly as Shelley started to sob quietly.

'Don't, Mum.' One of the boys came over to stand help-lessly in front of her. 'Please don't.'

'No, it's better to cry, Adam'. Stella thought it was Adam. He was one of the middle ones. 'Let it out, Shelley. You'll feel better for it.'

'Why, why, why, why?' Shelley was rocking, backwards and forwards, her face in her hands. 'Why, why, why? He didn't even tell me he was taking the gun.'

Why? Stella went cold. She had asked herself the same after Cody had died.

Why on earth had she gone out that night?

Why hadn't she got home earlier? Checked her before she'd gone to bed.

They'd been told that everyone carries the bacteria. Why did it attack Cody? Why did she die?

May as well have asked the man in the moon. There'd been no answers for her.

Stella took Shelley's hand. 'It's too early for answers, Shell. You've got to rant and rail, feel despair, get angry, be hurt ... and then later, much later, you'll be so glad that he was part of your life. You've had a good marriage. He was such a lovely man. We all loved him. Pete got so much pleasure out of his boys, and he adored you.'

'Why?' whispered Shelley brokenly. 'Why? We've been having some trouble with a dingo, we think, on our boundary near the national park. But why did he take the gun and not a rifle? It doesn't make any sense'

'I don't know, Shell.'

'I knew he was depressed, this bloody drought. Year after year. We were going to have to ask the bank for refinancing again. But he wouldn't, he couldn't ... I know he wouldn't.' Shelley closed her eyes. 'He'd stopped talking to me, he was so angry. I've got no idea what he was thinking.'

Hell. 'Don't do this, Shell, of course he wouldn't. Don't go there,' Stella said urgently, taking both her hands. 'Do you feel like going to have a rest? I've bought a casserole and I'm going to put it in the oven, for later. I've brought you some of my pills. I rang Will Talbot and asked if it would be all right and he said one would be fine. Here, take it with your tea, and you can go and lie down for a bit.'

It was happening far too often, that's what Stella did know. Too many men, the farmers around her, were dying for no good reason.

The atmosphere was beginning to get to her. Cody had died twenty-five years ago, but it was exactly the same—the milling around, the confusion on everyone's face. The soft muted voices as though the recently departed might be listening. Maybe he was.

Oh my God, she thought, stricken, it had been like this for Diana too. So far away, she'd sounded so remote, so in control when she'd rang. Stella and Tom had been quite intimidated. 'No need to come,' she'd said. It had been terrible not knowing how to help and being so far away. She wiped the tears angrily from her eyes.

Well, if Pete was watching, she just hoped he could see how upset everyone was. The stupid fool, accident or not. What a mess. Stella banged the oven door shut, the noise echoing in the empty kitchen. Where in the hell had Tom got to? He should be here.

CHAPTER TWENTY-EIGHT

'Would you all like to come over for a quick meal on the way home? We've got to go past the gate.'

They were in Patrick's car, loaded with all their purchases, on the way home from the sale. And he certainly didn't have to detour.

'Your parents would have probably gone with Mal and Rosie, wouldn't they?' he said. 'There'll be no one at home. Stay,' he urged.

'Thank you. We'd like that, wouldn't we, kids?' Diana turned to the three passive faces in the back. They must be exhausted; it had been a long day. But there were no mutinous looks. Besides, she was curious to see Lost Valley. She had only vague recollections of the house. It was an old rambling sandstone place, and there'd been a long run of absentee landlords while she was growing up. 'Are you sure that's all right?'

'I think we can manage,' he replied confidently, not that she thought the little matter of whipping up a meal for five on the spur of the moment would be beyond him.

They swept through the entrance into the tree-lined gravel drive, with a curved sandstone wall on either side, ending in two stone pylons holding up the black, wrought-iron gates.

'What beautiful trees,' Diana murmured, observing the bare branches. 'A drive of elms?'

'Yes, they're magnificent in spring.'

Diana looked at the green lawns, massive trees and shrubs, and garden beds neatly edged. 'What happened to your drought?' she asked dubiously.

'I put in a couple of bores, year before last, and they've kept up the water fairly well. I've been lucky.'

'Mmm, well, I'm not sure about lucky. Fortunate maybe.'

Patrick smiled.

They had circled round in front of the house. It was a beautiful old homestead made of brick and stone, only one storey, but it had a slate roof and solid round stone columns lining the spacious front verandah. French windows, opening onto the verandah, shone square, golden eyes in the late-afternoon sun. A lot of work had been done to it since she'd last been here.

'Oh Patrick! It looks fantastic.'

His smile was broad. 'Yes, it does, doesn't it?'

She couldn't help smiling back at him.

*   *   *

Diana suggested the kids go outside and play. She watched as they ran outside, immediately running and shouting, making up some game.

'You have no idea, they're so different from the day we arrived. You'd hardly recognise them. I was so worried I'd done the wrong thing, bringing them to Australia. I feel awful for the Summers, but the kids have run and played all day like normal children. I'd appreciate you not talking about it in front of them, though, because of their father—' She stopped. God, she was rattling on.

'Of course I won't. I think you were right to take them away, change environments. What would you like to drink? Beer, wine, whiskey … I think I have most things.'

'A beer would be good, thanks. I feel thirsty.'

They were in the enormous kitchen. Diana was impressed. Patrick, or whoever had decorated the place, had kept faithfully to the age of the house. No granite benchtops and stainless steel ovens here. It had a comfortable look—smooth pine counters, white cupboards and splashback, and a black and white tiled floor. An Aga stove had been fitted into the big old fireplace.

'I love these things, we've got one at home.' Diana walked over to the stove and swept her fingers over its smooth enamel surface.

'You're a very tactile person,' Patrick said, handing her a beer.

'Yes, that's an accurate observation.' Diana smiled 'My fingers sometimes run away with me. They have a life of their own.'

'I suppose an artist can be excused on that front.'

She was looking at his hand holding the beer, at the muscles of his forearm before they disappeared under his shirt, that was rolled up to his elbow. The strength of that arm— he must roll around a few beer barrels in his spare time.

The thought of his fingers touching her stopped her breath. 'Where are my children?'

'The kids are fine. I can see them through the window.'

She followed his line of sight. The children were immersed in some game. Milo was gesticulating wildly and the girls were following him.

'You must think I'm a crazy woman, holding your hand the other night in the car.'

'No, I appreciated it very much. Sharing my grief with you. If it helps, I'd be perfectly happy for you to do it again. I know you're going through hell right now.' Patrick came to stand beside her at the Aga. He took the beer from her hand and put it down beside him on the benchtop. He just stood there patiently, his arms by his sides.

She couldn't help herself and reached out her hand. It was like touching a bronze come to life. His arm was solid and muscular with a fine sprinkle of black hairs. He was so still, so controlled, watching her intently. Her insides quivered— damn, she had a sudden urge to ruffle his composure. She reached up and kissed him.

It was a simple kiss, straightforward, a meeting of lips, a mingling of breath, that was all. But the shock that rocketed through her was unexpected. The guilt, huge … wrong, wrong, wrong. Charlie was there all around her. Bad move, when would she ever learn?

Man, woman, right time, opportunity and all day the curiosity had been building. She knew that.

Not very bright, Diana.

Charlie, would you go away?

Diana drew a trembling breath and took a step sideways, away from Patrick. He was just watching her. No smile, no grin, no flippant comment. He wouldn't get one from her either.

She walked away from him, inspecting the kitchen. 'I love what you've done to the house, the kitchen.'

'It's been a labour of love,' he said, and went to the fridge for another two beers. 'A wonderful way to get away from my life in Sydney.' He paused. 'After Rory, well, I immersed myself in work and Van did the same thing. She was a solicitor.'

'Everyone deals with it differently.'

'We grew apart, not together.'

'Why are you telling me this?'

'The next time you kiss me, I want this to be behind us. I may not be able to put dead ghosts to rest but at least I can allay the live ones.'

Diana gave him a quick look. Surely he couldn't feel Charlie? She swallowed. She watched him take a tray of steak out of the freezer and put it into the microwave to defrost, and then pull out a loaf of bread and some tomatoes.

'Will your children eat steak and bread?'

'Will they ever! I can't get enough meat into them. It's like chocolate is for most kids. Have you any tomato sauce?' Her hands were shaking. She held on to the back of the chair in front of her. 'I shouldn't have done that, I'm sorry. I can't quite believe Charlie's dead. I keep thinking he'll walk in or ring up with some new zany project. I have no right to go around kissing people. I don't know what's the matter with me.'

Patrick faced her across the table.

'Looking back, I seem to have been travelling a single road,' Diana went on. 'A few twists and turns, but my road came to a dead end when Charlie died. Now I don't know what to do. My children are half English. Do I deny them their English or their Australian heritage? I didn't realise how much I missed Australia until I came back. How being Australian is so powerful. It really means something to me.' She shrugged. 'Then, my work has always been important. Well, more than important, but so are my children. But you see, at the moment I can't pot. It's never failed me before.' She looked up at him.

'Give it time.'

'Don't say that, I'm so sick of that excuse. I've never really wanted to do anything else except pot, or maybe be a farmer.'

Patrick smiled. 'Your dad talks about how you and he would argue about what to sow, how you read *The Land* newspaper from front to back, and you were always coming up with some new idea.'

'Did he really? I'd forgotten that. How embarrassing,' said Diana. 'How long were you married?'

'Four years.'

'That's not very long.'

'Compared to ten with Charlie?'

'When you say it like that, it isn't very long either.'

Did you want more, Diana? You could have fooled me.

Suddenly Charlie was there, all around her. Why did it hurt so much, the remembering? When she'd come out here she'd wanted to forget. Have her old life take over. Fill up the empty spaces with her family and Mog's Hill. It had almost worked. Then Charlie would pop up at the most odd times, like when she'd held Patrick's hand. Was she going crazy?

She didn't think she'd do that again.

Charlie wasn't here anymore, she had to get that through her thick skull. But how do you suddenly stop being someone's wife? He'd been such a huge part of her for the last ten years. Even dead, he was still a part of her. Kissing Patrick was confusing.

No more kissing.

'Would you like to see the house?' Patrick asked.

Walking first into the old-fashioned dining room, Diana spotted an Arthur Boyd hanging over the huge oak sideboard that was almost the same size as the table.

'Oh my, that's beautiful. Isn't it interesting how modern paintings can look so right in an old house?'

'Probably it's because the rooms are large enough to show them off. Look at the high ceilings.'

'I guess,' she agreed. 'I love wood—look at these window frames.' She ran her fingers over the beautiful oiled cedar.

'Mmm. They nearly drove me demented. Do you know how much stripper and sandpaper it took to get them back?' Patrick shook his head.

'Did you do them?' Diana was surprised.

'Yes. They had coats and coats of cream paint when I started. I took the doors off and had them stripped in Sydney but I did the windows myself. It took me ages.'

'You've certainly done a great job.'

'It was worth it, wasn't it?'

Diana looked at him curiously. Charlie would never have had the patience to do something like this. She followed Patrick into the hall where a bronze sculpture stood on the hall table.

'A Remington! How fabulous.' She raced over to the group of galloping cowboys and horses and gazed in admiration. 'How did he do it?'

Patrick chuckled. 'It's a copy. But it's lovely, isn't it? I found it in a gallery in New York when I was there.'

'That's enough surprises, I don't think I can take any more.' She grimaced theatrically.

They walked back into the kitchen.

'I can't stop thinking about Pete Summers. Dad will be so sad. They used to go off to ram sales together, sometimes. I don't know whether they still do.'

'Dinner's nearly ready,' said Patrick. 'Just have something to eat and I'll get you home.'

*   *   *

The kids were subdued when they called them in to eat. It had been a long day for them all. Diana frowned at Milo as he squirted tomato sauce over his steak. 'On the side, remember. Saskia, do you want me to help you cut that up?'

'I can do it.'

Diana watched as Saskia awkwardly tried to cut through her thick piece of steak with her fist around the fork. She was going through a very independent phase at the moment.

'Sam and Alex should be up to visit soon.' Patrick said.

Milo looked up, his mouth full, suddenly remembering to put down his knife and fork.

'You could come over and ride the motorbikes. Better still, I can send one over for you to practice on, while you're here. Tom can teach you, or your mother. I'll get Mal to run it over.'

'Mum, that's great. We can, can't we?'

Diana looked helplessly at Patrick and shrugged. 'If you're sure, I think so. Thank you.'

She really didn't know about the offer of the mini bike, but Milo had looked so excited, how could she say no? It was hard to keep from telling the children to hurry up. Patrick must have sensed her unease since the kiss. It had been a mistake. The sooner they got out of this situation, the better.

CHAPTER TWENTY-NINE

Just five weeks they'd been here, these beautiful grandchildren of hers. Stella sat surrounded by gifts from them. There was a large lump in her throat and she was having some difficulty controlling the tears.

'Don't you like it? We had to wait 'til you were home, but you didn't get back 'til after we'd gone to bed.'

Milo looked anxious, like he was hoping his water pitcher wasn't the thing that was making her unhappy. He was incredibly like Frank, Tom's father, in his manner. How had that crossed a couple of generations? It was a wonder Peg hadn't noticed. Though not all that strange, considering she didn't know who he was half the time.

'I absolutely love it, all of it. It's just that I can't believe you all thought of me and bought me something.' She blew her nose and sniffed. 'Goodness, what booty!'

'What's a booty, Stella?' Saskia had propped the stuffed dog on the chair next to her. She turned and grabbed it by both ears and looked deeply into its one eye. 'I think Spot is hungry. Actually, I wouldn't be surprised if he was very hungry.'

'It must be lunchtime then. Sienna, can you get the bread and margarine out of the fridge? Tommo will be in soon, and Mummy's having lunch with Granny. Milo, you can do the drinks.' Stella rose, gathering herself together. 'Saskia, booty is the word pirates use for treasure. It means lots of treasure.'

'I don't think it looks like real treasure,' Sienna said doubtfully. 'There's no jewels and money.'

'I just mean that it's treasure for me. Thank you so much, all of you. I'm just happy, so happy you've come to Australia.'

'If you're happy, why are you crying?' asked Milo, puzzled.

'Sometimes people cry when they're happy.' She went to get some knives from the cutlery drawer.

'Mummy cries when she's sad,' Milo said.

'Mummies and grandmothers are allowed to cry if they are happy or sad,' Stella said firmly.

Tom spoke from the doorway. 'Milo, you'll find women cry quite a lot of the time. Best not to ask why.' He paused to kiss Stella on her forehead before going in to wash up.

'Stan rang and they're going to be a few days late,' Stella called after him. Stan was their shearing contractor.

Tom came back into the kitchen. 'What do you mean a few days?'

'Well, a week really.'

'Bloody hell. That's just not good enough. I've got to get the ewes shorn before lambing. They know that. What on earth's happened?'

Tom had such a short fuse these days. Stella busied herself filling the kettle. 'Apparently WorkCover came into the shed they're in at the moment, the Palmers, and said the board was unsound and shearing was cancelled until they got it right.'

'Damn them. We finally get rid of the unions and now WorkCover makes life impossible. As if the board at Palmers hasn't been sound enough for the last thirty years.'

'Well, can you find anyone else?'

'You've got to be joking, who can find shearers these days? Milo, if you're looking for a career I advise shearing. Shearers are going to be extinct in the next few years!' With that, Tom stomped off to the bathroom.

'What's a shearer, Stella?' asked Milo.

Stella had to laugh. 'You've been to the shearing shed. The shearers come to take the wool off the sheep, before lambing.' And hoping to put Milo off from his next question, which she had a feeling she could predict fairly accurately, she addressed Tom, who had come back into the kitchen and was standing in front of the Aga.

'How is the state of your suit?'

'Hmm,' he grunted, 'it's been so long since I've used it, I've no idea.'

'You'll need it for Thursday.'

'Is that Pete's—'

Stella's warning glance stopped him. 'Yes, it's on Thursday. Eleven o'clock.' She didn't want any references to funerals in front of these three. 'You'll be meeting your cousin soon.' She told the children.

'Is our cousin Phillipa?' asked Sienna.

'Yes, that's right. She'll be coming home soon, for the holidays. Have you any English cousins?'

Milo looked to Sienna and Saskia and then answered for them. 'No, Daddy didn't have any brothers or sisters, and you have to have them before you can have cousins.'

Once again Stella felt a pang for the English grandparents. She'd forgotten that Charlie was an only child. They would be missing this lot unbearably. She would get them to ring again tonight. Again, she wished they had a computer so they could email and Skype, which everyone was talking about—free international telephone calls. If only, she sighed.

'Stella, why does the wool have to come off the sheep before they lamb?'

'Because we are lambing in winter, the shorn ewes find a nice sheltered spot to have their lamb—so they both stay warm and protected.' Stella smothered a smile. That being exactly the question she'd expected.

* * *

'Granny,' Diana called, closing the door gently behind her. She stood for a moment stretching the muscles in her back, before going straight to the kettle and filling it.

'Would you like a coffee? Granny?' She paused at the doorway to the sitting room. Her grandmother was sitting in her chair, as usual, eyes closed. She must be sleeping. She did, Diana was relieved to notice, appear to be wearing her hearing aid.

Diana suddenly noticed a large smudge of dust on the front of her T-shirt. She hadn't bothered to change before coming into town. 'Blast I'm filthy!' she said, under her breath.

'Well, no one's going to pull up a galloping horse because of that!' Peg said, opening her eyes and peering at her.

Diana laughed and went to sit on the arm of the chair to give her a swift hug. 'How I've missed you, Granny.'

'I'm so glad you're here, Diana!' Peg beamed at her. 'I have the most beautiful memories, you know. I was just thinking what fun we had with the horses. Your grandfather was a magnificent horseman. We had a sire called Tinker—he had another name, but we always called him Tinker. He threw a lovely line, very sought after, they were, his foals. People came from all over the place.' She shook her head sadly. 'It was a terrible day when your father sold all the horses. Would have broken Frank's heart, Tom replacing those beautiful horses with his wretched motorbikes. I was just remembering riding up and down the hills, mustering. We'd take our lunch with us in tins in the saddlebags and bring in the sheep. It was very gentle, everyone knew the way, horses, dogs and the sheep, too. I'd just loop the reins over the saddle on the way home and be so relaxed. That was until my wretched horse propped when we got to the creek and I sailed straight over his neck and into the water, much to your grandfather's amusement! You'd think I'd learn. All the same, I think it was a better pace we lived. Not all this hurry, hurry, hurry.'

'That's bizarre, Granny, I've just been telling someone all about Gramp's picnic racehorse. I can't remember his name, but he had huge teeth and he looked at you as if he could talk.'

'That was Sputnik. He was a dreadful-looking foal and had been gelded. But he turned out to be a wonderful race-horse. Not surprising, because your grandfather was a much respected judge of horseflesh. Anyway Sputnik won quite a few races. We grew quite fond of him. He ran over a cliff and killed himself in the end, got spooked by lightning, we think.' She paused. 'I never forgave your father for not teaching you girls to ride.'

'Ah, but we rode motorbikes—they were much more fun and you didn't have to catch them first,' said Diana. 'Would you like a coffee or a cup of tea?'

'Tea, thank you, darling.'

Diana caught sight of Rosie passing the window on her way to the back door. 'Rosie's here.'

'I haven't seen Cody for a while. You must tell her to come and visit.'

Diana looked aghast at her grandmother

'Hi everyone,' Rosie said as she walked in. 'How are you, Granny?' She looked curiously at Diana's expression. 'What's wrong?'

'Rosie, isn't it lovely to have Diana home?'

Rosie and Diana exchanged looks.

'Yes, it is.' Rosie said. 'You've got a mark on the front of your shirt, Diana.'

'I simply don't know why Cody doesn't come to visit me anymore,' said Peg.

'Granny, Cody died a long time ago. You must be getting muddled up with Sienna or Saskia, Diana's daughters.'

'Diana's got daughters? No one told me.'

'Granny having a bad day today?' Rosie asked Diana, eyebrows raised. 'I can't bear it when she talks about Cody as if she were alive.' She picked up the pile of books on the shelf near the door. 'I've come to get your library books, Granny. Are these the ones?'

'Oh Rosie, I've already done that,' said Diana.

She put the books back down and sighed. 'You could have said. I usually do it on Mondays.'

Diana shrugged. 'She didn't tell me you changed her books on Mondays.'

'What about the washing, is that ready?'

'Diana's done it already, haven't you, dear?'

'Right. It looks like everything's in order then. I've got to get back to work. Enjoy your day. There's no doubt about it, Diana, when you come back you're a wonder.'

Diana grimaced as the door slammed a little too loudly behind her sister. 'Granny, you're stirring up trouble. You should have told me about the library books.'

'Now, now. It must be comforting for Rosie to know you're here to help me and there's not so much for her to do. She works so hard up at the hospital. I think I'm nearly out of whiskey. Do you think you could get me a bottle when you're out shopping?'

Diana couldn't help smiling. Her grandmother could change from weird to perfectly normal in an instant, and she did enjoy her whiskey at the end of the day.

CHAPTER THIRTY

Peter Summers' funeral had been terrible. Tom was very quiet on the way home. Stella wished they'd stayed a little longer, but Shelley did have family from Wollongong there. Tom went to park the car and left her at the bottom of the kitchen steps. She became aware of raised voices in the kitchen.

'You are not the boss of me.'

'You're only a girl and you don't know how to.'

'I can ride the bike, Tommo's going to teach me.'

'You can't even reach the handlebars.'

Stella rushed up the steps. 'Hey. What's wrong?'

'Sienna has to realise she can't ride the bike.' Milo was adamant.

'Sienna is too small.' Saskia piped in.

'I am not. It's not fair, Stella. I'm almost as tall as Milo anyway.'

Stella hid a grin. That much was true. Sienna was growing so fast. 'I think it might be an age thing, Sienna. Mummy was driving a car when she was ten, but we didn't let her before that even though she was tall like you.'

'Mummy drove a car when she was ten?' Milo was incredulous. 'Which car?'

'An old paddock car. She and Rosie used to drive down to the bus in the morning and then drive home in the afternoon.'

That silenced Milo, but he swiped at Sienna on his way out the back door.

'Milo hit me.' Sienna started to cry.

'Milo!' Stella called after him. 'Come back here.'

But he kept going down the stairs and unfortunately almost ran into his mother as she came round the corner on the bike.

Diana braked hard. Milo kept running. She called once, looked with amazement after him, then parked the bike, took off the helmet and came up to the kitchen.

'What's happened?'

'Milo and Sienna were having an altercation.' Stella grimaced.

'And Milo hit me.' Sienna proffered her arm as evidence. 'I can ride the bike, I can, I can. Tommo said he would teach me.'

'Why did Dad say that? He hasn't asked me. And I think you're too young.'

Sienna burst into tears. 'It's not fair, it's not fair, Tommo said I could.' She raced to her bedroom, slamming the door.

'Dad didn't say that, did he?' Diana turned to her mother.

'I don't know. He must have led Sienna to think something.' Stella shrugged.

'Don't you think he should have asked me?'

Stella didn't know what to say. 'I'm sure he was going to.'

'Was going to! Mum, these are my children. I'd appreciate some support here.'

'We wouldn't undermine you. It's a mistake, calm down.'

'I'll find Milo and then I'll calm down.' Diana ran out the back door.

Saskia came over and wrapped her arms around her legs. 'Don't worry, Stella,' she whispered.

Stella bent down and picked her youngest grandchild up and hugged her. 'Thank you, sweetheart.' She sniffed. 'Saskia, you do smell beautiful.'

'Mmm, I like the way you smell, too, Stella.'

'What! Is that my perfume?'

'Mummy calls me the perfume thief.'

Stella burst out laughing. 'Well, don't do it again,' But she hugged Saskia just that little bit harder. 'Come, we'll go find Sienna.'

*   *   *

Milo was sitting in the cab of the old Aveling Barford grader, very high up. Diana slowed to a walk.

'Hi, you should watch where you're going.'

Milo said nothing, just sat there with his hands on the wheel, his face set.

Diana leant against the huge tractor wheel. 'So why are you annoyed about Sienna learning to ride the bike?'

'Sienna is only eight and her arms aren't long enough.'

'You're right. I totally agree with you.'

'But she said Tommo said—'

'I think you have to trust that I wouldn't let Sienna do something that would harm her,' she interrupted.

'You weren't there. Daddy wasn't there. I had to.'

'Thank you, but you don't, Milo, you mustn't—'

'You don't understand.' He wrenched himself out of the seat, jumped down and ran back to the house without waiting for her.

* * *

Diana had been expected at the club half an hour ago for dinner with Mal and Rosie. Pushing the door open, she noticed it was quite busy before spotting Rosie at one of the tables in the corner.

'Hi Rosie, sorry I'm late. Just had a bit of a problem with Milo.'

'Don't tell me the wonder child is causing trouble.' Rosie looked up with a sceptical look on her face.

'No, just normal stuff. The kids are getting on each other's nerves a bit, maybe they should go to school. I feel for Mum and Dad. It's a big ask to suddenly have three kids dumped on you, not to mention a crazy daughter. Then Mum thought we should ring the other grandparents. She'd been trying but couldn't get on, but we got through to them tonight.'

Diana sat down gratefully. It hadn't been an easy conversation. There had been an awful lot of 'When are you coming back?' questions. Questions she wasn't prepared to answer at the moment. They adored the kids and were missing them badly. She wasn't ready to even think about it.

'Why are all these people here? It looks busy for a Thursday.'

'Pete Summer's funeral has brought everyone in the district out of the woodwork,' said Rosie.

Of course, the funeral. Diana had forgotten how the town turned out in force to farewell one of its own. 'Where's Mal?'

'He'll be here later. He's been with Alan Summers all day.'

'Oh I'm sorry. Was it awful? I didn't have much time to talk to Mum and Dad about it.' Talking had been a bit strained after Milo's outburst. She didn't understand why Milo had got so upset, or why she had. But her parents had to know there was a bottom line.

'Pretty dreadful,' said Rosie. 'Everyone looked shell-shocked, mostly. Enormous turnout.'

Really, her parents hadn't said anything about the funeral because she hadn't asked. They knew it was a topic she wasn't comfortable with yet.

Diana went to the bar to get them a drink. A wine for Rosie and a beer for her. She tried a different craft beer that she'd never heard of and carried them back to the table.

She blew the head to one side and sipped the icy brew appreciatively. She hoped they weren't going to discuss Pete Summers all night. It gave her the creeps. This was not a good night to have come into town. She could feel the funereal gloom all around her. It hadn't been like this for Charlie, she'd made sure of that. Charlie's parents had been a little shocked but he had so loved a party. He was always waltzing in, swinging her around and saying, 'Party time, Di! Let's have a party!' And a whole stream of friends—even people she'd never met before—would suddenly appear at the door, carrying a few bottles and chips, and the party was on.

Charlie was given a good send-off. It wasn't like this—Diana looked around at the muted conversations and solemn faces. A terrible sadness overwhelmed her.

'Sorry, Di,' said Rosie, watching her. 'Once again I didn't think. This must be awful for you.'

'It's okay. Charlie's was different to this. He did love a party and I did my best to send him off in style. Something he'd have appreciated.'

'I remember when you wanted a party,' Rosie leant forward, 'for your sixteenth birthday. Do you remember? Now that was a party and a half.'

'Are you joking? It was a total disaster. I got drunk. Some of the boys snuck in some alcohol. And Dad was incredible. He showed me how to put my fingers down my throat and throw up.'

'Did he really? He never showed me.' Rosie was astonished.

'Probably didn't need to. It was way too soon after Cody. We should never had it so close.' Even now she had a problem saying death.

'I think Mum and Dad wanted to do anything that would help life get back to normal for us all. Dad anyway.'

Diana had celebrated her twenty-first with a bottle of Jacob's Creek Shiraz in her bedsit. Charlie had insisted on throwing her a thirty-first, because she'd missed out on a twenty-first, he'd said. They'd been married a couple of years and it had been a surprise. She hadn't got drunk at that one because she'd been nursing Milo.

And all you could do was ask how we were going to pay for it. I was doing it for you.

Enough!

Rosie got her attention again. 'I've been meaning to talk to you about Granny. Mum and I've been thinking, she could qualify for some help, things that would help her to stay home—shower rails in the bathroom, someone to help her with shopping or to have a shower. I've been thinking we should sign her up to Vital Call? What do you think?'

'That sounds wonderful, Rosie, before something terrible happens.'

'She would have to be assessed by ACAT. I'll get some forms. Dad will have to fill them in. We have some good nurses in town who do this "at home" service. I know you've been doing your bit, but Granny needs more help now. What we'll do when you go, I'm not sure.'

'Rosie, I'm really worried about Dad. Do you think he'd ever ask for help?'

'No. And he's the one who has to ask for it,' she said. 'It's like a holocaust at the moment, which is mostly because farmers are very bad at admitting there's anything wrong. They won't ask for help. I've got an idea though. I wonder if I could get Will Talbot to go out there and talk to him?'

'You're about the only one who could. Have a go, will you, Rosie? I wish there was more I could do,' said Diana. 'Will Mal be long?'

'I don't know. He doesn't communicate much these days. I'm worried about him, too.'

'Why?'

'I don't think he's happy.' Rosie sipped her wine.

'Midlife crisis?'

'I guess. No, more than that. I think he wants out. But I'm afraid it includes me and our marriage and I'm too scared to have it out with him.'

'Oh Rosie, no, he loves you. I'm certain,' said Diana. 'Having said that, I wouldn't have been surprised if Charlie had wanted out of our marriage. Which makes everything that happened so much worse.'

'So you think I could be forcing my husband into crashing his car?'

'No, I definitely don't. Rosie, don't jump to conclusions.'

Mal suddenly appeared and sat down heavily at the table. 'What a day.' He looked from one to the other. 'What's wrong?'

'Nothing,' Rosie said quickly.

'Good. I've had enough drama for today. Who wants a drink?'

*   *   *

A week later Stella and Diana were peeking out the open front door as Will Talbot leant against his car, hands in his pockets, his long legs stretched out in front of him. Tom had one elbow propped against the gate post. They had been talking for quite a while.

Diana and Stella returned to the kitchen, and Diana resumed her favourite position, leaning against the warm Aga, while her mother washed up cups in a saucepan in the sink.

'Rosie did this, when?' whispered Stella

'We were talking the other night in the pub and she must have got right on to it.'

'How long have they been chatting?'

'At least ten minutes. Why are we whispering?'

Stella chuckled. 'I don't know. It was so wonderful of Will to come out here in the first place to talk about all those aids for Peg. But when your father went out to open the gate for him and they started talking … I couldn't believe it.'

'Does Will usually pay home visits?' Diana asked curiously.

'Never, at least not out here. He often visits Peg in town but they've always got on so well.'

'Good on Rosie. She said she was going to ask Will to talk to Dad, on the pretext of talking about Peg.'

'Diana, you didn't?' Her mother was horrified and stopped as she was about to pour the kitchen bucket into her new pitcher.

'Look, Mum, something had to be done about it. Dad's not the same as he was.'

'Don't be ridiculous! As if any of us are the same as we were twenty years ago. And he has pressures. I know he's finding it hard to come to a decision.'

'A decision! He's not making any decisions.'

Milo appeared at the back door. 'Mum, Tommo said I could have a lesson on the bike, if it was all right with you. Can I ask him now?'

'How about you wait a little while, just until Dr Talbot goes?' Diana said. 'I'll come and get you when he's ready.'

'Okay.' Milo disappeared again.

'It's really hard to work out where Granny is at the moment, isn't it?' said Diana.

'Home, I hope,' her mother muttered.

'No, that's not what I meant. I mean mentally.'

'Hallelujah! Welcome to our world.'

'Would you stop being so sarcastic?' Diana groaned. 'She can never remember I have three kids but the past is as clear as crystal. And you never know what she's going to come out with next. Do you know she was telling me the other day about going to the wool sales in Sydney with Gramps. How they were picked up in a hire car courtesy of Pitt Sons in O'Connell Street and taken to the wool stores to inspect their wool. Can you believe it—a hire car! Then they were handed white coats to wear, the agents discussed their wool—*at length*—and told them the price they'd thought they could get. Then they were driven back in the hire car again, and entertained for lunch in an enormous room that Granny said had a marble floor and a huge glass atrium. Then they went to the actual sale, where they always got more for their wool than it had been valued at. "Always" she said, tapping her nose and nodding, you know how she does. And then they would have a few nights in Sydney staying at The Metropole before coming home. What a life!'

'Well, I must admit those times had certainly disappeared before I came on the scene,' said Stella. 'I remember falling to the ground and kissing the earth when they put a Reserve Price on wool, which saved our bacon, I can tell you. Anyway they moved selling the wool to Yennora, it wasn't nearly as glamorous.'

'But I mean, is it all true?'

'Is what true?' asked Tom as he came through from the front.

Diana and her mother jumped.

'Granny's days of high living at the wool sales that she was telling me about,' said Diana.

'Probably. I went once with them, I remember. It was pretty amazing. Everyone wore suits and ties. I wore a tie and I was only eleven. I remember being handed a very large lemonade. I think the most exciting thing for me was riding in the limousine. I got to sit in the front. Where's Milo? I promised I'd take him for a lesson on the bike.'

Diana and her mother watched as her father walked on through the kitchen and called for Milo.

Sienna followed them back into the kitchen and looked disconsolately at her grandfather and Milo disappearing down the back steps. 'I don't know why I can't go, when Tommo said I could.'

Sienna was good at not letting anything go. 'I explained to you, darling, you're just not old enough.'

'I'll never be old enough.'

Diana raised her eyebrows at her mother as Sienna flounced from the room.

CHAPTER THIRTY-ONE

There was someone in the doorway. Diana was awake instantly. A little figure shivered in the pool of light that came from the hall.

'Sienna? Sienna, what's wrong?' She extricated herself from the bedclothes as carefully as she could to avoid waking Saskia, and wrapped her arms around the stiff, pyjama-clad body. The wet, pyjama-clad body.

'Oh, Sienna you haven't done this for ages,' Diana whispered, stripping off her daughter's pyjamas as quickly as she could. She took a T-shirt from her drawer and pulled it over Sienna's head, and then climbed into bed with her.

She could feel Sienna was still trembling and trying not to cry. 'It's all right, sweetheart, it doesn't matter.' Diana rocked her in her arms. 'Is anything wrong? Did you have a bad dream?'

'Yes, I had a bad dream.'

'It's okay, we all have bad dreams. Can you remember what it was?'

'I dreamt we stayed in Australia for the rest of my life and we never went back to Gospel Oak.'

Oh lord. 'That would never happen. We'll go back.'

'And I never saw Grandma and Grandpa again,' She hiccupped. 'Or Polly, or my school, or my friends.'

'Of course you'll see them again.'

'But Stella told Tommo we weren't going back. We were going to go to school here.'

'That was only a maybe, and only for a little while, just for you to have something to do. But we have to make those decisions—you and Milo and Saskia and me.'

Now wasn't that the truth. It wasn't going to be just her decision, was it?

'Right, now think about something lovely and happy, close your eyes and this time your dream will be a happy one.' Diana kissed her daughter and held her, realising suddenly how much Sienna had grown. It must be all the meat they were eating.

Sienna closed her eyes. 'I'm thinking about Saturdays,' she whispered. 'Saturday's my best day.'

'Why Saturday?' Diana couldn't help asking.

'Saturdays Grandma takes me and Saskia shopping. We go to Brent Cross and I have a babyccino and a pink cake.'

'And I have a poppa and pink cake, too.' Saskia chimed in, wide awake.

'And she always buys us something, just a little something, and we look at all the shops.'

Saturdays had been Diana's day off. Charlie took Milo to football—draped in every bit of Arsenal paraphernalia they had acquired over the years, hats, scarves and jumpers—and disappeared completely for a few hours, and the girls would go with Charlie's mother.

Diana could pot, if she needed to catch up. What heaven that was. She could go and get her hair cut or just hang out. Saturdays. Brent Cross was an enormous shopping mall a few miles away from where they lived in Gospel Oak. Every shop and retail item known to man could be found there, she was sure. Diana usually avoided it like the plague. She much preferred the local shops, just around the corner.

'Stella takes you shopping,' she said.

'Stella doesn't have time when we go shopping, we have to hurry and the shops aren't very big.'

She had that right.

'Sometimes we'd meet Polly there with her mum.' Sienna's voice trembled.

'Shh, just think about Saturdays. And being with Grandma and Polly again and all the things you'll have to tell them when we get back.'

'I'll tell them about Spot,' Saskia piped up. 'When we go back do you think Stella will look after Spot, or will I have to bring him with me?'

Diana was pretty sure Stella wouldn't miss Spot all that much, but Saskia would be devastated to hear it.

'Right now, I think Spot needs you and Stella. Close your eyes and go to sleep.'

Diana thought of the new supermarket in town, with its four adjacent shops. Not exactly Brent Cross, was it? Should she take them away for a few days? Go to visit Megan for a little holiday? They could hire a car in town, Bruno's always had one or two. She definitely needed a car.

Her daughters settled into sleep on either side of her. Diana rolled Saskia's leg away to give herself a little more room in the overcrowded bed.

*   *   *

Diana met her mother in the hall as she was coming out of Rosie's old bedroom with Sienna's sheets in her arms.

'I'm sorry. We've had a little accident. Can I do a wash today?'

Stella looked stricken. 'Oh! Who?'

'Sienna, but don't say anything. She hasn't done it for ages. She gets paranoid if you say anything.'

'Of course I won't. Diana, it worked.'

'What worked?'

'Well, something worked. Your father has suggested we should get Peg assessed by an ACAT team, you have to wait six weeks. At least he's decided on something. And he's agreed to take some of these tests Will's talked to him about. One step at a time.' Stella looked relieved. 'Here give them to me.' She whisked the sheets from Diana's arms and went down the hall humming something unrecognisable.

*   *   *

Diana put forward her plan at breakfast that morning.

'Let's go down the coast for a few days to visit Megan.' She looked expectantly at Sienna and Saskia, then round to Milo.

He frowned back at her. 'Tommo said I could have another lesson on the bike today.'

You couldn't keep all the people happy, all of the time. She sighed.

'You can do that before we go.' She turned to her father. 'I want to hire a car from Bruno's. He still has them doesn't he?'

Tom was busy filling out a form. 'Mmmm, I think so. What's my mother's maiden name, Stell?'

The phone rang. Her mother got up to answer it. 'Williams.' She picked up the phone and disappeared into the hall.

'What's her date of birth?' Tom looked up, registered Stella had gone, and went on filling out the form.

'What are you doing?' Diana asked.

'Applying for the assessment Will told us about yesterday. At last it seems there is something we can do. It'll help her stay in her house for longer, that's got to be a positive. Can you children stop that noise? And no, I won't have time to give you a lesson today, Milo.'

Diana opened the back door and signalled with her eyes, giving her children no choice but to move outside. Her father had been a little miffed after she'd confronted him about his plan to teach Sienna to ride the bike. He'd admitted no wrongdoing. 'Absolute nonsense.' he'd said. 'There's nothing wrong with giving her a go with me on it. How's she ever going to learn, otherwise?'

Maybe a little distance would be good for everyone. Some time out.

CHAPTER THIRTY-TWO

Diana had forgotten how beautiful the South Coast was. Inlets, sandy beaches, national forests with huge gum trees stretched endlessly before her. She'd have to take one of the logging tracks and show the kids one of the forests, with their patches of regrowth and hillsides of felled logs and the tall, dark deep bush ringing with bell bird song, so different from the stands of gums at home with their knobby branches and interesting shapes. They'd have a picnic. Megan would know where to go.

'Soon we'll be swimming in the Pacific Ocean.' She turned down the volume on the radio so she could be heard over 'It's a Hard Knock Life' from *Annie*, the girls' favourite at the moment.

'Can we swim in winter, Mum?' asked Milo dubiously.

'It depends on the day, but we have been known to swim in the winter, or at least paddle. I can assure you it's no colder than England can be in the summer.'

'Have you been here before?'

'Not to Megan's house, but we had a holiday near here once in July and I remember swimming.' Summer hadn't been a time for holidays because of harvesting or haymaking or bushfires, or all three. It hadn't really mattered, since Diana had loved being at home on the farm and doing things with her dad—sheep work in the dusty yards, mustering on the bikes, swimming in their creek. Who needed to go away? It was fun being at home.

'Who is Megan?' Sienna asked.

'Megan is my friend. I met her when I went to college. She came to England a few years ago and met you all then. You'll probably remember her when you see her. She's tall, with lovely long blonde hair that she puts up in a bun. She's good fun, you'll like her.' She was also energetic and organised and practical. They'd always got on so well. Hopefully Megan would take them all in without a worry; if she was anything like she used to be, it would be okay.

'Swimming won't be the same without Daddy.'

'No, Sienna it won't.' But she couldn't help thinking rather resentfully that it was she who used to take the kids to swimming lessons and insisted that they learnt to swim. On the other hand he'd loved playing with the kids in the water. Still, this was the first time Sienna had mentioned her father in ages. That had to be good, didn't it?

'Will Daddy be there?' Saskia asked.

Diana nearly ran off the road.

'Daddy's dead, you dummy.' Milo turned on her.

Saskia started to cry.

'Milo, don't talk to your sister like that.' She couldn't cope with this. She had no idea what to say. She turned the music on again.

Perhaps it was because she hadn't let them see his body, she hadn't wanted to see it herself, not lying in a coffin. They hadn't really talked much about Charlie, not for a while now. The little game about what Daddy was doing in heaven hadn't lasted long. Then coming home she'd been so engrossed in her own and her family's problems. She really must get a book about grief, there must be thousands of them.

At the next sizeable town, Diana pulled up at a bookshop. They all went in and re-emerged with a book each, and one for her—how to explain to your kids about the death of someone close. Perfect.

*   *   *

'This is fabulous, Megs,' Diana said from the window seat. She looked out the big plate-glass window to the sea, velvety grey now in the fading light. The house, part of an old dairy farm, had white weatherboards with dark green windows and doors, and was nestled in a little valley that widened as it reached a small beach, where a creek meandered through the sand bank and spilled out to the sea. Megan had a few boar goats, in their swinging white skirts, their brown faces quietly munching away on the long coastal grass and, she had been assured by Megan, the blackberries and everything else in reach. They seemed so happy inside their old-fashioned post-and-rail fences. But Megs said that contentment was misleading—she spent half her life chasing them all over the adjacent farms.

The sun had disappeared completely and the red flowers of the coral tree fluttered in the cool breeze. There was hardly a house visible, except in the distance a few lights twinkled over to the south.

Megan had taken them on a tour of the property. She'd done a whole lot of renovating without losing the original feel of the old farmhouse. Her pictures hung along the walls of the gallery—a glassed-in verandah along one side of the house. They'd inspected the old dairy, now a studio where Megs did her potting, weaving on her huge loom, and sculpture too. It even had a bed, so when she was lost in a project she didn't have to come back to the house.

There were views of the ocean from every one of the windows upstairs. They'd been exploring down to the beach, although no one had ventured into the water. Having settled their bags on their beds they were now all down in the big, warm kitchen with its terracotta tiled floor and long-planked dining table. A delicious beef casserole simmered in the oven, with the promise it would marry well with the scent of the cab merlot rising from her glass.

'How long have you been here?' Diana asked.

Megan sat on the window seat. 'My parents died about seven years ago. Mum had cancer and Dad drowned two months later in a fishing accident.'

'I remember. That was a terrible year for you. That was after your trip to visit us in England when I was pregnant with Sienna, if I remember correctly?'

'Yes.' Megan shook out her long blonde hair and secured it with a clasp.

'You're looking good, my friend.'

Her blue eyes crinkled into a smile that lit up her face. 'And you're not so bad yourself—middle-aged mother of three.'

'Thanks.' Diana rolled her eyes and took a sip of red wine.

She looked over to the table at the end of the kitchen where Sienna and Saskia sat absorbed, threading shells and brightly coloured glass beads onto a leather thong, making themselves a necklace. Milo was concentrating on doing a charcoal rubbing. Peace reigned with the muted sounds of the ocean in the distance.

'This is the first time I've felt relaxed since Charlie died.'

Megan watched her friend closely. 'It can't have been easy for you.'

'I've been so immersed in my own troubles, sorting things out with Mum and Dad, I've been neglecting the kids. Saskia scared me silly today. She asked if Daddy was going to be here. So I bought a book on grief counselling.'

'They don't look too bad to me.' Megan gave a little laugh, shooting a glance at the three at the other end of the kitchen.

'No, they don't. They're good kids. Maybe if they did a bit more ranting and raving ... The problem is that my parents didn't know Charlie, there's no reality for them in his death. And I can't talk about it.' Diana grimaced. 'I know I should be talking about Charlie more. The trouble is I don't know where to start. Every time I want to talk about him I get so cross and angry. I want to remember the good times, then all this resentment comes flooding out. I can't lumber the kids with that. So lately I've tended not to say anything.'

'Maybe they have some resentment they want to get rid of, too? I wouldn't worry too much. Kids are pretty adaptable. Look at me. I had a mother who was always wandering around in a Valium haze and a father who was a workaholic. They spent most of their time talking to each other *through* me—when my dad was around, which was hardly ever. But I survived.' And then she added with a smile, 'Although I think it was mostly due to you and Johann and Paul. Those were good times, weren't they?'

Diana thought about the first time she met Megan. 'Quite bizarre, how we met.' She took a breath. 'Do you ever see Johann?'

'He drops in sometimes. He travels a lot, ever since Paul died,' she said. 'Paul was so gentle. It was so unfair—he was such a promising artist, so talented.'

'AIDS was the most unfair, horrible killer.'

'Johann nursed him, through it all, almost three years. You were in England then. Since then he's become quite the eccentric. You knew he held one of his exhibitions here last year?'

'Yes, I read it on the web. So tell me about this place, you hold exhibitions and working camps or weekends for artists?'

'You name it, I do it—even kid's camps. The only good thing my parents did was leave me this place. I love it here. I have two exhibitions here myself, during the year.'

'Don't you get lonely? What about ...' Diana trailed off.

Megan gurgled with laughter. 'My love life? It's fine. When there's a balance needed between my art and company, the art comes first. I can always find company when I want.' She winked at Diana.

'You haven't changed, Megs.' A tiny twinge of jealousy was quickly dispersed. What if she could put her pots first ... No, she wouldn't change her life. Not remotely.

'Oh honey, we've all changed.' Megan put down her wine and got up to check the cast-iron pot, a thick cloth wrapped around her hand. 'Mmm, I think it's ready. Come to the table, my children, and eat. We have a big day ahead of us tomorrow.'

*   *   *

Diana walked into the kitchen the next morning, fully dressed, rubbing her wet hair with a towel. 'I find the sound of the ocean soporific. I can't believe I slept so long,' she said. 'What on earth are you doing?'

Megan sat at the kitchen table with a few art books scattered across the table. She was rapidly sketching Saskia, who was sitting opposite her, a snapshot of Diana and Charlie propped up beside her on the toaster. The photo was an old one, probably dating from the time Megan had visited them in England. They were standing outside their house in Gospel Oak. Charlie was laughing into the camera, while she looked quite put out.

Megan didn't look up. 'I'm giving the children a book each for them to put things down that they remember about their dad. I'm doing a portrait of them doing something they liked with Charlie. Then they can fill the rest of the book with whatever they want—pictures, writing. Saskia said she wanted her portrait to be of Daddy reading her a story before she went to bed.'

Diana watched Megan's fingers flying over the page, Saskia was already taking shape. She was an amazing artist. Diana didn't know what to say. Such a simple thing, why hadn't she thought of it?

'Megs, I don't know how to thank you.'

'I'll find something.' She looked up briefly and winked. 'Why don't you put the kettle on?'

'Where's Sienna?'

'Waiting outside, I think, for her turn. She's opted for going for a walk with her dad.'

'Going for a walk?' Diana was stupefied. 'Yes, Charlie was all for taking the kids for a walk, if it got him out of hanging the clothes out or helping me clean up.'

'That's not the spirit, Diana. Careful.'

'I know, I know. Do you see what I mean? I just can't seem to let it rest.' She sat down at the table. 'What about Milo?'

'Ah, there you have trouble I think. I couldn't get him to suggest anything.' Megan fixed Diana with a quick look. 'Pour yourself a coffee and take it with you. Why don't you and he go for a walk?'

When Diana stepped out the back door, Milo was sitting disconsolately on a garden seat with Sienna.

'Do you think Megan could put Polly in my picture with Daddy?' Sienna asked.

'I'm sure it would be no trouble at all.' And Diana wondered again why she resented the fact that Charlie held such great memories for them all. He had been a great dad. She took a deep breath. 'Milo, do you want to come for a walk?'

Milo looked very much as though he wanted to say no but he reluctantly got up. His hands were in his pockets and he scuffed the dirt in front of him. They went down the winding path to the beach and Diana asked him, 'Left or right?'

'I don't care.'

'Well, let's go right.'

Right was towards where the little creek emptied into the sea, the glorious ocean spread out before them, sparkling in the morning sun. Down on the beach they sat on some rocks sheltered from the breeze. A seagull glided to a stop in front of them, regarding them quizzically.

'Are these the same seagulls we have in England?' Milo asked.

'I don't know. I mean they are the same breed but it's a long way over here.'

'I want to go back.'

'To England? Why's that?'

'I don't know, I just do.' Milo was scuffing holes in the sand in front of him again. 'I mean, I know Dad's dead but he's closer there. He might be a seagull and not be able to get here.'

They both watched the seagull. He did have the look of Charlie about him, strutting about, cheeky and inquisitive.

Diana gave a little smile. 'I think your dad would manage it. He'd do anything for you.' But she couldn't help thinking that he hadn't made the least effort to come back here while he was alive, bring the kids over. Why wouldn't these wretched, angry thoughts go away?

'Why did he die then?'

'I don't know. The road was wet and he'd been drinking, so it was a little bit no one's fault and a little bit his fault.' She hadn't told Milo before about the drinking, but maybe he needed to know the truth now. She watched to gauge his reaction.

'I feel safer at home, with Grandpa and Grandma. They're missing us,' he said simply. 'It would be better, wouldn't it?' Finally he raised his eyes to look at her, his face creased with worry and a question in his eyes.

'Lord, Milo, I'm so sorry. I've uprooted you all and brought you here to Australia because I was hurting so much. I didn't realise you guys would feel like I've taken you away from the reality of your dad, and all the things that help you to remember him. Problem is, we can't go back right now, Stella and Tommo need us, just for a little while. There's shearing next week. But after that, we'll go back.'

They sat there while white fluffy clouds sailed across the blue sky and the waves creamed foam up the wet sand towards them. The seagull lost interest and walked down to the water's edge.

Diana put her hand out to pull Milo up. 'Come on, you've got to think of something fun you used to do with Daddy. What about going to the football all dressed in your Arsenal gear? You brought your scarf with you, didn't you?'

He stopped. 'But he's never going to do that again, is he? That hurts too much.'

Diana knelt down and put her arms round her son. 'Oh Milo, it does hurt, doesn't it? I'm hurting too. Would it help if you gave me a hug when it's hurting, and I can give you one when I'm hurting badly?'

He nodded briefly and they turned and followed the path back up to the house. Diana realised she had some thinking to do.

*   *   *

'I've told Milo we're going back, when shearing's finished,' Diana told Megan that night once the kids had gone to bed. 'Then they can feel closer to their father. And they love their grandparents very much.'

'Both sets, I daresay.' Megan regarded her steadily.

'But as Sienna reminded me, mine have Rosie and Mal and Phillipa. It'll be different this time. We'll all keep in touch. I intend to have long telephone conversations with my mother. She's the one I worry about, but she'll understand, I think.'

'As I remember, you used to be such a close family. I was violently jealous—my dysfunctional lot looked much worse after yours came up to visit. What on earth happened?'

'People say things, do things, and if you're not careful the little sores, they grow like cancers. And I was half a world away, which didn't help. You know, you've got to keep talking.'

Megan passed her a plate with slices of brown bread, thickly covered with smoked salmon and a little grated lemon zest. Dinner for the two of them. Neither felt much like cooking.

'Well, I hope that includes me,' Megan replied swiftly.

'Megs, you've got no idea what a tremendous help you've been. I've got to go back for me, too. There's a lot to sort out. Mind you, I don't find the thought of another winter in England particularly enticing. Winter here is so different, refreshing not miserable.' Diana sighed. 'Sebastian is champing at the bit. I'm supposed to be preparing for an exhibition in September. There were at least twenty emails from him. Probate is about to be sorted. Life is chock-full of irrelevant necessities, isn't it?'

'Well, I've always regarded money as necessary and not in the least irrelevant.'

'You're right, as usual.'

Megan laughed and got up to fill her glass again. 'A little more?'

Diana looked at her half-full glass and then held it out. 'Why not?'

'It's not as though you're driving anywhere.' Megan chuckled.

'Don't talk about it. I told Milo today that Charlie had been drinking before the accident, and he hasn't stopped asking questions since. How much? What's too many drinks? And finally he made me promise I would never drink before I got into a car, ever again. I hadn't realised how worried they are that I might disappear too.' Diana put her drink down and rested her chin in her hands. 'Oh Megan, Charlie was drinking far too much. I didn't know what to do. He was unhappy, but he wouldn't talk about it. Start a painting and not finish it. Stack it against the wall. *Damn. Bloody. Hell.* And I didn't do anything.'

'Hey, what could you do? It's very difficult. At least you didn't disappear in a Valium haze like my mother..'

'Hmm ... and I'm worried about Milo. He's not happy here. I think he feels safer in England because he can look after me, after all of us, in the world he knows. I have no idea why he's developed this crazy sense of responsibility for us all.'

'It could be a number of things. Maybe Charlie used to tell him to look after you when he left, or maybe his grandfather said something. He's very sweet, you are one lucky mother.'

'I know. There's something very honourable about him, isn't there?'

Megan nodded. 'So, what's next for you, Diana?'

She shook her head. 'My life is so complicated at the moment. Mog's Hill is a nightmare—Rosie, Mal, Mum and Dad all at each other's throats, or mine. Perhaps it would be better if I got out of everyone's hair.' Diana grimaced. 'Will you come over and see us?'

Why did she feel so sad when it was the right thing to do?

CHAPTER THIRTY-THREE

Diana returned from Rosie's where she'd booked their return flight on the internet.

'When?' Her mother was not pleased with her decision.

'Tuesday week, after shearing's finished.' Diana didn't feel all that happy herself. 'You really should get a computer and the internet.'

'I can't see that happening in a hundred years.'

'Hey, it's okay,' said Diana. 'We'll ring. Blow the cost. Every week.' She draped an arm around her mother's shoulders and gave her a squeeze.

'I think you should stay longer.'

'I'm sorry, Mum, we can't.'

Diana went outside and sat on the back steps. It was certainly colder than the coast had been. She pulled her jumper tighter and wondered where the children had gone, they'd been here just a minute ago. Hearing voices, she followed the sounds and discovered them all behind one of the sheds, where Tommo was giving Milo a lesson on the bike. Looking like a miniature superhero character, the helmeted figure of her son was both terrifying and ludicrous. Two adoring fans sat on the ground a safe distance away. It looked as though Sienna had accepted that she wasn't going to learn solo just yet. Tom stood with his arms folded.

'Where's the accelerator? Brake? Okay. What do you do first?' The bike lurched off and stopped, Milo nearly going over the top of the handlebars. Diana didn't know whether to cry, laugh or leave them to it. *Relax.* She remembered her first lessons on the motorbike and that she'd ended up in the fence more than once. And she'd learnt on an adult bike, none of these mini bikes for her. He'd be all right. Backing off around the corner, she wandered off in the direction of the dogs.

Patrick had rung her from Singapore on the pretext that he was inviting them all to come over next weekend. Sean, Marnie and the boys would be there. And then he'd said he was missing her.

This wary dance they were executing was uncharted territory for her. She'd never been courted before, not really. Charlie asked her one night to marry him and she'd said yes. He'd been sitting at the bar in his usual place while she was working, his pint in front of him and his chin in his hands. It was worth it just to see the look on his face. He'd jumped up and shouted to everyone that she'd said yes. Charlie had wanted to get married immediately and they had, as soon as conceivably possible. He didn't tell his parents, and she didn't tell hers either. They had a civil ceremony at the local council chambers, conducted by a dapper little man with a

moustache dressed in a pin-striped suit. At four-thirty in the
afternoon. He was better dressed than either of them. Charlie had worn his sports coat and an open-necked shirt and
she wore a yellow shirt she'd found in an op shop, over her
good jeans. His best friend Simon and her friend Emma,
a fellow barmaid, had been witnesses. Charlie had bought
her a bunch of yellow roses. They'd gone back to the pub
after and had an uproarious night with lots of free rounds
supplied by her boss and some of the regulars. Then Charlie
had moved in with her.

It had been her idea to exclude both their families from
the wedding. Charlie's parents had been furious and so had
hers. But Diana had still been so cross with her own family.
She'd hung grimly on to the hurt. For so many years.

Her reasoning was they should be ecstatic that they'd
married at all. None of their friends were tying the knot.

Diana looked around her now. Drought was all powerful. They wanted rain so badly, it hurt to see how stressed
the country was, count the trees that were dying, or dead.
Along with the chilly wind, grey clouds were gathering on
the horizon. A storm, maybe, that would bring the follow-up
rain everyone was waiting for so anxiously. Time would tell.
The weather forecaster apparently couldn't but her father
had said it would rain. He really was the eternal optimist.
Little willy-willies twirled dust around the bare paddocks.
This must have been the paddock her dad had ploughed and
sown down to oats. She looked at the straight even lines following the contours of the hill. It sat waiting for rain. She
wished her life was as ordered as this, with lovely straight furrows running in the one direction. But her life was a mess.
Maybe she needed the rain too, before she could grow again.

Shaking her head against the ridiculous vision of her life as an oat crop, she realised she had walked quite a way. It was time to get back before it did, hopefully, rain. Head down against the wind, Diana retraced her steps.

Where was her core strength? It seemed to have disappeared, her ability to plough on, no matter what, and this had never happened to her before.

The potting shed door was closed. It had been locked the last time she'd been in, when she'd first come home but it opened when she pushed. She slowly walked over and pulled the old wool bale cover away.

She sank down onto the narrow wooden seat and placed her feet on the treadle. Pushed gently, placed her hands around the imaginary lump of clay. Felt her body fold into its familiar position with her elbows braced against her knees and watched the plate start to spin. Maybe she could.

Clay was amazing. So many uses, things you could make, from jewellery and plates and bowls, to the beautiful terracotta chimney pots she loved so much that dotted the skyline in Gospel Oak. Even now she was still fascinated by it. Perhaps she could order some clay. She felt a little drizzle of adrenaline trickle through her veins.

What if they did stay? Cancel the tickets. They could give it a year. If it came to a vote, it would be two against two. Saskia would have no problem with staying and being spoilt by Stella.

Idle speculation, Diana, and it's not going to do you any good. It's too late to change your mind now.

I know. Milo won't change his mind and Sienna would be miserable.

Restlessly, she got up and covered the wheel and walked back to the house. She paused on the wooden steps leading to the back door, listening to the conversation inside.

'Who was your favourite, Stella, when they were growing up, Mummy or Rosie?'

That was Saskia.

'Don't forget Cody. Or did you like Cody best?' Sienna piped up.

'Stella's not allowed to like any one best.'

Thank you, Milo, Diana smiled.

Perhaps she'd better break this up. They say eavesdroppers never heard good of themselves. She opened the door and took her boots off.

'Hi, everyone.'

'Well, everyone likes Saskia best, so I suppose you liked Cody,' Sienna said.

Her mother flushed, suddenly realising Diana was in the room. 'We all loved Cody.'

'And she stayed six and wasn't ever a horrible teenager or someone who needed to be shunted off to England.'

'Diana.' Her mother was horrified.

'Why did you say that, Sienna, that everyone likes Saskia best?' Diana sat on a kitchen chair and pulled Sienna onto her lap. 'It's not true.'

'Yes it is, but I don't mind.' Sienna settled comfortably into her arms. 'It means I get to do what I want.'

'Escaping under the radar, you mean.' Diana laughed. 'Rosie did that often enough. Being invisible does have its upside. You know, you're so lucky there are three of you. If there were only two, I'd have much better control. Have you doing exactly as I wish, just as my mother did.' She hugged

Sienna hard, and she couldn't help the look she threw at her mother being a little combative.

'Yes, you are lucky there are three,' Stella answered lightly, folding the last towel. But it felt like a slap in the face. 'Could you take these to the linen cupboard, Saskia? Sienna, these are yours, and Milo, these go to the linen cupboard too. Diana, these go into my room.'

Effectively dismissed, Diana took the pile of clothes from her mother and walked down to her parents' bedroom and placed them on the bed. New curtains, she fingered the silk. Pretty. Her mother usually had the last say. And she had asked for it. She wandered over to the dressing table. It was cruel to have mentioned having three children. Why had she said it? A sudden, sharp jealousy rose, along with the overwhelming knowledge that her mother had never loved her like she had the other two. Diana picked up the little white doily with 'Mum' embroidered in blue. Cody had made it for Mother's Day when she was in kindergarten. It wasn't some competition they were having. How could anyone understand it when she couldn't work it out herself? Suddenly she scrunched it in her fingers. Just two weeks left.

Cody, Charlie. Oh, it hurt so bad.

CHAPTER THIRTY-FOUR

Diana yawned as she heard her father's soft footfall go past. She eased herself out of the bed and pulled the covers over Saskia. Shearing started today. She grinned into the mirror as she brushed her hair. There was always this buzz of excitement when the shearers came. She pulled on the new jeans and blue wool jumper she'd bought in town on Friday. On consideration she'd felt her skinny London jeans weren't appropriate for the week ahead and there'd been nothing of her old wardrobe left. Long gone, her mother had said. Dressed, her face splashed with cold water, she finally felt awake enough to face breakfast.

It was still dark outside. Her father had put the kettle on and bread in the toaster. They fell into the usual routine—Diana got the cereal out while her father made tea. Milo appeared at the door, his hair standing up on end and fisting his eyes. They both smiled at him.

'Milo, go and wash your face, clean your teeth and brush your hair.'

'Oh Mum.' He heaved with exasperation and disappeared.

'You're a hard mother.' Tom chuckled. 'At least he was fully dressed and ready to go.'

'Did you wake him?'

'No, I did not, he woke himself up. He's keen to come and see what it's all about.' Her father's smile was wry as he buttered the toast.

'Amazing what will get him out of bed at—what is the time?' Diana yawned.

'Six-thirty. Exciting time, shearing.' Tom poured milk into his cereal and started eating.

Milo was back and joined them at the table. 'What time do they come, Tommo?' he asked as he stuffed his mouth full of Weet-Bix.

'Sometime after seven, sport, start at seven-thirty on the dot.'

'Stan is still the same Stan who used to come?'

'Sure is. He'll be pleased to see you again, Diana. He usually asks after you, wants to know how you're doing. The team's changed. There's a couple of young ones, God knows, they're as scarce as hen's teeth these days.' Tom ruffled his grandson's hair as he walked past on his way to the sink. 'I'll see you over there.'

It was just light at seven. Diana shivered with the cold but you could tell it was going to be a beautiful day, with the sunlight sparkling over the dewy paddocks.

'Diana, could you take these over with you?' Her mother appeared and handed her two towels and a fresh bar of soap.

Two utes were parked haphazardly outside the wool shed. Together, she and Milo climbed up the steep steps. She looked around with some satisfaction. Yesterday, they'd tidied and cleaned the shed. Washed the floor with disinfectant, scrubbed the board clean of blood stains and muck, filled the little oil cans, and swept the outside loo free of spiders and cobwebs and installed new toilet paper rolls. Last thing, they'd shedded the sheep, penning them up under cover for the night, before making sure the swinging doors out onto the board were firmly closed. Diana could remember times sheep had escaped and created havoc in the pristine shed before they'd been found the next morning.

They found her father inspecting the old Lister engine that powered the old shearing machines. Her grandfather had installed it before the power was connected in the fifties and Tom had never bothered to replace it. He cranked it and it hummed into life.

'There, old girl,' he said with a satisfied little grunt. He wiped his hands with a rag and looked up. 'Oh Diana, there you are. Come and say hello to Stan.'

Stan Hockey had been their shearing contractor for as long as she could remember. Short, big-bellied, with a shock of white hair. His smile was as wide as she remembered too.

'You haven't changed a bit, Stan.' Diana's hand was enveloped in a mighty handshake.

'Can't believe that, Diana. I'm an old man now, nearly as old as this fella.' He jerked his head towards her father.

'Both of you need your heads examined. You should have passed the reins over to the next generation by now and be living the life fantastic on a beach somewhere, with plenty of sun and plenty of rum.' Diana was well aware Stan was fond of his rum, perhaps a little too much on occasion. 'Stan, this is Milo. Say hello to Mr Hockey.' Diana was pleased to see her son stick out his hand.

'Well now, pleased to meet you, young fella. Had to stick around to meet you, didn't I?' He gave Milo's hand a hefty shake and gave him a wink. 'Reckon your grandpa and I can rest easy now you're here. We might just put our feet up and let you take over here.'

'I don't think so. Milo has a lot to learn about a shed,' Diana cut in. They were all laughing at the horrified expression on Milo's face. 'I can't believe you're letting him in the shed. You're sure he won't be in the way?' she asked Stan.

'No, he'll be right. I know how important it is to the boss. Milo can pick up the locks and put them in the old press. Learn a bit about pressing the old-fashioned way.'

'Don't you dare let him anywhere near that old press. It's far too dangerous.'

'Mmm, I heard a little boy got pressed in a bale in one of my other sheds. They didn't find him till they got to Italy and opened it up. Quite a shock for them.'

By now Milo's eyes were out on sticks.

'Don't you believe everything Stan tells you, Milo. He used to tell me that story too. Just do everything Tommo tells you, and you'll be okay.' Diana looked at her son anxiously.

'Come on, Milo. Come and meet the shearers.' Her father propelled him away. She hoped he'd be okay. Girls weren't all that welcome in the shearing shed when she was Milo's age.

'Oh Diana, I forgot.' Tom turned back. 'Stan asked me if you could get some tranquilliser from Tim Spelling when you're in town.'

'Some what?' Diana was not sure she heard her father properly.

'Tranquilliser. They're going to shear the rams for me, maybe this afternoon, and they'll want it by then.'

'You're not serious. They tranquillise rams now?'

'Yes, it's much easier on the rams apparently. Who am I to say? As long as I don't have to shear them.'

'I can go into town later and be back for smoke-oh. Anything else?'

'Maybe get me five extra wool packs at Spellings.'

He turned away again. Diana stood watching them go, rather forlornly, before making her way back to the house as the sun broke over the horizon.

*   *   *

Diana had just finished backlining the race of shorn rams, and had let them out into the holding paddock beside the shed when she heard the cry 'Smoke-oh' and the sudden silence as the final shearing machine switched off. Stan appeared round the corner to count out the run of snowy-white, newly-shorn ewes. She wiped the sweat from her face.

Lunch. Good idea—she was hungry, she'd missed smoke-oh this morning as she hadn't got back till ten and she'd been working fairly solidly since then, mustering the next mob ready for tomorrow's shearing. Quite easy work, back lining. Just a pass down each sheep's back with the spray gun, but getting them into the race was hard without a dog, and the old dog was not going to work for her. The pup was too mad. So she'd had to do without. Tranquillising might be good for the shearers but it made the rams awfully doughy moving around the yards.

Her father was doing the wool classing. She hoped he was still keeping a good eye on Milo. She went over to the tank and washed her face and hands before the guys came out. With great difficulty she'd stayed away from inside the shed. She knew there'd be no trouble now; heavens, they had girls working all round the shed these days. Milo was only ten but he was good at doing what he was told. She was dying to know how he'd gone on his own, without an overprotective mother in sight.

True to form, the shearers were about to partake of a magnificent feast. Stan had brought a grill and set it up outside on the loading ramp, and there was the delicious aroma of steak cooking. There was no doubt that hadn't changed. Shearers always ate well.

Diana went to the basket she'd brought over from the house and took out their sandwiches. She set out the bottles of soft drink she'd bought in town and opened hers and took a long swallow.

She spied Milo walking towards her. 'Hey, wait for the shearers first, then you go and wash up. Over there.' She pointed. Milo was walking out with the same stride as the men. He looked as if he'd aged four years. In four hours. But he looked happy. Deliriously happy. Tom was grinning from ear to ear. She couldn't help laughing at them. 'Okay, I don't think I need to ask.' She handed them each a Coke.

Milo took a long appreciative swallow. 'Thanks, Mum.' Diana was trying not to laugh. She was so proud of him. He sat down on the wool bale and started eating. With a mouth full of bread and vegemite, he said, 'Mike's going to show me how to shear a sheep after lunch.'

'Really!' Diana swallowed. Exactly how far should she let her son off the leash? He was only ten. She exchanged glances with her father who was just as thrilled with his progress as was her son. He couldn't be serious.

'He's done well,' he said proudly. 'Filling a bale with locks, learnt how to stencil our mark and done an immense amount of sweeping.'

'There's Mike and Olly and Phil and young Stan,' said Milo. 'That's four shearers beside Stan, but he's only the contractor. Then there's George, who's the rouseabout. I really want to be a rouseabout, Mum, but I probably want to be a shearer better, but I have to be a rouseabout first.' He helped himself to another vegemite sandwich.

'Do you,' Diana said faintly.

Three heads appeared at the top of the stairs. Stella with a girl in each hand.

'Hi there. Thought we'd see how you're all doing, and we've brought you some fresh tea.'

Sienna was holding the thermos but wasn't moving from Stella's side.

Diana held out the three mugs they'd used at smoke-oh. 'Fantastic. Sienna, could you rinse these out under the tap? The tap under the tank. I simply cannot move.'

Reluctantly Sienna disengaged from her grandmother and took the cups.

'I've been using muscles I didn't remember I had,' said Diana. 'Tomorrow is going to be awful.' She smiled up at her mother. 'How have you lot been getting on?'

'We're off this afternoon to see Granny. Will you last the distance, do you think?' Her mother was smiling too.

'Mmm, I hope so. I can't imagine how Milo is still keep-ing going. Why don't you all come and help me put the sheep in the race after we've had something to eat? Not having a dog is a nightmare. Stan's dog won't even look at me, and our old dog is hopeless—a few barks and she sits down and won't move.'

'I knew we'd be conned into helping if we came over,' said Stella, but she was laughing.

'Milo.' A voice came from where the shearers were sitting having their steak. Milo disappeared and returned a minute later with three giant, iced cupcakes covered with hundreds and thousands.

'Look what Mike gave us!' He proudly handed one each to his sisters. They were impressed. They weren't sure what to think of the large men dressed in blue singlets and soft reinforced jeans and funny shoes, but the cakes looked good.

'What do you think of the wool?' Stella asked Tom.

'Not bad, considering the season. They're cutting well. Although I'd say that dust storm we had last week is going to affect the yield. Better than I thought anyway.'

'That's high praise—we must be going to have a bonanza of a wool clip.' Stella sounded more than a little surprised with the unusual rave review.

'We would if the price was any good. Bloody hopeless. We're getting the same price for the wool as we were getting ten years ago.'

Stella rolled her eyes at Diana as though to say 'Well now, that's more like it.'

* * *

Stella and the girls had helped for a while and then gone into town. Things had changed in the sheep industry since Diana had gone away. Sheep breeding and wool growing was now an exact science. Even the language was totally different—all microns and newtons and yield. When Tom had taught her about wool it was all about colour and brightness and length of staple. He'd shown her how to open the wool horizontally down the sheep's side and flick the staple for tenderness, check for softness.

Diana was just finishing the last of them before the final count out for the day, when her phone rang. Looking behind her down the race she could see she was at least three quarters of the way through.

She thankfully shrugged the backpack, containing the chemical, on to the ground and leant against the railing. 'Patrick. Where are you?'

'Singapore and it's raining.'

'It's not raining here.' She looked over the backs of the sheep to the low scrub-covered hills in the distance. Could anything be more different?

'We're all quite comfortable. I'm at the Race Club.'

'Good for you. I will have just finished backlining four hundred and fifteen sheep and twenty rams by the end of today.'

'I'm impressed. Are you managing?'

'Well, I have to admit I'm not as fit as I should be.'

'What about getting Mal over tomorrow?'

'No, I don't need Mal to help. I'm just so pleased I haven't forgotten how to do it. A dog is what I need. Dad will help with the last run, anyway. Enjoy your lunch.'

Diana rested against one of the posts in the yards. There were butterflies in her tummy. She hadn't told Patrick she was leaving. Shouldering the backpack again, she finished the last few.

Diana balanced the backpack on top of a post so it wouldn't get stamped on in the rush, and then opened the gate to let the sheep out. She zipped up her jacket and made her way stiffly over to the bike.

*   *   *

Mal was at the back door the next morning, leading a dog on a piece of baler twine. A rather strange looking dog, it was mostly black with half its face white. A bit of border collie in there somewhere, Diana decided.

'I was talking to Alan Summers last night and he was mentioning that his dad's dog needed some work, and I thought maybe you could do with some help this week.'

Diana looked at the dog. It looked straight at her with sad eyes and a hopeful expression. 'How could I resist that?' She laughed, squatting down to pat his head. 'Will he work for me? I am having little success with the dogs round here,' she said doubtfully. 'This has nothing to do with Patrick, has it?' She straightened and looked at Mal.

'No, well, he mentioned something about a dog and I thought of the Summers. They usually have quite a few dogs round there, and sure enough Alan said we'd be doing them a favour. He's missing Pete, they think.'

There was simply no way she could turn down that dog. Something about him went straight to her heart. Getting up this morning had been hard enough with each muscle screaming in agony. She'd be a fool to turn down some help, if he would work for her.

'Thanks Mal, it was very good of you to think of it.'

Mal looked a little embarrassed. 'I wish I could help myself but there's so much going on at the minute. We're sending another load of cattle up north on agistment, today. Oh, his name's Jelly.'

'Jelly? What sort of a name is that?'

Mal grinned. 'Apparently when he was a pup he ate a whole bowl of jelly that Shelley put out to cool, and then you know Jelly and Shelly, they rhyme, and Pete was always saying it meant he didn't have to remember an extra name, they were so similar.' He cleared his throat. 'Anyway, give him a go. I can always take him back tonight if he doesn't suit.'

'Thanks so much, Mal. Are you sure Shelley is happy to let him go?'

'Um, apparently she can't look at him, and he keeps on going to the place they found Pete. Just sits there. I think everyone would be pleased if you could find a use for him this week.'

'Okay, come on, Jelly.' Diana took the end of the baler twine from Mal and tied him to the verandah post. 'Just you wait there and I'll get you a drink. Oh, and say thank you to Patrick for me,' she added dryly.

Mal mumbled something and was out of the door and down the steps.

Diana turned around. Sienna was behind her, still in her pink pyjamas. Milo and Tom had already gone over to the shed. 'Hello, darling. Look what we've got. His name's Jelly'.

CHAPTER THIRTY-FIVE

'Where did he come from?' Stella looked in amazement at Sienna, who was trying to coax a strange dog inside the kitchen door. The dog, in true working-dog form, was not coming inside.

'Mal brought him over. His name's Jelly.'

'Sienna, he won't come in. He's not used to it.'

'But I want him to come in and have his breakfast.'

'He doesn't have breakfast. He gets fed tonight like all the other dogs.' Stella noticed the bowl of Weet-Bix on the floor. Her advice was a mite too late. 'Here, take it outside.' She shook her head and handed the bowl to Sienna. 'And close the door. It's freezing in here.' The temperature had dropped and the stiff breeze outside was contributing considerably to the chill factor. She went to look at the Aga—damn, it had gone out, no wonder it was so cold. When she'd come as a new bride it had been fuelled by coke but they'd had it converted to gas some time ago, much cleaner. She'd have to check the gas bottle. Surely they hadn't run out of gas? In the middle of shearing, it was just what she didn't need. Outside, she groaned. Sure enough, the gas bottle had an echoing ring right down to the bottom. She would have to take the ute and go and get one later.

* * *

Diana helped her lift the empty gas bottle and roll it into the ute.

'Don't take too much weight,' Stella said.

'I'm stronger than you.'

'Those two have certainly palled up.' Stella watched Sienna and Jelly as they slowly made their way over to the shearing shed, stopping every few feet for a pat or a scratch behind the ear.

'I know. Doesn't make for a wonderful, sharp working mind though, does it? Oh well, it's got to be better than yesterday. I'd better get going and try to get rid of these kinks before I get there. Thanks for taking Saskia. Bye, Mum.'

Diana followed Sienna and the new dog over to the shearing shed, then Stella picked up the keys and called Saskia.

'Come on, poppet, we're off.'

Saskia had her head down over some drawing and was reluctant to stop what she was doing.

'If we don't go now we won't be back in time to get lunch ready. Quick! Coat on.' She fed in her arms and zipped her up, kissed her on the nose and bundled her into the ute.

To think so much had changed in these last few weeks. The house was full again. Alive with noise and people. She couldn't bear the thought of them leaving. Next week, Diana had said. She'd actually booked their flight.

Shearing was so busy. A tense time for everyone. Stella guessed it was the strict timetable. It wasn't as though they worked harder at this time than others, it was still dawn to dark most days. Why was this so different? There were people on the place. Having family in the house was the same. It was busy but she had to say she was enjoying the rush. Milo had almost fallen asleep at the dinner table last night, poor little chap. He was exhausted, but it was amazing watching his face when he described shearing the sheep to them all. Not that he'd actually shorn any sheep. Tom had been so proud of him. Milo had been up early this morning to go with Tom again.

Stella just couldn't bear the thought of them going.

She pulled in to the service station that supplied them with their gas bottles. 'Hi, Joe, can I exchange this bottle for a full one?'

'How're you going, Stella? No worries. Run out of gas at shearing. Not good.' Joe shook his head sympathetically as he rolled the bottle out of the back of the ute and stood it up.

She wasn't surprised it was common knowledge that they were shearing.

'Saskia, do you want to buy some chips or lollies? Come and choose.' Stella had learnt her lesson. Little treats were important to these kids. No matter, she loved buying them things.

'Get something for the others too. Can we book it up, Joe?'

'Sure can do, Stella. How's the fuel out at the farm? Do you want me to run out with some more fuel soon?'

'No, we should be right for a few more weeks, thanks Joe.'

Rosie's little white Honda pulled in beside her. Smiling, she put her window down.

'Feel like a coffee? We could go round to Granny's?' Rosie asked.

'Sorry, got to get the bottle back before lunch. It's bedlam there this week.'

'Okay, but I'm missing our coffees.' Rosie looked a little sad.

Stella felt terrible; she hadn't had time to see Rosie for weeks now. 'Next week, okay? They're going, Monday week.'

'I suppose they've got to get back. We'll miss them, though.'

Stella pulled out of the service station and turned for home. No, she did not feel guilty for not visiting Peg. And she had a good excuse—no time. Besides, Peg had plenty of visitors at the minute. Will Talbot was so good to drop in on her, working out ways she could stay in the house. Where were all the people working out ways she could stay in hers? Mal and Rosie were breathing down their necks. Talk about empty-nesters, *they* were the ones being pushed out, and if she wasn't careful the landing would be quite traumatic. Guiltily, she remembered Frank had died when he was sixty and they'd all moved out to the farm when the girls were little. Peg had moved into town. It had been so easy.

Peg was an amazing person. Never stopped working, it was exhausting being in the same room with her. She'd run the farm in the war years, thought nothing of cooking enormous meals for lots of people or hand-sewing all her baby clothes, loved riding out with Frank and mustering or anything else that needed doing on the farm. And moving into town hadn't stopped her bottling jars of tomatoes and preserving thousands of apples. Stella couldn't help feeling as if she hadn't measured up in some way. At least in the beginning. Tom had brought her home for dinner to meet his parents. Peg had looked her up and down and said, 'Not much of her, is there?'

So she'd had to prove herself, and she had.

Peg had taken Diana away from her. She'd watched her tall, awkward, prickly daughter working through the agonies of adolescence, pouring her heart out to Peg. Her daughter, who so wanted to be a son. Until she'd discovered her artistic bent. Now that had to have come from Stella's side of the family. It had missed her completely but with two uncles who were artists, surely she'd given that to Diana.

Stella looked over at Saskia, belted in beside her, her face almost buried in the packet of chips. No, she wasn't going to give up on this and stand aside, let them go back to England. Not without a fight.

After picking up the mail and the papers from the mailbox at the ramp, Saskia got out eagerly again to open the gate, but Stella had had to help her eventually or they'd never have lunch ready. She wished Tom would fix that gate. Inside the house, she put the mail down on the table and put her energies into getting the gas bottle back in.

CHAPTER THIRTY-SIX

It had rained in the night. Twenty-three millimetres, and that was nearly an inch. There were smiles all round. Shearing finished and a little bit of rain. Extraordinary the effect it had on everyone. Her mother was humming and her father was almost happy.

Tom looked up from reading last week's local paper. 'Ninety points is enough to get the oats going. As long as we get some follow up, and the sheep don't all die because they're just off shears.'

'Honestly, Dad, you're very hard to please.'

'I'm the easiest fellow in the world to please, hey, Stell?' he asked.

Stella shook her head and walked over to answer the phone. 'Diana, it's Patrick.'

Diana took the phone and resisted the urge to walk out to continue the conversation in private.

'I was wondering if you might like to bring the kids to Sydney for a few days before you go,' Patrick said. 'You can all stay here. They haven't seen Sydney yet, have they? There's plenty of room. I'll be in and out so you'll have to look after yourselves. What do you think?'

Diana looked at her children eating breakfast. How did he know they were leaving? Mal must have told him. Or her mother. It would be a shame not to see a bit of Sydney before they left. Shearing was finished. Her parents might come too. Have a holiday.

'Thank you, we'd love a couple of days in Sydney. Is there room for Mum and Dad, too?'

'Of course.'

'Fantastic, thank you. I'll check with Mum. We'll see you tomorrow night.'

Oh dear, maybe it wasn't the most sensible decision she'd ever made, but when had she ever done the sensible thing?

*   *   *

Diana was the last to climb onto the train. Her father handed her the bags one by one, and before she knew it, he was just a small dot on the railway station.

Milo had the window seat beside Diana. They had been able to get the two seats that faced each other at the end of the carriage. Her mother was sitting opposite with Sienna on one side and Saskia curled up beside her, reading them a book.

Diana had asked both parents to come to Sydney. Her father had just said no, he couldn't possibly, with the sheep just off shears and rain about. What rain, she had to ask herself. Twenty-three mils. Now it was all gone, there was no sign of any more rain. So she'd said to her mum, 'You have to come and see us off and spend a few days in Sydney.' Her mother had pinked with pleasure, and after demurring a few times and checking with her father at least six times if he didn't mind and would he be all right, had finally said yes, and had been the first to have her bag packed. She was more excited than any of them.

It was altogether a very strange situation. Diana had said goodbye to her father at the railway station. He was distant and she was hurt, so they'd been cool with each other. He could have come if he'd wanted to. But no—the sheep, the bloody farm and he hated Sydney.

The damn tears were starting up again.

'Diana, it's the way it is.' Stella reached over and gave her a squeeze.

Diana raised her eyes and managed a sort of a smile. She didn't have to say any more. By an unspoken mutual consent they didn't talk about Diana leaving.

Saying goodbye to her grandmother was awful. She'd probably never see her again. Granny hadn't realised it though. It was as though she was going away for a day and would be back tomorrow. What a bugger it all was. Peg had been such a strong woman, and to see her disintegrating like this was breaking Diana's heart.

The train rocked gently and racketed along, the murmuring conversations of the other passengers only faintly discernible. Diana checked her watch. Four hours to go till they got to Sydney. Sienna was poring over a few brochures they'd picked up at the railway station before they left. Milo, self-appointed tour director, his nose pressed to the window, announced each tiny station as they hurtled through.

'Will we see Alex and Sam?' Milo turned to them both.

'I don't know. They'll be at school, I guess.'

'Where does Patrick live?'

'Bronte. That's all I know,' Stella answered. 'Now we must make a plan. We can't afford to waste a minute. What do you want to do, Sienna? There's a red double-decker bus that takes you round to lots of places so you can see Sydney.'

Milo looked around. 'We have those in London.'

He didn't sound very impressed. Diana hid a smile.

'I remember you taking Rosie and me on that bus,' said Diana. 'Should we do that first? I really want to go on the ferry to Manly, and that,' she frowned at Milo, 'you don't have in London. I also suggest we have Maccas as soon as we hit Sydney.' She grinned at her mother. 'I think these kids are all suffering from withdrawal symptoms, they haven't had any junk food for two months. That has to be a record!'

'Oh!' said Saskia, breathlessly. 'Can I have a toy?'

'Yes.' Diana laughed at her. 'Happy Meals all round. What do you like to eat at McDonalds?' she asked her mother.

'I don't know. I haven't been for a very long time.' Stella looked round delightedly, at her grandchildren, at her daughter. 'This is going to be so much fun.'

Diana gazed over Milo's head at the countryside flying past. The grey-green gum trees, and cows and sheep and horses pasted onto grass, like a series of still life pictures.

'Now the sun's gone.' Saskia's nose was pressed to the window.

'Typical,' her mother said, 'it'll probably be raining in Sydney.'

'The zoo.' Sienna was still reading pamphlets. 'Can we go to the zoo?'

*   *   *

Diana poured a coffee from the thermos, passing it over without spilling a drop. The kids had fallen asleep.

'They are lovely children, Diana. A credit to you and Charlie.'

'Charlie was a good dad,' she said softly.

'He definitely was a charmer.'

'Oh, I'm so glad you saw some of that side of him.' Diana bit her lip and swallowed her coffee. 'He was different there, in London, wasn't he? Did I ever tell you about the day I came home and discovered he and the children had decided to paint a huge mural on the living room wall? Everything was covered in paint—children, carpets, chair coverings. And there on the wall was this huge jungle scene with lions, swooping cockatoos, monkeys swinging on vines.' Diana started to laugh. 'Honestly, if you could have seen them standing there with these massive grins on their faces. It took me weeks to get the paint out of their hair and off the carpets. Oh, Charlie.'

'Life with Charlie sounds like it was fun,' her mother said. 'I would have liked to have got to know him better.'

'There you were in London for the first time, and I was suffering from exhaustion and baby blues, so it was lucky Charlie was nice to you.' Diana frowned. 'It was such a pity your first meeting was a total disaster.'

'We got such a shock with you ringing and telling us you'd just got *married* and you'd be out on your honeymoon in just a few days. There was no time to take it all in. No time to organise anything here properly. I guess we were a little annoyed with you.' Stella did look somewhat ashamed. 'It was like we were going to lose you completely, when we'd always thought you'd come back, eventually.' Both hands around the coffee, she sipped it carefully, against the rock-ing of the train. 'Those were very black years after Cody died; she was so special, coming so late. After she died I just pushed everyone away.'

Diana stilled. This had to be the first time they'd talked about Cody together. 'I felt it was my fault. I was looking after her and I just put her to bed.' She paused. 'I thought you blamed me.'

'No, no, no, Diana, I blamed myself, and the guilt was too much. I'm so sorry. I just didn't think enough about how you were all feeling.' Stella looked out the window. 'I felt if I could punish myself hard enough it would get better. It didn't. Poor Shelley, the other day all she could ask was why, too. It brought it all back. It was such a terrible time for all of us. Then all I could think about was you coping alone when Charlie died and wishing I could have been there for you. You mustn't punish yourself.'

Tears swimming in her eyes, Stella turned to study Diana. 'You've got no idea how happy I am you came home. I don't suppose you'd think about coming back, to live?'

'Mum, it's impossible. The kids are hurting too much. This grieving thing—it's going to take time and work. They've got to go back. Me too. I think I got myself redi-rected when I went to Megan's. She really is a brick.'

'I'm glad, honestly, you get to accept death for what it is. There's nothing you can do about it.' Stella reached out and touched her knee. 'And you have to stop blaming yourself. I had to stop blaming myself. I get sad sometimes, like when I see you and Rosie together and remember Cody running after the two of you all the time.' Stella fell silent and turned to look out the window again.

'I know,' Diana said softly. 'It wasn't until I'd got through quite a few childhood illnesses that I realised I just wasn't old enough, I didn't know enough to have picked up that she was really sick. Then I stopped blaming myself so much. But I thought you—'

'No, no, Diana. No, I didn't. I'm so sorry.'

'Rosie said something, too. We kind of excluded her, we were so busy taking the guilt on ourselves.'

'You can't make me feel worse than I already do. We deal with hard things in a way that protects ourselves.'

Diana thought that over. Self-protection. Yes, she knew all about that.

Soon they were in Sydney. Backyard after backyard after backyard. Paling fences, hills hoists, both houses and yards diminishing in size as they got closer to the centre of Sydney until they seemed minute, doll-sized. The train went rocketing past.

'Where did you live, Mum, when you were in Sydney?' Diana hadn't ever heard much of her mother's early pre-marriage days.

'Kirribilli, in a poky little flat, quite close to the ferry.' Stella laughed, remembering. 'I worked in the city for four years on a women's magazine, it's not around anymore. I ended up in the fashion section. I did a bit of everything. It was a great job, I loved it. Then I came back for a holiday and met your dad at a dance, and that was that, really.'

'So what was your dream, Mum?'

'To be in fashion?' She laughed dismissively. 'But I've no idea as what. To travel maybe. I almost had my ticket saved when I went back for that dance. But that's past history now.' Stella smiled at Diana. 'I got to go when Saskia was born. I only wish your father had come too.'

'Dad's never wanted to travel, has he?'

'He always says he's going to, so maybe one day.'

'Well, you've just got to make him.'

Her mother looked a little wistful, gazing out as dark descended quickly, as it did in June, and the lights in the carriage came on.

Waking children, gathering rubbish, pulling the suitcases out, stuffing books and toys back into bags as the train pulled into Central made Diana appreciate having her mother there. There wasn't a need to rush, she told herself, the train wasn't going anywhere—it finished its long journey at Central. She pulled Sienna to her feet, helped her into her backpack and handed a bag to Milo.

Patrick was waiting on the platform for them. He wore a full-length cashmere overcoat over a white dress shirt and black tie. It wasn't hard to deduce there was a dinner suit underneath the coat. He'd meant the 'in and out' comment. And Diana wasn't put out.

'Hello, I hope you haven't been waiting too long?' Stella reached up to give him a kiss on the cheek.

'The train was only twenty minutes late.'

Patrick turned to her and bent to kiss her. He smelled good. Her cheek burned where his lips touched her.

'Hello, Patrick. We're sorry to hold you up. Why don't we get a taxi and let you go on?'

Patrick's eyebrows rose slightly as he studied her. 'No problem, I'm not in a hurry.' He picked up Saskia who suddenly went from half asleep to wide awake.

'Hello, Patrick. Mummy said we could have a McDonald's.'

Diana had to admit he took it all in his stride. Within a few minutes they were sitting at the McDonald's at Central Railway station with two trays piled high with burgers, kids' meals, coffees and cokes, and making plans for tomorrow, not that anyone was consulting her. Patrick seemed to have everything under control.

CHAPTER THIRTY-SEVEN

Diana had jumped nearly a foot the first time Patrick touched her in front of her mother, and it had just been a hand at her elbow. Three days, surely she could manage that.

And the house! The view was breathtaking—a vast blue ocean, a creamy-orange beach protected by rocky sandstone cliffs and hardly another house in sight. That was amazing for anywhere in Sydney.

The house itself was fairly unremarkable from the outside. Built in the fifties probably, red brick with square, white-painted timber windows, the house was two storeys high, perched on the side of a cliff overlooking Bronte Beach. Inside, it had been completely gutted and redesigned. His brother owned the bottom floor and Patrick had the whole of the top. No wonder he said there was plenty of room.

'My brother bought it years ago.' He told them as he escorted them upstairs to his apartment. 'He lives downstairs with Marnie and the boys. They're away for the weekend.'

'The kids were wondering if they were going to see Alex and Sam. That's a pity, they all got on rather well.'

'I'm sorry. I have a dinner to go to, but I will see you in the morning. Just give me a ring if there's anything you need to know or if you're worried.'

*   *   *

Patrick took them out on the boat the next day. Boat—it was a forty-five foot, sleek navy and chrome cruiser. The children were overawed. Diana sat on the long white leather couch, glass of Sav Blanc in hand, and tried not to feel too impressed. To cap it all, the day was perfect—considering it was the middle of winter—sunny and clear. There was just enough breeze to ruffle the water and heel the yachts. It was definitely a day to be on the harbour, everywhere you looked there were people on boats, from lone fishermen in tiny dinghies to the crowds on the green and yellow ferries.

'Londoners would kill for a day like this in the middle of summer, let alone the middle of winter.' Diana laughed to her mother as they left the wharf. Patrick was wearing shorts and a navy polo shirt and looking far too good for Diana's liking. She did try not to look but as he was everywhere— untying ropes, racing to the wheel and pulling up fenders— that was a difficult one.

What was a total surprise was her mother. Stella came alive on the boat, pointing out landmarks: pretty Kirri- billi House, one of the Prime Minister's official residences, with its pointy roofs and painted wooden shutters, the velvety-green lawns stretching down to the water; and then racing over to the other side to show the children Government house, home to the Governor, with its square sandstone towers, almost hidden in the trees, and the extensive gardens surrounding it.

'That's where I lived, over there.' She was back pointing to the north side. 'I caught a ferry to work every day.'

Stella smiled at Diana. No wonder she knew her way around. Her enthusiasm was infectious. Diana was fascinated to see this new side of her mother emerging.

Then the shadow of the Sydney Harbour Bridge, the great grey coathanger, loomed over them. They examined it thoroughly from the east side, from the west and underneath it, all of them calling up to hear the echoes. They rounded the Opera House, dodging ferries, and Patrick headed his powerful craft over to North Head. All the children were given a turn steering *Flyaway*. Diana had been offered one too, but had wisely turned it down. She didn't need Patrick, standing as close as that. No, thank you.

Patrick had bought food from a delicatessen, just salamis and packets of chips and tomatoes and bread rolls. A no-fuss picnic, Patrick called it, Sydney style. They anchored just off the beach and ate as the roll from the small waves moved the boat gently up and down.

* * *

'Anyone for a walk on the beach?' Patrick came into the lounge room with a cricket bat under his arm. They'd returned half an hour ago and Diana and Stella were sitting with the children on Patrick's comfortable sofas.

'Yes.' Three children jumped up.

Diana smiled at their enthusiasm. 'No one would recognise you lot for the three that arrived in this country just eight weeks ago.'

'Eight! It's gone so quickly.' Her mother made a face. 'I might stay here I think, and start getting resigned to some peace and quiet.'

'You won't know yourselves when we've gone. Thank God for our lives back again, you'll say.'

'I think you may be wrong about that. But I might ring your father.'

Diana stood up. 'Don't do anything about dinner, Mum. We'll order some fish and chips.'

'Yeah.' The children threw their arms up in the air and danced round the room. They all laughed at their exuberance.

'Lord, you're easily satisfied.' Diana smiled over at Patrick.

'It's the best way for preparing you all for the return to English cuisine,' he said. 'We'll pick up the stumps on the way out. Sam and Alex leave them in the room at the bottom of the stairs.'

Diana and Patrick followed more sedately as the three children raced down the stairs to the narrow back garden and then wound their way down the steep steps to the beach.

'I don't know how to thank you. We've had a wonderful day.'

'So have I.' Patrick grinned and threw the bat and stumps onto the sand, and reached up to guide her onto the flat rocks at the bottom of the steps. Taking his hands, she jumped. His grip was strong and she would have stumbled if he hadn't held her steady.

Laser blue eyes met green and held briefly before she brushed past him and jumped down onto the sand. What was she reading in those eyes? He wasn't saying much. He could see the situation was impossible both for her and for him. A woman with three kids. Wrong time, wrong place, no matter what the attraction. Surely he understood. He'd be sensible. How she hated that word. Patrick picked up the bat and stumps and followed her.

A hectic game of beach cricket followed. Patrick was bowling when Milo hit the ball clean over Diana's head into the water behind her. Without thinking she dived in to get the ball.

She came up spluttering and teeth chattering, 'It's absolutely freezing,' she cried, as she ran out of the water. 'Milo, you'll pay for that.'

'Sorry, Mum.' But he was giggling and Diana just tackled him, wet clothes and all, on to the sand. The two girls joined in and they were all suddenly a heap of arms and legs and wet jeans and howls of mirth.

They didn't last much longer. The light was fading and Diana had managed to wet all of them to some extent. Shaking the sand out of her hair, she gasped, 'First one home gets first shower.' And the three were off; Saskia, as usual, doggedly trailing way behind.

Patrick reached down to give Diana a hand up and she stood brushing at the sand that covered her face and hair. 'I can't believe I went in the water. Why didn't you tell me it was so cold?'

'You didn't ask.' Patrick laughed at the astonishment on her face. 'You just dived in.'

'Story of my life,' she muttered. 'Come on, they'll put sand all through your house if we don't catch them.'

* * *

'It's so lovely to be warm and dry.' Diana sank into one of the white leather lounges.

'You are totally mad,' said Stella. 'You know it's winter. Thank heavens you didn't hurt yourself.' She shook her head and got to her feet. 'I'm going to read Saskia a story, Milo's got his phone and Sienna is engrossed in her book.'

'Thank you, Mum.' Diana settled back and looked around the room. The decorating theme was white on white: square white furniture, white walls and white floor tiles. Of course the view was fantastic, but the room lacked the warmth of Lost Valley. Missing were the many personal touches—it all was a bit sparse. They'd managed to clutter the place up a bit with her kid's paraphernalia—heaped towels, books and all their bags. She wondered how Patrick felt about the mess. He walked in with a bottle of wine and three glasses.

'If I didn't know better I'd say a different person lived in this home to the one who lives at Lost Valley,' Diana said, reaching to take the glass offered to her.

'Perceptive of you. I'd say you were right.'

Diana looked at Patrick over the top of her glass as he stretched out his legs in the chair opposite her.

'Sean kept this for me to use after Van and I broke up. Marnie had it decorated. For me it's just a place to stay.'

'So your heart's in Lost Valley?'

He sat up and looked at her. 'Lost Valley was my salvation. My cows are pretty straightforward. Give them enough water, grass and a bull once a year, and they're grateful and happy. I quite enjoy pottering about at the farm,' he said. 'So what have you got planned for tomorrow? I'll be leaving pretty early but I'll be back for dinner.'

Diana was more than a little frustrated. Just when things were getting interesting he veered away and closed doors. There was a lot more she wanted to ask.

*   *   *

They did the zoo the next day. Caught the ferry from Circular Quay across to the zoo and had nearly walked half the way up the steep hill before Diana and Stella realised there was a cable car that would have taken them up. They lunched at the zoo and found some more wallabies for Saskia. Sitting on the ferry on the way back, the kids were quiet, looking at the water burbling past. Diana and Stella exchanged glances.

'That was pretty successful,' Stella said.'

'Brilliant.' Diana grinned at her. 'I don't think they'll ever forget this time with you.'

Her mother didn't answer.

Later that afternoon shopping was the aim and they found a magnificent shopping mall in Bondi, all light and space.

Sienna looked around in wonder. 'They're bringing the outside in, Mummy!'

It may not have been quite as big as Brent Cross, but nearly, and they found babyccinos and cakes with pink icing. Diana was just returning from the toilets with Saskia and Milo, who were flagging a bit and very ready to go home.

'Surely everyone's had enough?'

'Please, Mummy, just one more shop, and then Stella said she'd show me where they did the shoot.'

'What shoot?' Diana looked curiously from her daughter to her mother, who took a large sip of her coffee.

'I was just telling Sienna about the time I had to find green shoes to go with a dress they wanted to photograph, and I searched high and low until I found a little shop not far from here that had one pair of green, hand-made shoes. I raced them back just in time to find the model had size ten feet and they didn't remotely fit.'

'What did you do?'

'They shot it all on the beach, barefoot.'

Trailing behind Sienna and Stella, who were debating the merits of big bags versus little bags and ankle boots over knee-length, once again Diana was struck by how little she knew of her mother's life in Sydney before she married. Going from working on fashion shoots to living on a farm, with three thousand sheep and a handful of dogs for company, must have been quite a change. Guess that was love for you. And her dream, she'd always said, had been to travel, for which she had waited thirty-five years. Diana let out a sigh and quickened her step. The shopping jaunt was mostly a success. Sienna had brightened up considerably, so it had all been worth it.

*   *   *

When they returned that afternoon, Alex and Sam were back. The children fell into each other's arms and within the space of thirty seconds had decided to go to the beach.

'No one's to go in the water,' Diana called after them, and looked exasperatedly across at Marnie at the lack of response from any of them.

'They'll be fine. My boys are besotted with catching crabs. Would they like to have dinner with us? I can throw a few more steaks on, or would they prefer sausages? I'd ask you all but I think Patrick's got plans. Your mum's very welcome.' Marnie's look wasn't sly exactly, but near enough.

That made Diana more uncomfortable, and more determined than ever to keep her mother firmly by her side.

'They'd love it. They haven't been with many children since we came over. I can see they're enjoying themselves immensely. It's my last night with Mum, so we'll cook dinner for Patrick.'

Diana followed Stella back upstairs. She went to the fridge and freezer and pulled out food enough for three and started cooking dinner.

'Hello.' Patrick lounged against the doorjamb, his jacket off and his collar loosened. He looked tired. Diana handed him a beer.

'Thank you. Where are the children? And your mother?'

'Mum's having a rest, and the children are being entertained by your two nephews.'

Diana found Patrick's concerned frown funny. 'I wouldn't worry too much. Don't forget, my children are tough little Londoners. They can look after themselves. It was in the country they were like fish out of water.'

'You didn't have to do this.' Patrick took in her preparations. 'I was going to take you out to dinner.'

'That's okay. I thought I could do something for you, to thank you. And it's our last night.' Suddenly it was real, they were leaving tomorrow. Damn. She did not want to go.

'That's very thoughtful of you, Diana,' he said, and bent to kiss her on the lips. She nearly dropped her beer. She would have, except Patrick caught it and put it down on the benchtop before kissing her again. She felt his body warm and solid against her. Real. She reached up and wound her arms around his neck. 'Stay,' she thought he whispered into her mouth, but when she opened her eyes he'd moved over to the fridge to check there was wine cooling. She must have been mistaken.

'Red or white?'

What? She had to think. Scramble her thoughts back together. 'Um, we're having steak, but I think Mum likes white, if that's all right.'

'No problem. I'll just go and get changed.'

CHAPTER THIRTY-EIGHT

Diana closed the bedroom door behind her and leant against it. This was ridiculous. Her real problem was that she had enjoyed that kiss far too much. and they were getting better. That is, if you considered better to mean her head going dizzy and that awful feeling of her knees going all weak. Now she was forty years old and not to be fooled by the chemistry. That's all it was—lust. What was really interesting was she could feel it all again. Feeling wasn't good at the moment. She needed to have control over her emotions. The next twenty-four hours were going to be terrible.

So, deep breath, Diana.

*   *   *

They'd finished eating and her mother had disappeared into her bedroom with the telephone to talk to her father. Diana was out on the balcony, listening to the chatter of the children below her and the crashing of the waves beyond that. It was dark, no moon tonight, but the stars were munificent, and lights twinkling on the water indicated ships passing.

'This is very beautiful.'

Patrick had come up and leant on the balcony beside her.

'You have no idea how lucky you are.' She felt him tense.

'You own this, all of it, the boat, this lovely house, the farm.'

'Well, yes …' He sounded uncertain, not understanding her.

'My father is home on his farm tonight because it owns him. He's obsessed with it, he won't leave it, can't leave it. It's like a millstone around his neck. He doesn't see it, of course. He feels he has this responsibility to keep it going, but it owns him. Now there's Mal, waiting for him to hand it over. He's been waiting for twenty years. Twenty years! That's a hell of a long time.' Diana moved away slightly, turning so she could look at him. 'Have you understood what a wonderful thing your grandparents did for you? By having the courage to break the ties to their history, their safe world, all to build a better future for their children.'

'I'm not sure my parents would agree with you. My dad has always felt deprived of his heritage, cut off from his roots.' Patrick looked down at her curiously. 'When I went back to Ireland, I understood we would have had no future there. I went up to the farm—or at least where it would have been, the country that my grandparents owned—and I stood there on that green hillside and I knew I wanted to own land, if not there, here. It was so beautiful. Very powerful. More than that, it was inside me, something I had to do.'

Stella walked out to join them.

'I can hear the children.'

There was noise on the stairs and the children arrived—exhausted, over-excited and not in the least wanting to go to bed. Patrick took over bath duty and had ended up as wet as they were. Her mother very nearly had a stroke seeing all that water going down the drain in Patrick's enormous tub. Finally, the children were in bed, but not asleep, Diana concluded from the muffled bumps and noises escaping from their bedroom.

'Coffee?' Patrick stuck his head round the door. Diana had gone back out to the balcony.

'Oh yes! Thank you. Mum excused herself. She's exhausted and she's gone to bed.'

He reappeared with two cups, with two chocolate biscuits balanced on top. 'I had to change my shirt,' he said.

'It looked like you'd have to change more than that, from where I stood.' Diana was laughing as she took her cup.

'How do parents ever manage to have an intelligent conversation?'

'Not very often. By the time the children are in bed they're too tired to talk. Often Charlie and I communicated with a series of grunts.' Diana felt her cheeks warm as she realised her comment might be misconstrued and looked out to sea.

'Do you want to talk about Charlie?'

'I do and I don't. No one out here really knew him and I'm finding that hard. I thought pushing him away and filling up my life with my old world would make it hurt less. But now Charlie's following me around. He's in my head. I don't like that either.' A shout followed by a squeal erupted from the bedroom.

'I'm sorry. Wait here. If they don't go to sleep soon they'll be impossible tomorrow.'

Diana was embarrassed. She put her coffee down and disappeared inside. Why did she say that? By the time she came back, Patrick had surrounded himself with a bunch of pamphlets.

'I wanted to show you these. I want to grow hops, with the idea of building a brewery. I'm thinking of putting in around six acres to start. I've talked about this with Tom, I thought he might give me some advice, that he may even want to plant a few as well.'

'Good heavens!' Diana was dumbstruck. 'What on earth did he say?' Their fingers brushed as she took one of the brochures. She thought she'd been burned.

'I might have to do some more talking. He's not convinced.' Patrick laughed. 'I'm not finding Mal very responsive to my ideas either. Look here.'

Patrick was too close. The hairs on her arm were standing on end. The very air around them crackled. The words blurred on the pamphlets he handed her. 'So when do you plan to start?'

'Next week. I want to begin ploughing and planting the hops.'

'You?' She needed to step away. Get some distance.

Patrick chuckled. 'No. I'm employing contractors.'

'That's an unusual thing for our district, isn't it? I can't imagine Dad doing it. He only wants to run sheep.' It was so hard to concentrate on what she was saying. Patrick's arm rested on the balcony railing beside her. She was fascinated by the hairs on his arm. Were the hairs crinkly, or as soft as they looked?

'He could lease it to me, I'd do all the work. At his time of life that may not be such a bad thing.' He paused. 'As for me, I only want to kiss you again.'

Diana looked up to find Patrick's eyes intently studying her.

'I want to kiss you too.' The truth was clear in her mind, it was no use denying it or pretending anything else. All her good intentions had flown out the window ... well, over the railing.

Patrick pulled her over to a darkened corner of the balcony out of sight of the living room, lifted her chin and bent his head to find her lips. Rockets, an explosion or two, her knees gave way and she was clinging to his shoulders. One of his arms was supporting her, the other hand pulling at her nipple. She groaned into his mouth and his hand went straight down to her jeans, flicking open the metal button at the top and sliding down the zipper and cupping her. Their mouths locked and she arched up into his hand. His finger slid into her. And the unbelievable happened. She climaxed. With an intensity that shocked her.

Patrick held her as the tremors died away, kissing her softly, her eyes, her lips her neck. He was smiling. 'Goodnight, Diana. Sleep well.' And he turned and left her.

What on earth just happened? Diana stood stunned, unable to move or think ... Well, she knew what had just happened. How and why was a little harder to understand. She also knew she'd been his for the taking and he hadn't. Not even asked.

Turning off lights, she made her way to her room and got ready for bed, slipped into her pyjamas, brushed her teeth and sat on the edge of the perfectly made bed, absently stroking the satiny beige doona and whistling softly to herself.

She'd done it again, lost all reason when his arms surrounded her and his lips touched hers. It wasn't even one of those slow building kisses. No, it was pure, explosive heat. Insanity, kissing Patrick with her mother two rooms away, her kids not asleep. Would that have stopped her? She didn't think so, it only occurred to her just now. But for *that* to have happened ... she didn't even know if she really liked him.

She was leaving tomorrow. Insanity.

'Sleep well.' It was on the cards that she wouldn't. She didn't know about Patrick.

*   *   *

Lunchtime they were packed and all ready to go. Patrick was taking them to the airport. Diana felt it was desperately important that she carry them all through this. The children looked lost and her mum was being so brave. Patrick was being a pillar of strength; he seemed to know how hard this was for her. When he was talking about London and teasing Saskia about not locking herself in the toilet this time, Stella disappeared into the bedroom.

She returned with Diana's phone in her hand. 'I can't understand why I can't get through to your father. I know he wants to say goodbye. He won't answer the phone.'

Patrick looked up from his computer. 'Would you like me to ring Mal and get him to try? He might get through on the UHF.'

Marnie and the two boys appeared at the door.

'Hi, we just have a little going away present for you all. Some pictures we took at the races of everyone.'

Diana stood there looking at the pictures of the children cheekily balanced on the wooden railings of the racetrack, her mother and Rosie, Patrick looking at her. *Oh crikey. She nearly dropped the photo.* Then there was one of Sean and Patrick, one of her dad in the tent, his head thrown back and laughing, with the girls draped around him.

'I'm speechless. Thank you, Marnie, they're beautiful.' She went over and gave Marnie a hug.

'It was a wonderful day, wasn't it? Now you have to come back really soon. The boys were thinking they might have a little run on the beach before you leave. Is there time?'

'We've got half an hour, haven't we, Patrick?' He nodded and took the phone with him into his office. 'Sure, would you guys like to go? Don't get dirty.'

Her kids looked as if someone had just handed them a lifeline. They raced after Sam and Alex, discussing where they found the best crab yesterday.

'Coffee?'

Marnie laughed and shook her head. 'No, thanks. You'll be sick of the stuff by the time you get to London. Airport coffee. Yuk.'

'Thanks for that.' She gestured vaguely in the direction the children had taken. 'I think everyone was getting a little tense. A bit of a run will be good for them.'

'How are you getting home, Stella?' Marnie asked.

'I'm going to catch the train. There's one about six, I can get it from the airport.'

'Why don't you come back here? The boys and I are going down to the farm tomorrow for a few days, and we'll take you.'

'Thank you all the same, but I want to get back to Tom. We haven't been apart this long since I went to London to see Diana, and I have a feeling I'm going to be pretty miserable company tonight.'

Diana's phone rang.

'It's my ring, but where is the bloody thing?' Diana was searching her handbag, pulling out the passports and packets of tissues she'd stuffed in there. Stella joined her, lifting up cushions and looking around the chairs.

'There it is.' Diana pounced on her suitcase. 'How in the hell did it get there?' By then it had finished ringing. She scanned the number. 'Damn, it was Mal.' The phone rang again in Patrick's study. 'It'll be Dad,' Diana reassured her mother.

Patrick walked back into the room, his face solemn. 'Sorry, Stella. It's Mal.'

One look at his face and Stella sank into a chair and took the phone with shaking fingers. 'Oh my God, no. Mal, how is he?' She listened. 'Thank you, let me know as soon as you can. Yes.' She put the phone in her lap unable to let go of it. 'Oh no.' She gulped. 'Diana, Mal has just found Tom, up in the sheep yards. He's unconscious, not responding. Mal didn't wait for an ambulance. He's driving him into town and he's rung on ahead and the hospital's waiting for him.'

Diana just stood there. It was happening again. This, out of the blue, unbelievable ... No, no. Patrick put his arm round her. She wasn't entirely sure she would be standing otherwise. There was a clatter on the stairs. The children were back.

CHAPTER THIRTY-NINE

Night was falling fast, as it did midwinter in the south. Diana looked out the window at the yellowing landscape as it faded into the purples and blacks and pinpricks of light from the oncoming cars. There was no wind and you could feel the frost settling already.

She should have been in a plane on her way to England. Now she was in Rosie's car following the helicopter that had taken her mother and father from their local hospital to Albury. She didn't know how her dad was doing. Or the kids. Perhaps she should wait a little before ringing them. They were at Lost Valley with Patrick and Marnie, and looking pretty vulnerable and lost when she'd last seen them. How they'd got her mother home had been entirely due to Patrick's efficient organisation. Diana had been no use. The last time she'd seen her father kept cropping up in front of her. It would be so unfair if anything … *Not this time.* Please. She couldn't bear to go through this again.

Rosie shivered. 'It would help if you put the window up.'

Diana closed off the inch or so of air she had been hoping would clear the fug from the overheated car. 'What's up, Rosie? Have I done something to annoy you?' She looked at her sister's profile across from her.

'Only what's usually wrong after you've been around for a while.'

'Well, I was nearly gone. I should be halfway to London by now.' Diana looked out the window again. Saw the sinister shape of a kangaroo lope away from the side of the road. 'Oh, watch it, there's a kangaroo.'

'There are millions of the wretched things. They're always here at this time of night, they love the green pick beside the road, I think. But don't worry, I'll be careful. We wouldn't want to risk your precious neck, would we?'

'Oh, for Christ sake, Rosie. Dad's in emergency, in hospital, with we don't know what. Lay off the sarcasm, will you?'

'Diana rides to the rescue again, goddess in shining armour. How did we all get on without you, these last twenty years?'

'I can't imagine. Pure luck, I guess.' Diana was so sick of these jealous confrontations. They had more important things to worry about, surely.

'Right, lucky. You are one lucky girl, aren't you? You couldn't just be a poverty-stricken artist, could you? You swan in with three perfect children, and within a couple of months have Patrick salivating all over you.'

'I can't believe you said that. Have you no concept of what I'm going through? Charlie's dead, Rosie. It bloody hurts.

The pain is so great sometimes I can't breathe, and I think good, stop breathing. Then I remember I have three children depending on me and I *have* to keep on breathing. Then there are the nights when I think, what if I die too and there's no one for them? *No one*, Rosie. That's why I had to come out here. If something happened to me, my kids have a family— you and Mal, and Mum and Dad. People to love them. One thing I've discovered is that death happens. And what's more, it is final, Rosie, no second chances, no "let's try again" ... No chance to say I'm sorry. You don't get to make up. Oh hell!' Diana swallowed. 'When's the last time you saw Dad?'

'Sunday.'

'Did you give him a hug? Tell him you loved him? How much he meant to you? At the railway station I just said goodbye and thanks for having us all. I was in such a snit 'cause he wouldn't come to Sydney to say goodbye. How do you think I feel right now?'

Rosie was silent for a minute. 'Dad's not going to ...' Swallowing, she just couldn't get the word out. 'I'm sorry, Di, I'm so sorry. I don't mean it, well, I do, but it's coming out all wrong.' Her eyes filled with tears.

'That's ridiculous. Surely you can't be saying that you resent the fact that all these years I've worked my guts out, without my family backing me all the way ... And aren't you forgetting one thing? That you're the one getting Mog's Hill, lock, stock and barrel. Come on.'

'Yeah right, when?'

'It might be sooner than you think. Be careful what you wish for ...'

'Well, it might be nice if you looked at things from my perspective. How would you like to be hanging on, waiting

for twenty years? Twenty years, Di,' Rosie said through grit-
ted teeth. 'How would you like that?'

Diana was silent. She seriously didn't think she'd have
waited around for twenty years. And how was that her fault,
anyway?

'That's right, you got on with your life,' Rosie answered
for her. 'I'm watching sons of farmers all around us, waiting, marking time, not going ahead and doing what they
really want. All because they're in line to inherit the farm.
In these twenty years everything has changed so drastically
in the bush. Farmers aren't retiring. Mal is going crazy. He's
thinking he might want to do something else, feels he's running out of time. And now all Patrick is thinking about is
hops. It's just not his thing.'

'You know this isn't my fault.' Diana looked over at Rosie.

'I know, of course it isn't your fault, but it's good to blame
you.'

'Oh Rosie,' Diana started to laugh, 'at least you're making
me laugh.'

'I'm glad someone thinks it's funny.' Then Rosie started to
laugh, too. 'You're right, it's better than tears.'

* * *

The little car motored on down the highway through the
black night with both sisters lost in their own thoughts.
After a while, Diana decided to ask Rosie something else
that had been on her mind for some time.

'What's the deal with you and Mal?'

'I don't think he knows what he wants at the moment. He
won't talk to me. My trouble is I don't know if it's me or our

situation. I've tied him down with false promises and he's resenting it, I think. If we're exchanging confidences, what's the go with Patrick?'

'Nothing. Nothing at all.'

'It didn't look like nothing back there at Lost Valley. I'd be careful there.' Rosie cast a glance over at her sister.

'Why?'

'He suffers from commitment phobia. Mal thinks his heart belongs to his first wife, Vanessa.'

What did she know about the man? She hadn't told Rosie the truth though. It mightn't be something, but it sure wasn't nothing. She didn't have a clue what was happening. She felt like scattered pieces of a jigsaw puzzle. Bits of her that were Charlie's, bits that belonged to her children, her parents owned a couple of pieces, even— infuriatingly— Rosie. Now Patrick was angling for a piece, maybe a little piece she'd been holding on to all these years. She just didn't know how to put them all together, how to make them fit so she could be a whole person again. Fractured, that's how she felt. They all wanted a piece of her.

Silence clamped down in the little car as both sisters stared straight ahead down the darkened four lane highway. 'I want Marnie to ring. I'm too scared to ring her.'

Diana remembered the scene before she left. Three white, stricken faces, clinging to whatever part of her they could hold on to.

'I've got to go to Stella, I promised,' she'd told them.

'We can come too.' Sienna was almost hysterical. 'We'll be very good. We can give Stella a massage and buy you coffee. We can.'

Diana stooped and picked up Sienna and hugged her. 'I know. I wish you could come, but there'll be lots of waiting around. Here you'll have fun with Sam and Alex.'

She looked over Sienna's head to Marnie with her boys at her side. 'I'm sorry. This is the first time we've been separated since,' she swallowed, 'England.' Even now, mentioning Charlie's name was a no go; she just choked on the word.

'It's okay, they'll be fine. We'll take good care of them, won't we, boys?'

Diana reluctantly passed Sienna, who was now sobbing brokenly, to Marnie and tried to pick up Saskia who had wound herself round one of her legs.

'Come on, sweetheart. I need you to be strong and brave. It will only be for a couple of days. I promise I'll be back in two days, no matter what ... Oh God.' Diana buried her head in the soft curls. 'I'm not sure I can do this either.' She knelt down to hug Milo.

'It'll be okay, Mum, I'll look after them.' Milo said doggedly. 'Stella needs you.'

Diana rose, gave Saskia's hand to Milo and got into the car. As she was doing up her seatbelt, Sienna broke free and ran to the car pulling at the handle. Marnie ran to her and pulled her back. Through the glass Diana could see the tears running down her face, the soundless, broken sobs.

'Quickly, Rosie, let's go.'

Maybe she'd ring Marnie later.

CHAPTER FORTY

Stella had never been in an intensive care ward before. Twenty-five years ago, in their local hospital, there hadn't been one. This had a quiet sense of purpose about it. Not like those dramas on TV in the ER when everyone was screaming and running with trolleys in different directions. Here there were soft footfalls over the lino and rustling nurses, checking all the time; the machines with their satisfactory beeping, and Tom sedated, attached to all those tubes and monitors, just lying there. She watched his chest rise and fall and rise.

'Don't you dare leave me,' she whispered for the thousandth time. She hoped he was getting the message. A couple of the other cubicles were occupied. Busy nurses disappeared behind the curtains and then reappeared with instruments and little trays. No one she knew. She wanted Will Talbot and the nurses from home. People she could

trust. Diana and Rosie weren't allowed in. They'd arrived
last night about eight. They were outside somewhere. She
was the only one allowed in and she couldn't leave Tom.
They'd lost Cody. She wasn't about to lose Tom.

More tests. The young Indian doctor was thorough, she'd
give him that; if only she had some idea what he was talking
about. It was all so like the last time with Cody, jumbles of
words that ended with 'doing everything we can'. This time
it would have to be good enough. Tom was going to get better. She so wanted out of here, this strange foreign place. She
just wanted to take Tom home.

The specialist had been, once. Now all she had recourse
to was the young Indian, and he was so busy. Everyone was
busy except her. *Tom, Tom, Tom, what's happening to you?*
Stella sighed. Perhaps Diana and Rosie understood it better.

'Don't you leave me. Don't you dare.' She touched Tom's
fingers for reassurance.

There was movement behind her but she didn't look up.

'Mrs Crawford? We're just going to take your husband
for a scan, we won't be long. Why don't you go out and get
some air, go for a walk? Your daughters are waiting outside.'

These were two new faces—one young with pink
scrubbed cheeks, and the older one whose grey eyes looked
at her sympathetically. The shift had changed. They took
Tom in no time at all and she stiffly made her way out to
the waiting room.

Rosie sprung up as she entered the room where they were
waiting. It must be dreadful for them on those hard vinyl
chairs. She felt so drained and useless.

'Mum, come and sit down.'

'No, I don't want to sit. Let's go outside.'

They walked out of the hospital. It was freezing. The wind must be coming right off the snowfields. Diana put her arm round her, for a hug or just to keep warm. She realised it was her that was shivering.

'Do you want to eat?' Diana asked.

'No, I do not want to eat, I want to know what's going on. Have you two any idea what's happening?'

Diana shook her head and they both looked at Rosie.

'Not really. Why don't we ring Will? Have you been reading Dad's notes?'

'What notes?'

'The ones they keep at the end of the bed. We could tell Will what's in them and he could decipher them. I'll duck in and have a look.'

Rosie turned and left them in the shelter of a brick wall. At least it was out of the wind. If only she didn't feel so tired.

What a fool she was, not familiar in the ways of a hospital. It was just like before. 'No, Mrs Crawford, nothing yet, we don't know anything. Just wait till Cody's tests are back.' Or, 'I don't know where the specialist is, he'll be in to see you when he's seen Cody.' Or worse, 'Don't you worry, love, we're doing everything we can.' And that was exactly nothing at all.

'I should have listened to you,' said Stella. 'Your father's been under so much strain with the drought, wool prices, sheep prices, you name it—and if he was suffering depression as well, maybe it's done this.'

'We don't know for sure that Dad has depression,' said Diana. 'I mean full-blown depression. It could be stress, or it could just be one of those things. Wait till they tell us some of the results of the tests. It was probably us, me, all the added pressure.'

'Don't be ridiculous, Diana.' She couldn't seriously be blaming herself. 'Why won't anyone tell us what's going on?' It was so frustrating. 'How are the children getting on? They must be terribly worried without you.'

Diana laughed. 'I think the children are being looked after beautifully. I spoke to them just a little while ago. They're having a whale of a time.'

She was trying too hard. Stella could hear the worry in her voice. It was an impossible situation. She was so glad her daughters were here with her but it must be awful for the children.

Rosie came back out, shoulders hunched against the wind. 'Hey, I've written down some of the names of these tests. Let's ring Will.'

The three of them walked back inside and after talking to Will, Stella felt she knew a little more. Not that it was doing her much good. As Will had said, they had to be patient and wait for the results. Everything was being done that he could think of. Trust them, he said. If only she could. She examined Tom's face lying on the pillows. He had such a nice face, kind and strong. He looked pale. There were some more little skin cancers on his forehead to come off; she must get him to see Will about them. When they got home.

'Oh! Tom, don't you dare leave me.'

She hadn't wanted to marry a farmer. Escaped to the city as soon as she could, then she'd met Tom again and fell like the proverbial sack of spuds. She'd known him for years but they'd never gone out. She supposed she'd had to get the city boys out of her system. It was such a different world in the city. Everything moved so quickly; people seemed to skim over the essentials. There was no time to do anything except play catch up with everyone else.

Tom wasn't really a farmer, he was a sheep man. All he'd ever wanted to do was grow fine wool on beautiful big-framed sheep. He loved his sheep. He'd inherited the flock of Saxon blood sheep from his father and every year they'd bought rams from Merrigal. He'd only been saying the other day how he'd love to take Milo with him next time. That would be the fourth generation of Crawfords to buy rams from them. *Oh Tom, there's so much yet to do!*

Forty-two years together. They had a real-life marriage with ups and downs as everyone had, but they'd always had each other. She'd never have got over Cody's death without him. Tom hadn't cried when Cody had died; she hadn't either, not for a long time.

He'd cried when Phillipa was born. When he held her, wrapped in the flannelette hospital blanket, and she'd blinked up at him with that knowing look of the newborn. He'd had tears in his eyes then.

'Don't you leave me now, Tom. Hold on, my darling, hold on.'

She had strength to draw on somewhere. She would find it.

Enough for the two of them.

CHAPTER FORTY-ONE

A little later, her mother came back out to join them as they sat eating cardboard sandwiches at the hospital canteen. Diana had opted for a juice rather than face another tasteless cup of coffee. They were making plans. At least Rosie and her mother were.

She wasn't sure how much more of this she could take.

'Philly will be quite useful. She's getting holidays soon and she can stay with you. Or I can. Between us, we could manage, I think.' Rosie looked over at Diana as if throwing down a challenge.

'They're talking about putting in four stents tomorrow during the angioplasty. Four, that's quite a lot, you know.' Her mother was sounding a little too bright. 'I couldn't believe it when the doctor told us. Four! We're so lucky Tom is still alive.' Stella returned to the subject at hand. 'Diana and the children can be with us. I don't want Diana to go.'

'Diana said she had to get back to an exhibition in September,' Rosie said.

'Well, it's not September, yet.'

Diana just sat there. They were talking as though she wasn't even there. One thing was becoming quite clear—Rosie wanted her out, and her mother seemed not to want her out of her sight. Well, she was getting sick to death of it.

'I'm expected back in England, Mum.'

'The last time you walked out we didn't see you for twenty years.'

A minor exaggeration. Her mother wasn't above stretching the truth to make a point.

'I was upset. You and Dad just told me to get on with my life and there was nothing for me at Mog's Hill. Pretty tough stuff.'

'Diana, Diana, we were only wanting the best for you.' Stella sounded as if she was going to burst into tears.

'Didn't seem like it from where I sat. You bought my ticket.' She shouldn't have said that.

Her mother just looked at her. Opening her mouth and then closing it again, she seemed to be having trouble finding the right words. 'It wasn't like that, Diana. Please. We went to the final exhibition for your year, do you remember? Two of your lecturers collared us and told us you had a really bright future ahead of you. To make sure you went overseas. You were so lucky to get the residency in London and you—you were hell-bent on coming back to the farm. We didn't know how to stop you. So your father and I decided,' she paused, taking a shaky breath, 'what we decided. We didn't know you were going to take it so hard, walk out the door and never talk to us for six months.' She blinked away the tears. 'And then we didn't see you for ten years. I hope, now you have children, you can start to imagine how much that hurt us.'

'I'm not sure I'm hearing this right. That was all for my own good? Rosie and Mal getting the farm was just because you wanted me to go to England? Don't be ridiculous. What was wrong with sitting down to a discussion, like people generally do?'

'You're forgetting what you were like then. You were hard to get through to, strong-willed, stubborn. You wanted to come home and you were impossible to talk to.'

Diana looked from Rosie to her mother. Rosie appeared stunned. It must have been news for her, too.

'Well, thank you very much. You were right. I have made a success of my career, so I guess I should thank you.' Actually, thanking her parents was the last thing she felt like doing.

Diana was shaking as she rose and left the canteen, blindly walking down the corridor. If she wasn't careful she'd hit out at the next person she met. Physical violence had never seemed so attractive, right now.

Starting with her family. So much pain. For so many years. And it was for *her own good*? Come on.

'Diana.'

She didn't hear the voice as much as notice the hand on her arm, restraining her. She turned ready to lay into whoever it was.

'Patrick.' She looked blankly at him. 'What are you doing here? Are the kids …?'

'The kids are fine. What's wrong?'

'You don't want to know. I've just had a session with my mother and Rosie. I'm out of here. I don't suppose you have a car handy?'

'Absolutely. I thought I'd see Stella and Tom first.' His smile was rueful. 'I wouldn't like them to worry. Are you sure you want to go?'

'I am certain I want to go, and if you want to talk to my mother, she's down there, and my father is still in intensive care and not permitted visitors. They're doing the angioplasty tomorrow, and he'll be home the day after, apparently.' Her voice felt raspy.

Patrick handed her his car keys. 'Turn right as you go out the door.'

She felt his eyes follow her down the corridor, knew she was walking stiffly but she couldn't do anything about it. She passed the darkened flower shop and the empty front desk. Outside, in the cold black night with thousands of stars twinkling above her, she felt a rage so deep it was making her tremble.

*   *   *

She wasn't sure when Patrick rejoined her. It was damn cold in the car but at least it was out of the wind. He started the engine, but just sat there, not putting the car into gear.

'They're worried about you.' He wasn't smiling, just watching her carefully.

'It's a little late for worry, I'd say.'

'What happened?'

'My mother just told me the reason I was shoved out of the nest, very forcefully I might add.'

'And?' he prompted.

'For my own good. How about that? I'm very angry. All those lost years.' She closed her eyes and leant back against the soft leather. 'I know I started growing up after I left

Australia, but it was a bit like being thrown in at the deep end.'

The heating started to kick in and the frost on the windscreen began to melt away. Patrick put the windscreen wipers on once, twice, then turned them off.

She picked at the stitching in the leather trim under her knees. 'I thought it was because Mal had just got engaged to Rosie and they finally had the son they'd always wanted.'

'Your father has never given me the impression he was hankering for a son. I think that's your problem.'

She whispered, 'Take me home, Patrick.'

'I can't. Your mother really wants you to be here tomorrow when Tom has the operation.'

'Well, I can't face them at the moment. I can't go back to that motel room I'm sharing with Rosie.'

'We'll find you another. I will be with you tomorrow and then I'll take you home.'

'Promise?'

'Promise,' he answered softly. He put the car into gear and reversed out of the parking space and turned into the main street. He pulled up at the first motel they came to that had a vacancy sign shining out front.

'Okay?'

'What are you doing here?'

'I was worried about Tom, but mostly I was worried about you. Marnie and the kids seemed to be getting on fine.' He got out of the car.

Diana felt strangely light-headed. Was it her anger or exhaustion? It was a bit hard to tell. Patrick came back with two keycards and handed one of them to her.

They had to go up a flight of stairs and her inaction had Patrick taking the keycard back from her to insert into the lock. They stood and looked at each other outside the door.

'Oh, for heaven's sake, come in.' She took his hand and pulled him after her.

It was your standard motel room. A narrow wooden bench stretched along one side. Standard prints on the walls of what appeared to be country scenes—a bridge over a creek and a hut on a mountainside—and a very big bed in the middle of the room. For some reason the bed seemed to double in size and levitate before her eyes. Patrick pushed her stiff figure down on to it. He found the bar fridge and pulled out a miniature whiskey bottle. 'Want to share?'

Diana nodded. It didn't matter to her one way or another, just that it was alcohol. 'It just makes me so mad they didn't have enough respect for me to talk to me like an adult. Nobody asked me what I wanted. And then to take twenty years to tell me? I simply don't believe it.'

'Maybe they were afraid of the reception they would get. They'd made the decision with their eyes open. I think they were taking the responsibility that came with that. Maybe they thought everything would sort itself out.' Patrick handed her the tumbler with the amber-coloured liquid. 'No ice, sorry.'

Diana drank, enjoying the strangely warm, smooth taste of it. She didn't normally drink whiskey.

'At least if we'd talked about it, it could have been my decision. Now I'll never know … I shouldn't have walked out like that. I'm behaving badly.'

'No.' He laughed. 'Well, yes. But it's a normal reaction. I don't think you realise how much your parents are in awe of you.'

'What?' she turned, round-eyed.

'They adore you. They're so proud of what you've achieved, and they live for news of you.'

Diana was speechless. 'You're crazy.' Then she added, suspiciously, 'How do you know?'

Patrick sighed. 'I've been here for the last four years. I was shown the photos you sent. I passed your pictures in the hall each time I walked in the door. They never stopped talking about you. And then you came back ... and I met the real-life Diana. I saw what they were talking about.' He came to sit on the bed next to her, took the drink from her hand and kissed her.

All she could think was how right it felt. That it was good. Like coming home should feel.

When Patrick lifted his head the next time she was lying beneath him on the bed and managed rather breathlessly, 'You're not serious.'

Patrick laughed and stretched out beside her, his head on his hand, tracing light crazy patterns on her arm. 'I like surprising you.'

'Ha. Very funny.' She hit him on the arm and then she kissed him. A heart-stopping kiss, with her hands moulding and enquiring. Learning his body as a blind man would. Not a stitch of clothing removed, the only bare skin she was touching was at his neck, his cheek bones and the skin on his forearms. She knew it was driving him crazy.

Diana held his hands at bay but she let him roll her over so that he was on top again. She stretched back and looked up at him. 'What's next in the surprise stakes?'

'I take it all back. No more surprises. I want you, Diana. There's nothing surprising about that.'

She pushed him away. 'I'm sorry.'

'You're sorry about what?' Patrick took her hands in his. His beautiful hands.

Oh God. 'I can't do this,' she said brokenly.

'Listen, go to sleep, stop worrying. We'll take tomorrow as it comes, one thing at a time. All you need to know is I'm here. Okay?'

He said goodnight, leaving her lying on the bed, and walked out of the room. Reaching for her phone, she texted Rosie that she'd see her in the morning.

*   *   *

When Diana woke, her head was rolling with images of her mother and father telling her to leave home, intertwined with Patrick pulling her along the road and lifting her onto a big black horse. The children were standing in a garden behind locked iron gates, their little arms outstretched, entreating, begging … She woke in a sweat, registering the knock on the door. Groggy, she grabbed her jacket, as she had no night clothes with her, and put her head warily round the door.

'Breakfast. Good morning.' The blonde-headed girl in a tracksuit on the other side of the door was far too cheerful for this time in the morning.

Diana gave a mumbled thanks and took the tray, with what looked like a cooked breakfast under the anodised cover.

Half an hour later, and considerably more together, Diana answered the knock on her door, sliding the chain-latch free. Patrick, a half smile on his face, took her in his arms and kissed her.

'I definitely like surprising you.'

'You promised, no more surprises. Anyway that wasn't a surprise, after last night.'

But that wasn't true. She was surprised, every time he put his arms round her. By the way her heart raced and her legs folded beneath her. By the way she unconsciously reached for him and wound her arms around his neck and lifted her head for his lips. This morning he was all lemony aftershave and toothpaste. Lucky him, hers was still in her bag with Rosie.

She took a step back. 'Thank you for breakfast. That was thoughtful, I forgot all about ordering last night.'

'I hadn't had anything to eat, I was starving.'

'Oh no! Patrick, I'm so sorry.'

'Well, I had a feeling you may not have had much to eat either. Sleep well?'

'I ... not really, I had these weird dreams. Actually, all last night seems a bit of a blur.'

'That's a pity. I'll have to start all over again.' Patrick smiled and reached for her.

'No, you don't.' But she was laughing as she fended him off. 'Did you really mean what you said last night?'

'Which bit? That I'm here for you?'

She shook her head.

'That your parents are in awe of you, or that I am?'

'My parents.' She didn't want to go to that other space.

'The first time your father talked to me about you, we were facing flames twenty feet high. I was on the back of your fire truck wrestling with the hose, and the pump was being particularly difficult to start. Your dad said you were the only person he'd ever known who could get the wretched thing going, first pull.'

Her knees gave way and she fell backwards on to the bed, Patrick on top of her.

'How he wished Diana was still here, she'd been his best mate for fires. He said how much he missed you at times like that.' Patrick's hand wandered down her side. 'He'd always remember you, clambering on to the back of the truck, the first time he took you. You'd have been twelve or something. Do you want more?' He nuzzled her neck.

'No, I was fifteen before he let me go with him,' Diana whispered, closing her eyes. 'I've always thought I was never good enough, not the son they wanted. I don't think I want to know this.'

'Don't you want to know how excited your mother was to get photos from you? She'd race out to me and say "Look …"' Patrick kissed her neck and started a slow journey downwards.

'Stop it. Stop it. No, I don't want to know. Mum was always so critical of anything I did.' Diana struggled to sit up and Patrick sighed and stretched out to lie beside her.

'Your mother adores you, but then,' He fiddled with the button on her shirt. 'Not as much as I adore you.'

'Patrick, will you hold me for a minute? Just hold me.'

'Now that's the sort of question I like, only I could hold you for a lot longer than that. It will be the letting you go that's going to be the problem.'

'Very funny. Ooh.'

He took her in his arms and they lay on the bed as he pulled her close. It was so comforting. She felt truly cared for. Then Diana realised Patrick was using his fingers to make those crazy patterns on her arms and pressing little kisses into her neck. She lifted her mouth to his lips. They were firm and warm. She closed her eyes.

Who would have believed this meeting of lips, touching of tongues, could be so amazing. His hands wandered about just above her waist, pulling her body to him till it felt like a piece of her soft clay, slowly getting closer to the underside of her breast so that it positively ached for his hands. She paid him back in kind, re-learning his body, waiting for his groan or intake of breath before moving her fingers away.

If only everything would go away and she and Patrick could ... Dream over, Diana.

'You are a heck of a kisser.' She groaned. 'Hey, it's time to go.' Reluctantly she tried to disentangle herself. 'Patrick, I've got to ring the kids.' She pulled his face down so she was looking him squarely in the eyes. 'Why me? Why now?'

'I've asked myself the same thing. No idea. Maybe you are a fantasy come to life. I do know I don't want you to go back to London.'

'I've got to go back.'

'I know.' He sighed and sat up.

'What if the real me doesn't stack up to the fantasy? I can be very difficult to deal with in real life.'

'Tell me about it.'

'Ha.' She sat up and punched him lightly on the arm, and gave him a piercing look from under those straight black eyebrows. 'I don't really know where we're going with this.'

Patrick grinned. 'I told you. Let's take one step at a time.'

Then let's hope they're baby steps, not giant ones, Diana thought. She was so not ready for this.

'Let's go.'

CHAPTER FORTY-TWO

When they got to the hospital Phillipa was there in the waiting room with Rosie.

At least Diana thought it was Phillipa. She was the right age, but this girl had black hair and black leggings with a loose top and two rings in each ear.

Diana looked again. 'Phillipa?'

'Aunty Di!' The girl jumped up to give her a hug. 'Poor Tommo, poor Stella. Isn't it awful?'

Rosie was in tears. 'They're about to take him in, Mum's still with him. It's going to be hours before we know. By the way, thanks for letting us know where you'd got to last night. Mum was nearly going demented.'

'Sorry.' Diana closed her eyes briefly, she wasn't going to bite. The only way to deal with yesterday was to forget it. Forget it all. Or at least shelve it. It must be horrible for Rosie as well. She turned to Phillipa. 'Well, what's been happening to you? Tell me all. Start at ten years ago.'

'It's going to be a long story.' Phillipa laughed. 'How about I get you both some coffees? How do you like it, Aunty Di?'

Aunty Di? Diana looked at her niece. 'Perhaps we could start with you calling me Diana.'

'Sure, and I'm Philly.'

They both laughed and Philly took the twenty dollar note her mother held out and danced out of the room.

'Black, Philly, black,' Diana called after her and then she turned to Rosie. 'I can't believe it. She's all grown up.'

'I know. And I don't know when it happened either.'

'She's lovely, Rosie.'

'Yep.'

Diana moved over to the hard blue vinyl sofa Rosie was sitting on. 'Do you want a hug, little sister?'

'Yep.'

Diana put her arm round Rosie. 'We can do this, you know. We've done it before.'

Rosie nodded but didn't say anything.

Time vanished and she was crawling into Rosie's bed that awful morning, cuddling up to her, hearing the car with her parents and Cody roaring down the drive.

The silence stretched out.

There was an innocence stamped on that memory. That was before it all happened, before Cody died. She'd so wanted to go back to that time before. Play it out again, only with a different ending. She'd tried so hard, so many times.

She looked up. Phillipa was back, juggling a cardboard tray of cups and a packet of donuts. At the same moment Rosie's phone rang.

Diana sprang up to help. 'Here, I'll take those. Thanks.

'Hi Mal. No we haven't heard anything. Yes, Diana's back. I'll ring, I promise.'

'Here you are, Rosie.' Diana handed her a cup and then fished into the bag for a donut. 'Very good thinking, Philly.' She smiled at her niece.

'I've got a phone call to make. I'll be back in a few minutes.' Philly disappeared out the door.

'What are you going to do, Di? When are you going back to the UK?' Rosie asked.

Diana slid further down her end of the sofa. 'I don't know. If we can help, I'll stay, but Mum may not want us cluttering the place up when Dad comes home.' She frowned.

'I'm sure Philly and I can manage. Charlie's parents will be pleased to see you, won't they?'

'Yes, I suppose so.' Diana looked out the window. Sebastian would be pleased to see her, anyway. He'd be rubbing his hands in glee. Of course the Suttons wanted them back. And Polly, of course. Patrick had thrown her into a tailspin. He was very kind and thoughtful. He'd said they could stay at Lost Valley, she and the kids.

It was easy to look at the obvious road to take. Put the kids first; she couldn't ignore her career and the money, either. But what did she want? Australia came with its own set of problems. Surely she and Rosie could work things out.

She'd told Rosie on the way down that death did happen to people you loved. Cody, Charlie. So if something happened, the worst happened, Mum would be okay. She'd have Rosie and Mal and Philly.

But not to see her dad again … Diana couldn't bear the thought. Even though she wished they'd handled things differently all those years ago.

'When are the kids due back at school?' Rosie asked.

'They've got another few weeks holidays. This is their big break, you know, their summer holidays. Missing a bit of school for them has been worth it. I was so worried about them, Milo in particular.'

'Oh.' Rosie picked up a magazine, idly flicking through the pages. 'You're so lucky, living in London.'

'You must come over and see us.'

'And how exactly do you think that's going to happen?'

'You're both working.' Diana really didn't understand her sister. Everything was so negative with her.

'Unfortunately we're still supporting Philly, for another year and a half. Kids don't seem to cost less as they get older,' Rosie said stiffly.

'I hate hospitals,' said Diana. 'I'm going out for a walk.' And she picked up her jacket and left.

She picked up her pace and walked down the brightly lit street behind the hospital. At least her sister belonged somewhere. Belonged to someone. Diana felt rootless and unwanted. She and her kids were like tumbleweeds stuck up against a fence for a while and then rolling on. They were probably the reason her Dad was lying there in the hospital. She kicked at a small stone and watched it bounce against the wall. She'd left England because she'd felt so alone. Alone is different from lonely. You couldn't be lonely with three kids at your heels. Alone was what she couldn't cope with. She'd needed her family. She'd needed to come home. And where had that got her? Here in a place where her sister was furious, quite rightly, her mother was acting psycho and her father had a heart attack probably because of her. Great. She pulled her coat closely around her and stepped out into the wind.

Home was different to what she'd remembered. Her parents had changed. Or had they? Maybe she was the one who had changed.

Then there was Patrick. There was no future for them. She had to go back. She wasn't that naive child this time, twenty years on. She could look after her own, and herself, for that matter. When they heard what was happening, as soon as she could manage it, they were going back to England.

Diana squared her shoulders. Feeling more in control than she had in ages, she made her way back.

Rosie wasn't in the waiting room. Diana tiptoed to the entrance of the intensive care ward. Her dad was back from theatre. Rosie, Philly and Stella were sitting beside Tom's bed. His eyes were open. Her mother smoothed a strand of hair off his forehead. There was a powerful lot of love in that simple gesture. Diana stood there, not sure she could go in. The tubes, and the awful beeping monitor attached to her father were fairly daunting. Her mother looked up and saw her. She smiled and waved her in, finger to her lips.

'Shh, just for a moment. Look who's here.' Stella turned back to Tom. 'The surgeon's just been in and the diagnosis is good. We were lucky, very lucky—three arteries were nearly completely blocked. And the amazing thing is they did it without a general anaesthetic. We can be home in a couple of days.'

'Dad, I'm so glad. That's wonderful,' Diana whispered, wiping the smart sting to her eyes with the back of her hand.

'Hi Dad, how are you feeling? Philly's here too.' Rosie leant forward.

Diana stood back.

*   *   *

Patrick had come to pick her up and they were about to head back to Lost Valley.

'Well, if you want, there's plenty of room for you at our place,' Rosie offered, standing beside Stella and Phillipa to say goodbye.

'Thank you, but I think we'll be heading back off to London, as soon as I can re-book our flights.'

'Why?' Stella asked.

'Well, you'll have your hands full with this patient.' Diana tried to make a joke of it but couldn't help the tremble of her lips.

'Oh no, Diana, don't leave.' Her mother grabbed her arm and pulled her to the door. 'Don't you dare. It will kill him if you leave us now.'

'Mum, that's not fair. He'll need peace and quiet, not three kids running around.'

Her mother sounded quite fierce. 'Please, Diana, it will make such a difference for him knowing you're around to help out.'

'Mum,' Diana started to feel slightly desperate, 'you've got Mal and Rosie and Philly.' But she was no match for that desperation in her mother's eyes. 'We'll be at Patrick's for a few days yet. We haven't re-booked our flights. He's taking me home now. The kids ... I've got to go.' She gestured vaguely.

'Just leave it for a few days then, that would be perfect.' There was no mistaking that look of satisfaction in her mother's eye. Botheration.

Diana kissed her mother on the cheek and gave her a swift, hard hug. 'Okay. Don't worry, Mum, everything's going to be all right now, isn't it? It's good news about Dad.'

Her mother closed her eyes for a moment and gave her a little nod. She was coping, but this had been a terrible twenty-four hours for her. Her eyes were too shiny. Diana wouldn't do anything to make it worse for her parents. The question was, what was for the best?

She started off down the busy corridor. Hospitals were always full of people, nurses and doctors, physios and admin scurrying along, and the visitors who were much slower moving, looking as though they would much rather be anywhere but there. Where was home? It was where her children were. Pretty simple really.

*   *   *

Stella checked the beeping machine for the hundredth time. 'Stop worrying. If you don't stop asking after things at home, I am walking out of here now. Right now.'

'Oh Stell.' Tom closed his eyes and groaned as if in pain.

Stella leant back over him. 'What's the matter? Are you feeling all right?'

Tom opened one eye and couldn't resist half a smile.

'You wretch, stop doing that to me.'

'You wouldn't walk out on me now, I knew it.' Tom chuckled. 'Sit down, Stella, and tell me you love me again and not to leave you.'

'What? You heard me?' she whispered fiercely.

'Yes, and the nurses, they told me, said how you kept on saying it. Over and over. I'm not leaving you, Stell,' he said quietly, enveloping her hand in his large one.

'Well, it was a close call. I wouldn't like to see a closer one. We're going on a holiday when you get over this and we are going to take things easy. I think it's time to go, Tom, move on somewhere. Let Mal and Rosie take over. Why don't we move into their house?'

'Not much room there for Diana and the children, if they decide to come back?' He raised one eyebrow.

'As soon as you're right, Diana's going back to England. She thinks this is all her fault.'

'Stupid girl. She really takes the cake for blaming herself for every blessed thing.'

'Tom, I told her why we decided to give the farm to Rosie.'

'Jeez, Stella, I thought we weren't going to tell her, not after all this time. We agreed to let it lie.'

'I was trying to get her to change her mind and stay. She was so angry, Tom. It may not have been the right thing, but it's done now.'

'Not much you can do about it then.'

'No, um, Rosie was there too.' Stella looked uncomfortable. 'I just didn't think, I was all fired up to get Diana to stay.'

'Rosie won't like that much.'

'So where *are* we going to go?' Stella felt so frustrated.

'We're going home, Stell. We're going home.'

She looked into his blue eyes and shook her head slowly. 'I don't know what I'm going to do with you, Tom Crawford, I really don't. Bloody farmers. You enjoy pitting yourselves against the elements, don't you? And you really believe that if it doesn't rain tomorrow it *will* rain the day after, or next week. You're so patient and strong, and so stubborn I feel like killing you, but then I realise I'd miss you far too much.

You know, I really just love you all the more for it. I can't help myself. What a fool.' Stella lifted his calloused hand to her cheek and kissed it. They sat in silence in the small cubicle until they were interrupted by the arrival of Tom's first meal on a tray.

CHAPTER FORTY-THREE

Diana left the children in the big sitting room in front of the fire, playing a board game, and walked into the spacious kitchen at Lost Valley.

'Peace and quiet reigns. I think the morning's exertions have worn them out.'

'Well, you can hope, can't you?' Marnie laughed. 'I'll give them ten minutes.'

She was making pastry. Rolling and pulling it to her, and rolling it out again. Just like Diana with clay. She hadn't even thought about clay for days now. 'Mum and Dad and Rosie have just left Albury.'

'Oh that's so good.' Marnie looked up. 'I'm just making a chicken pie for you to take over.'

'Well, I thought I'd go over now and warm the house up, find some flowers, you know.'

'This will be ready to take in about five minutes. Why don't you go and pick some of the flowers here? There must be a few early bulbs out, I saw some the other day. Then you could put this in the oven over there. It should only take about forty-five minutes.'

'Thank you so much. You've all been so kind, I don't know what I'd have done without you.'

Marnie came over and gave her a swift hug. 'It's been absolutely no trouble at all, you know that.'

'Can I leave the kids? It's just that I think Dad will be exhausted after the car trip.'

'Sure, they'll be fine.' Marnie stopped, leaning on the rolling pin and wiping her hair out of her eyes. 'Why doesn't Patrick take you? He can chop wood or something useful.'

Diana laughed. Patrick chop wood? 'No, there's no need for me to inconvenience any one. I'll be fine.'

'It'll be no trouble.'

'What will be no trouble?' Patrick and Sean had just walked in.

'For you to take Diana home, to get everything ready for Tom and Stella,' said Marnie.

'I'm fine, really. There's no need.'

'Well,' said Patrick, 'I can take you over and you can pick up Tom's ute and come and go whenever you like.'

Damn, a car would be useful. 'If you're sure it will be okay,' Diana said stiffly. 'Thank you.'

Marnie handed her some secateurs and pushed her out of the kitchen. Patrick followed her and silently watched as she cut some of the early jonquils and some white sasanquas. The bush was covered in them. The scent of the jonquils was almost overpowering.

'I'm sorry,' said Diana. 'You must think me very ungrateful when you've been so kind.'

'Relax. This has been a worrying time for you. Tom's a good friend. Don't you know I would do anything I could to make this time easier for him and Stella?'

'Is that why you ... you have this *obsession* for me?' she suddenly flung at him wildly.

'Calm down. No, it's not.' He took the secateurs from her, then the flowers, and dropped them on the ground. 'You are entirely to blame for my obsession.'

And she was crushed in his arms. She could feel the zipper of his jacket digging into her side, smell the damp wool of his sweater, the cold on his lips and face, but she was warm. Tingling and warm.

'I don't want to commit to anyone,' she ground out.

'I can wait.'

'No.'

Patrick looked at her helplessly. 'Right. We'll leave it.'

* * *

They went in the back door of the empty house at Mog's Hill. It wasn't locked. It had never been locked in her memory. Diana laid the flowers on the kitchen table and put the pie Marnie had given her on top of the oven. She turned the Aga on to warm up the house and heat the oven.

Patrick had followed her in. 'Would you like me to start the fire in the sitting room?'

'Thanks. I'm just going to change the sheets. And put these in water.' She smiled at him. She was much calmer now. It was the right decision. For once she'd elected a cautious way forward. She'd let her emotions rule her head, far too often. Now she would go slowly. Surely she'd learnt something in forty years.

She changed the sheets in her parents' room, put a little bowl of paperwhites and jonquils on the dresser and went into her bedroom to change the sheets on her bed. Five minutes later she was still there, sitting on the bed, the clean sheets clasped to her chest.

'What's wrong?' Patrick stood at the door.

'I'm losing Charlie.' Her eyes were bright with unshed tears. 'Mum bought this bed for us when we came back for our honeymoon. Five days, we were so miserable. But mostly we were very happy, in England we were happy.' She sniffed. 'But he's going, I know he is. It's so sad.'

'It's not sad. It has to happen this way. Anyway, you'll never lose Charlie. Every time you look into your children's faces you'll see him. He's with you forever.'

'That's right, isn't it? Why aren't you jealous?' she asked him curiously.

'I fell in love with all of you. You were Charlie's wife. You have three children. You're Tom and Stella's daughter. You have a freckle there.' He touched her face gently. 'I can't separate any of that from the essence that is you. I just want you to realise that I am here, Charlie is not.'

'Well, why am I having such a problem? Why do I feel so terrified, so out of my depth?'

'I'm sorry, Diana. You're not ready. Maybe one day you'll feel like talking to me about it. Until then, we can be friends. How about that?'

Friends. Did she want that? What if she said yes, what if they could be together? What if she said yes?

'Oh Patrick, I can't substitute you for Charlie just because he's dead and you're alive. I know there's chemistry between us but as you said before, the timing's all wrong. I have to go back.'

'I know. I don't have to like it, but I know.'

'The children need to go home, and I need to return to England. We need to heal, Patrick. And we've got to do it by moving forward, not ignoring it. I'm pleased, in one way, we came back. But it wasn't the solution. Maybe we're ready now to move on, I hope so.' She pushed him away, frustrated. 'I'm not me, can't you see, it's like I'm only half a person. You deserve more than that. I've got to get myself back first. Do you understand?' she asked, searching his face.

'I can wait.'

'No, Patrick. I just don't know what the new me will consist of. Just friends, you said. Please be my friend.'

She'd done it this time.

Her head was pressed against his chest and his arms held her. Lights from a car swung round into the room.

'Oh, oh, I can hear a car.'

CHAPTER FORTY-FOUR

Her father was white-faced and looked old, really old. Her mother even seemed quite shaken. They looked so pleased to be home as they sat and drank their tea. Rosie looked a little anxious to be off, understandably, as she hadn't seen Mal for three days. Patrick had left already.

First, things had to be sorted.

'What kind of help do you want, Mum, for now?'

For the first time in her life, her mother looked a little uncertain. Diana couldn't believe she hadn't worked it all out.

'I think, maybe you could give us a couple of days first, by ourselves. Can you stay with Patrick for a couple of days? Then you'll be back to stay here, won't you? Dad will need some help, just for a little while.'

Stay. No, they wouldn't be back to stay.

'I'm sure Mal will be here if you want something.' Rosie cut in.

'We'll be right at Patrick's, and I can come over to help you with showers. I don't think you need the children around just at the moment,' Diana said firmly.

'I can do all that,' Tom spoke up crossly. 'I'll be right enough in a day or two.' He was so embarrassed with all this attention. 'I think I might go and lie down for a minute.' They all went to the bedroom with him. He refused to undress, pulled his boots off and lay on the bed with an eiderdown thrown over him. 'Stop fussing.' He glowered at them all and they retreated.

'I'm glad I've got you girls together for a minute. Just a minute, Rosie, sit down please. I need to talk to you both.' Stella waved the teapot at them. They nodded and sat down.

Stella hesitated. 'The only way is to jump right in. We've decided that we're staying here at Mog's Hill, health permitting, but the doctor sounded positive. He said with a little care, eating the right food and so on, your father will be fine. All those depression symptoms are more than likely health-related. High cholesterol. Really, the heart attack has been a blessing in disguise.' She took a shaky breath, and looked first at Diana and then at Rosie. 'I know this might be a shock for you, Rosie, but that's the way it's going to be. One thing I realised, sitting beside that hospital bed, was that your father loves this place so much. He loves his sheep, and this is what he wants to do with the rest of his life. So that's it. For the meantime, we're staying here.' She filled her own mug but Diana noticed her hand was trembling slightly. 'So we can offer you a home, Diana, for you and the children. Don't go back to England, please.'

Diana was rooted in shock. Rosie exploded.

'Well, I guess we've got our answer. Thank you very much for nothing. Twenty years of promises. I can't believe you can sit there and just calmly tell us that you're staying on here. That you're ruining my life—mine and Mal's and Phillipa's—just so Diana has a home! I don't believe it!' She shook her head violently at the proffered mug of tea.

Diana took her mug and went to her favourite place, leaning against the Aga stove. How could her mother have said such things? Rosie had every right to be furious. She'd probably never talk to her again.

'You don't understand, Rosie, this is about your father and me, what he and I need. We're just not ready to leave here. These last few days have defined what's important for us. He still wants to breed his sheep, and get up in the morning and stand on the back verandah with his mug of tea and decide what needs doing for the day. He wants the worry of whether it's going to rain. Life is a series of challenges for a farmer and he, we want to face them.' She shrugged. 'We aren't leaving.' She glanced briefly at Diana. 'I'm sorry if you have to put the Diana interpretation on it. She needs a home at the moment, and she has one here as long as she needs it.'

Stella turned to Rosie and looked at her steadily. 'You still get the farm, darling, when we die or when we have to move. Diana, you will eventually have Peg's house to do with what you want. I'm sorry there's not much of a fair share, but we did promise Rosie and Mal.' She grimaced. 'And to give you an equal share means Mog's Hill would have to be sold. And that would break your father's heart.'

'Mum, it was never about the money,' said Diana. 'I just always saw myself as the farmer in the family, and coming home to help Dad, it was all I ever wanted to do.'

'But you had so much talent. They all told us that and we wanted to give you a chance and we felt something drastic had to be done.'

'Damn it all, why didn't you tell me that?'

'We just didn't realise *how* hard you were going to take it. I only hope now you're a parent you can understand a little better. It's so hard to make decisions—the right thing for you, Rosie, and the right thing for Diana. But now this is the only right thing for us.' Stella looked pleadingly from Rosie to Diana. She put out her arm but Rosie shook it off and walked away.

'So, this has been about Diana all along. I should have guessed. Well, now she's back, you obviously don't need me here anymore.' Rosie had turned for the door.

'Hang on a minute.' Diana found her voice and reached out to stop her sister from leaving. 'You're not going any-where. I've had this situation up to here. Twenty years ago you and Dad decided, arbitrarily, that I was to have a career,' Diana accused her mother. 'Not that you seemed to care how I achieved it. I put my head down and did it anyway. Five months ago my husband died in an accident. It was okay none of you came over to the funeral—I understood that. All I asked for was a little time to have some support— dare I ask, loving support—for just a few weeks. To come home to my family, for just a few weeks, in twenty years. Jesus! And what happens? You're all embroiled in this family succession war that I never had a part in. Never. It's nothing to do with me. Do you understand, Rosie? Nothing!'

'How dare you say nothing,' Rosie said. 'Seventy, was the plan. Dad was going to retire at seventy. But you come home and now it's never, not until Dad dies. Try thinking what this has done to my husband. Mog's Hill has been like a millstone around his neck. We could have done so many things, and now it's too late.'

Rosie glared at both of them and then stormed out of the kitchen, the door slamming shut behind her. Diana and her mother looked at each other aghast.

'Diana, we really thought we were doing the right thing.' Her mother looked stricken. 'But you were so unforgiving. You pushed us away.'

'Mum, I got my strength from having to show you all I could do it. I'm not sure I'd have made it otherwise. In hindsight we can be very wise. Who knows what would have happened if you had told me the truth? The fact is you didn't tell me for twenty years. It makes me so mad. Patrick makes me mad, putting all this pressure on me to make decisions about him. I don't want to make decisions. I'm not ready to decide anything. I just wish Rosie would ... grow up some more.' Diana sat sprawled at the table and put her head in her hands and groaned.

'Mum, that was not the most politic thing you could have said.'

'I know. I just had to say it. She'll calm down, she's not as unforgiving as you.'

'I think Rosie just may have her work cut out forgiving the both of you. What is it about being a parent that gives you the right to make these life and death decisions for your child?'

Stella reached out her hand to cover Diana's. 'We wanted to do what's best for everyone, but that may not make everyone happy. I'm sorry, Diana.'

'I'm sorry too. Looking back, it was all mixed up with Cody's death somehow. I felt so guilty, and then I felt, or deduced, that you blamed me and were punishing me for not doing the right thing that night. So with a judge and jury of one, it was easy to convict myself. It was only natural I had to take the sentence—banishment.'

'No, oh no. That was never your fault, Diana. I'm so sorry.'

They sat for a moment in the warm kitchen. The memories were thick and swirling around them. Finally Diana whispered, 'If I'd only gone in and checked her.'

'No, I went out that night and I knew she was hot.' Her mother stopped. 'We're doing it again, aren't we?'

They both laughed, a laugh and a sob at the same time. 'Cody was such a beautiful child,' Stella said.

Her mother sat back in her chair, her eyes closed, but Diana could see two tears squeezing through the lids. Hers were burning. She got up and went round to her mother's side and put her arms round her.

'I love you and Dad so much. We'll work it out.'

And much to her astonishment, her mother burst into tears. She put her arms around her and held her. She felt small and fragile and old. Her mother in tears. Never. Well, never before anyway.

'Why don't you go and lie down in my room for half an hour? I'll put the pie that Marnie gave us in the warming oven, and it can just wait for you both to get up when you want and have something to eat. Do you want me to stay tonight?'

Her mother sniffed and shook her head, and looked so like Saskia for a minute, Diana almost smiled. She reached for a tissue.

'It's been a big few days. I think I might go and rest for a minute. No, you go, and thank you, Diana.'

Her mother squeezed her shoulder briefly and walked stiffly out of the kitchen, head up, shoulders straight.

* * *

Patrick was waiting for her at Lost Valley, outside on the verandah. She was barely out of the car before he'd crushed her in his arms.

'I thought if you hadn't come soon, I was going to come and get you.'

'I told you not to wait, and I meant it. Patrick, you're smothering me. You have to give me some space.' She remembered the last half hour's confrontation in her parents' kitchen and tried to struggle out of his arms. 'Leave me alone.' The last thing she needed was this.

'I just want to help.'

'You're going to have to give me some room. I don't need to be rescued every minute of the day.'

'I just want to be in the vicinity when you do need it then.' Patrick growled into her neck. 'Mates do that kind of thing. I'll be right there, beside you, any time you want me.'

'Oh Patrick, stop it.'

A small bundle of very aggressive boy came hurtling out of the darkness. Milo.

'Leave my mother alone. Leave her alone! Didn't you hear her?' He was pummelling Patrick with his arms.

'Hey, Milo, wait.' Patrick tried to catch him but thought better of it and moved away from Diana to the front of the car.

Milo stood protectively in front of his mother, tears not far away, his hands still fisted. 'We don't want you. I told you. We don't want you.' And he turned and buried his head in his mother's stomach.

Aghast, Diana raised her eyes to Patrick, beseeching him to go. She watched him reluctantly turn and go back to the house.

'Here, get in the car.' She pulled Milo in on top of her. He was all arms and legs. It had been ages since she'd had him on her lap. He'd grown. She eased the seat back as far as it would go.

'Milo, you're enormous.' They sat silently for a minute in the dark. She smoothed his dark hair and wiped the tears with her fingers before fumbling for the pack of tissues in the central glove box beside her.

'We need to talk, Milo. Why did you hit Patrick?'

His arms tightened around her neck. 'You said it was just us, just the four of us. We don't need him.'

'Patrick's been very good to us. He came all the way down to Albury to get me and bring me home. It wasn't very polite to hit him.'

'You said stop. I thought he was hurting you.'

'We, um, he wasn't hurting me. Patrick wouldn't hurt me.' She paused. 'Don't you like him?'

'No.'

Wonderful. 'Any reason?'

'He watches us all the time.'

'I guess he doesn't know much about kids. Sam and Alex like him, don't they?'

There was a grunt. That could be a yes or a no, but probably was 'I'm not agreeing with you even if they do'.

'Can we go home now?'

'Not really. Tommo has just got home and needs some peace and quiet for a few days. Then we can go back.'

'I mean London. I don't want to stay here.'

'I know, I mean London too. Just a few days to help Stella and Tommo, okay?'

'Then we can go back?'

'Yes.' She took a deep breath.

Milo was silent. She could hear his breathing. She could see it in the frosty air.

'Milo, you must apologise to Patrick. Say you're sorry you hit him.'

'I'm not sorry.'

'We are guests in his house. You can't go round hitting your host.'

'He was pushing you against the car and you told him to stop.'

Lord, he was a stubborn child. 'I was only kidding, having fun.' But she couldn't make herself go further with an explanation than that. 'I want you to go inside now and say you're sorry. All right?'

'I'll tell him I'm sorry, but that he must not push you around or I'll hit him again.'

Milo disentangled himself. Diana didn't know whether she should laugh or cry. Her wonderful son was going to look after her, by hook or by crook, and so was Patrick. She was totally overwhelmed by all this protection. She'd been so independent all her life.

I totally agree, you are very difficult woman to protect. I learnt that pretty early in the piece.

I am not a difficult woman.

But she couldn't think of anything that would verify that statement.

Together they walked into the house. Patrick was sitting on a stool in the kitchen. Everyone else, thankfully, had disappeared. It was all very quiet.

'Have you had dinner, Diana?'

'No, I'm fine, thank you.' She gave Milo a little shove.

'I'm sorry, Patrick.' His eyes were focused on the ground, and Diana turned him around and went to walk with him back to the bedroom before he could make good the rest of his threat.

'Milo, wait.' Patrick stopped them. 'I'm sorry, too. It must have looked as if I was hurting your mother. You need to know I would never do that.'

This time Milo raised his eyes and looked directly at Patrick. 'I know because I won't let you.'

Diana gave a little sigh of frustration and took her son to bed.

CHAPTER FORTY-FIVE

Diana and Milo parked the quad bike back in the machinery shed. She put both their helmets on the bench, and they walked back to the house.

'Lunch will be good, I'm hungry. I think you're getting quite good on that bike, Milo.'

'It's good fun. When are we going back, Mummy?'

She wished he'd stop asking her that. The last week had been busy and full but it hadn't shifted him. Patrick had spent the week in Sydney, their only communication had been on the telephone.

'As soon as Tommo's on his feet,' Diana said. 'He has to take things quietly for a while. Anyway, it's only July. What's so important to get back to?'

'I want to see my other grandparents. And my team is playing cricket now. They haven't got a wicket keeper.'

When they walked into the kitchen everything was in chaos.

'Where have you been?' Stella looked up briefly from the telephone, mid conversation. 'No, she's back. There was nothing you could have done, darling. We'll be there shortly.'

Diana felt the world spin out of control. 'What's happened? What's wrong?'

Stella closed her eyes for a moment. 'Bad news, I'm afraid. Peg passed away. Rosie just found her on the floor. She must have had a stroke, or it may have been her heart. At least it must have been quick. I hope so.'

'Where's Dad?'

'He's getting changed. We'll go in, now you're back. I'm thinking you don't want the children involved in all of this.'

'God no.'

It was happening all over again. Another death. Panic. *Breathe.*

'Granny was ninety,' she whispered to herself. 'It was what she would have wanted. This is okay.' Fat, salty tears started to run down her cheeks.

'Oh Diana, you mustn't be sad. Peg had a great life and she was hating this, this decline, for want of a better word.' Stella wrapped her arms around her. 'Don't be sad for Peg.'

'I'm not. I'm sad for me.'

Sienna, her face worried, came in and rushed to her mother and clambered on to her knee. 'It's all right, Mummy. Look, Saskia and I have made a book for you—to draw pictures of Granny, and you can write down some of the funny things she said. And look, I've already put her name on it for you—Peg Crawford.'

Diana looked down. Sienna had folded three pages of white A4 paper together and tied them in the middle with one of her ribbons.

'Thank you, thank you so much.' She looked at her mother, who now had two fat tears running down her cheeks. 'Oh dear.' She hugged her child to her. Then she reached for her mother.

* * *

'You're the only one, Diana,' her mother had urged. 'Peg would so love you to do it.'

Her grandmother had been dead only a day and they were discussing the funeral and choosing the hymns—arguing was probably a better description.

'Well, not that anyone thinks anything I've got to say is important,' said Rosie, 'but Granny always loved "Abide with Me".'

'Of course she did, Rosie. And Psalm 23, too.' Stella wrote it all down.

'I didn't do Charlie's eulogy,' said Diana. 'Bill Sutton did it beautifully. I think you should do it, Dad.'

They were sitting round the kitchen table—her father, her mother, Rosie and Mal—having a cup of tea. The children were finally in bed.

Her father waved away the teapot. 'No thanks, Stell.' He shook his head slowly. Everything he did was a bit slower these days. 'I can't, Diana. I barely saw Mum these last few months. It really upset me to see the way she was going and I let it all fall into your hands—Stella and Rosie, and now, since you came back, you, Diana. I'm not one for public speaking. Diana was always special to Peg. We would appreciate you doing it.'

Rosie picked up the cups to put them in the sink. 'Well, we're not really needed at the moment. Come on, Mal. Phillipa will be back tomorrow. Just let us know what you've decided.'

'Rosie, don't be silly, sit. There are two readings, and we wondered if you and Philly could do them?' Stella put her pen down.

'Why don't you ask Milo, I'm sure he'd be up for it.' Rosie couldn't help herself.

'I'm sure he would—if we asked him, but your father and I would love the two of you to do them. I'll copy the verses out for you. I've spoken to the Reverend Keith, and the Church Guild is doing a morning tea and sandwiches for afterwards in the church hall.'

'I hope there'll be plenty. Granny will not be happy if there is not an overabundance of food.' Diana grinned. 'We might all get struck by lightning.'

'It had better bring some rain with it,' Tom grumbled.

*   *   *

Diana decided to approach her father when he was out of the house. He, of all of them, had to know Peg best, by the sheer number of years. She found him in the machinery shed with a hammer and a cloth and a bottle of WD40, on his back, cleaning the boom spray.

'Now I've got you where I want you. I can't believe I know so little about my grandmother. This is terrible. Why didn't I ask her all these things before?'

'What do you want to know?' Tom slid out from under the boom spray and handed her the hammer.

'Where was she born, to start with?'

'Gunnedah.'

'Right.' Diana scribbled on her piece of paper. 'When?'

'Ask your mother, she knows dates better than me.'

'What do you remember?'

'She loved the horses, riding. Always keen to go out mustering with my father, nothing fazed her, very practical person my mother. On the other hand, everyone rode a horse in those days.'

'Where did she get her education? She was always reading something. And had an opinion about it.'

'Gunnedah, I guess. She certainly didn't back away from an argument. She could argue the hind leg off a donkey.' Tom grunted and put his hand out for the hammer again. 'I dunno where she went to school, or even if she went. I do know she ran Mog's Hill single-handed when Dad was away at the war.'

'Did she? I didn't know that. I remember the cooking—she cooked for my school fetes, and for church stalls and the local bushfire brigade. She was always cooking.'

'Go and talk to your mother. She had a funny relationship with Mum but they ended up friends, I think.' He disappeared under the boom spray again.

Diana stood and looked at his legs in the old blue overalls for a minute. 'Peg encouraged me to keep making pots, you know.'

'Mmm, she thought a lot of you, Diana. I think the two of you were pretty alike.'

'Really?'

Diana walked back down to the house and found her mother watering the abelia bushes with Milo's pitcher.

'What do you think I should be saying in this eulogy, Mum? How did you get on with Peg?'

Stella laughed. 'I don't think Peg thought all that much of me when we first met. I'm not sure who exactly would have been good enough for your father in her eyes. It took me a while before I worked that out. We got on a lot better after that. I think what I'll remember about her is that she never complained. No matter if there were bushfires or droughts or floods, she used to say "What do I have to complain about, there's plenty worse off than me." Amazing generation of women, that lot were. We Australians have a lot to thank them for, really.'

'Thanks, Mum. I think I've got what I need.'

CHAPTER FORTY-SIX

The church was warm: the familiar white-washed walls, sun streaming in the stained-glass windows and wooden pews filled to the brim with strange faces. Some she recognised. Her dad gave her a wink. Rosie was holding Mal's hand on one side of her and Philly's on the other. The kids were unusually restrained and in their good London clothes. The sea of faces before her floated en masse like a cloud of pink balloons. She was usually one of them sitting down there; she wasn't used to looking down over the congregation. She'd sneaked one look at the coffin. It was so tiny. Why, oh why had she ever agreed to this?

She was going to have to start. Her sheets of paper rattled. That was her hands trembling. She grasped the lectern more firmly. At a nod from the rector she took a breath.

Before she knew it she was nearly at the end. Just two more paragraphs to go.

Her eyes caught sight of Patrick, sitting towards the back. He'd been wonderful these last few days, everything you could wish for in a friend.

'The way she embraced life leaves behind an enormous legacy to us all. Don't waste anything. Not time, money, water or food. I think the most valued of Granny's possessions was the chest freezer where she was able to store huge quantities of food.'

Another sprinkle of laughter.

'Waste is the greatest sin, and living life to the full, the greatest virtue. That's what she always said. Not a bad motto.'

Diana looked at Stella, and her dad. And saw the love. That had been there all this time.

She gathered her papers together and made her way down the steps to join her mother and her father, squashing the kids into the pew to make room for her. They knelt to pray. It was time to wake up to herself. Her grandmother was perfectly right—time was wasting away and she had things to do and a life to get on with. The children needed to go back to Gospel Oak. There was healing to be done and it could only be done there.

She had to regain control of her life and her children's lives.

Well, Granny, time is a-wasting.

* * *

Diana sipped her tea out of the white china cup and looked round the church hall. *They've done you proud, Granny.* The church hall was full. Seventy years her grandmother had been part of this town. The children were clustered around her again. At each introduction, Saskia mostly buried into her groin.

'Well done, Diana. We'll miss Peg.' She turned. Sid and Una Herschel were smiling sympathetically. They were a lovely couple.

'Thank you. When are you coming over to visit me?'

'In August. We have your number. Una can't wait to get to the markets in Portobello Road.'

'Your family will be sad to see you going.' Una nodded in her parents' direction.

'I'm depending on you two to talk them into visiting. Dad's so much better now. I think they'll come.'

'Wild horses won't keep them from coming, I'd be guessing.' Rosie had joined the group. 'Got to go see their wonderful eldest daughter. Good work, Diana. Granny would be pleased.'

'That was a lovely reading, Rosie.' Una reached over and squeezed her hand before they both moved away.

'Ah yes. I'm used to taking second place.' Rosie's eyes followed them, 'Maybe after you've gone, Diana, everything will get back to normal. Not that I'm aware what normal is at the moment. My husband won't talk to me, my parents have decided to stay on the farm and no one gives a damn what we're going to do with our lives. I will be quite thankful actually when you've gone back to England. Any more chaos around here could be quite difficult to contend with.'

'Rosie, I'm really sick of being blamed for our parents' decision.'

'If you hadn't come out here with the grandson in tow.'

'Don't you dare, Milo has nothing to do with this. *We* have nothing to do with this. It's our father's decision, which he has every right to make.'

'Everyone seems to have rights except us. Damn you, Diana, I am so sick of this. Here I am, year after year, looking after Granny, but who gets to do the eulogy? Diana, of course.'

'You were perfectly able to get up and say something if you wanted to. Rosie, this is not the time or place to be having this discussion.'

Diana suddenly realised her children, wide-eyed, were listening to every word. They hadn't really seen her and Rosie go head to head before. Suddenly her mother was whisking the children away and asking Diana and Rosie to help take the empty cups into the kitchen.

Diana followed Rosie into the kitchen.

'I've had it, up to the neck,' she said. 'How dare you talk like that in front of the children. In front of the whole town. You can blame me all you like, you can take it out on me, but for pity's sake, don't do it in public.'

'You don't understand.'

'Oh yes I do, welcome to the world of the eldest, Rosie. Things are expected of eldest children. Now it's time you grew up. Stop crying over what you think you're missing out on and thank the heavens for what you do have. But I am not going to take the flack any more. I have finished taking the blame for everything that goes wrong. We're booking our flight back as soon as I can do it.'

Diana turned and walked out of the kitchen.

CHAPTER FORTY-SEVEN

Gospel Oak , London, July

Twenty-eight hours after leaving Sydney, Diana's hand shook slightly as she inserted the key into the front door of 22 Torrington Row. She shepherded the kids and bags inside. They were all exhausted. It was nine o'clock in the morning and it promised to be a hot day. China-blue skies, 23 degrees. Inside it was cool. Janet and Bill had promised to air the house occasionally, so it wasn't too stuffy. Bill had obviously been working in the garden. It looked beautiful, a riot of colour—pink roses and purple asters, the pastel hollyhocks towering at the back and the red geraniums in pots. She hadn't told them yet they were coming back. One step at a time.

They all just stood there in the gloomy hall.

'It feels different to what I thought.' Milo stood uncertainly with his bag at his feet. The two girls clutched their little koalas Stella had given them at the airport.

'We're all tired. It will be better tomorrow. Let's open some windows.'

They trooped into the sitting room with the jungle mural on the wall. Milo went straight for the remote. Sienna went to the telephone to ring Polly, Saskia was back to clinging to her hand or whatever part of her was free at the time.

'Hey, bags first. We won't unpack yet, just put them in your rooms.'

Diana struggled with the window sash, it was always sticky. She hefted it up. She and Saskia wandered into the other rooms, opening windows and pulling up blinds, Saskia holding a corner of her jacket.

Milo was right. It didn't feel the same.

'Can Polly come over?' Sienna had the phone in her hand.

'How about tomorrow? We all need a little down time.'

'Okay.' Sienna disappeared again.

Milo had picked up her bag and was struggling towards the stairs with it. Diana rushed to catch him. 'No, no I can manage, thank you, just get yours.' She ruffled his hair. She went on up to her bedroom, put the suitcase down at her feet and looked around. Charlie's slippers were tumbled on the floor, his dressing gown still on the hook behind the door.

Well, what had she achieved by her headlong rush across the world?

Things were better now between her mother and herself. But Rosie?

No. Rosie hadn't come to say goodbye.

Patrick? No, she couldn't think about Patrick.

She turned. Saskia stood at the door, still clutching the little grey and white koala.

'Mummy?' Her honey eyes were brimming with tears.

'Hello,' she said softly and picked up the round, warm body and held her, as her arms tightened around her neck and her head rested on her shoulder.

She was so lucky to have three such beautiful children.

You fool, Charlie, to be missing out on this, holding your kids, watching them grow.

But he wasn't answering her today. She blew some curls away from her mouth. 'Everything's going to be okay, little one. Just you see.'

'I want Daddy,' Saskia whispered.

'I know, darling, but Daddy's not here anymore, not in a way we can touch him. But I have an idea. Let's get your book out that Megan gave you and do another Daddy story.' She put her down and they descended the stairs slowly, hand in hand.

'Let's look for some pictures of Daddy. How about that time we went to the castle and he pretended he was a ghost? Remember, and he chased you all round and round and knocked over that suit of armour and it made such a noise!'

Saskia stopped on the step and looked up at her. 'You said that wasn't funny, didn't you, Mummy. And the lady came and got cross at Daddy.'

'Yes, that's the time.' But she couldn't help laughing at Charlie as he picked up the pieces of armour and tried to stick them back together, the children open-mouthed with horror and the very cross-faced guide. 'And isn't there a picture of Daddy trying to be a snowman?'

That had been funny. The kids had come rushing in one snowy day saying to come and look at their snowman. They'd packed snow around him; put a carrot in his mouth and a cap on his head. Why he hadn't frozen to death ... Diana swallowed. Then just two months later he was dead. He shouldn't be dead. And maybe he wouldn't be if she hadn't said for him to leave. Here she was, standing at the foot of the stairs, just where she'd told him to grow up.

Get out ... Get out ... Get out! she'd shouted at him.

That's what she had to live with for the rest of her life. She couldn't forgive him for leaving her, let alone ever forgive herself.

*   *   *

Diana's eyes flew open. Slowly she registered the familiar chairs in Gospel Oak. The weird jungle mural on the wall. She must have fallen asleep. What was the time?

Stretching out her arms and yawning, she suddenly remembered another fight. There'd been heaps of them.

The little pair of black undies definitely weren't hers.

Or Sienna's.

She'd pulled them out from where they'd been stuffed down the back of the sofa cushions. Whose were they? When had they been dropped behind the cushions? She frowned. Who'd been babysitting lately? Ah, Toni, a girl from one of the neighbouring houses down the street. Maybe she'd had a friend over? That was only a couple of weeks ago.

'Look at this?' She waved them in front of Charlie's face. Which turned an interesting brick red in front of her eyes. 'Look what I found.'

'What, where did you find them?'

'Down the back of the sofa. Pretty, aren't they? I think they're Toni's.'

She'd been so naive.

*   *   *

The kids were long asleep. Putting off her bedtime any longer was ridiculous. Diana made her way slowly up to their bedroom. Her bedroom. One look at the bed had her turning around and continuing upstairs. She'd never asked Toni if they were hers.

You're not going to do this to me, Charlie, not any more.

Funnily enough he didn't answer.

She sat at her wheel. For the first time she felt free of the depression. She got up and took out some clay she'd left in the fridge and removed the plastic. Slopped some water on it. Banged it down on her table. Banged it some more. More water, more banging. This felt good. It started to soften under her hands. With the rhythm and the familiar motion, the clay started to shift and mould under her fingers. More water.

Do you see Charlie? I can and I will.

Thumped and shaped, faster and faster. One hand behind her she switched on the wheel.

And in an instant the clay was fixed and the wheel spinning and the water flying.

She took a deep breath.

She could do this.

*   *   *

It was two weeks later that Diana attacked Charlie's belongings.

'There that's done.' Hands on her hips, she stood in her bedroom, balancing a pair of old sheepskin slippers on top of the box she was giving away to the Salvos. A couple of things she'd kept—his Arsenal jumper, and the soft blue cambric shirt she'd bought him ages ago that she'd always loved him wearing. She'd use that for work.

There, that wasn't so bad. The first thing on her list of things to do when she got back was done. The second may be a little harder.

Diana registered the knocking at the door. She really wasn't in the mood for visitors. Let them knock away.

Milo was second on the list. She had to smile as she remembered how he'd taken over at the airport and struggled to pull their entire luggage off the carousel. She would have to be careful she didn't lump too much responsibility on him. He was nearly eleven, but he was still a child.

Now there were only Charlie's art things. She looked despondently up the stairs. The knocking had started again and she stood in two minds about whether to go up to the studio or down to the door and give whoever it was a piece of her mind.

She didn't want to talk to anyone today. She wanted to get this done and have it all away before the kids came back at three-thirty.

The knocking was getting louder. Whoever it was wasn't going away.

Diana ran down the stairs and threw open the door, ready to tell the rude person to get lost, and stared blankly at the man on her doorstep.

'Johann!' She squealed and threw herself into his arms.

'Hey, steady on.' Johann, laughing, gave her a huge bear hug.

'I don't believe it. I haven't seen you for twenty years. How did you know where I live?

'Megan told me.' He stood there grinning back at her.

She pulled him in the door. She was so pleased to see him, and stepped back to look him over. Just the same Johann—black hair, silvered now, still long and pulled back in a ponytail; twinkling blue eyes with long lashes that she and Megan had always said were totally wasted on a man; his face tanned and healthy.

'This is wonderful. Was that you knocking before?'

'Mmm. Your phone's not working. I had to ring Megan to make sure I had the right place and she said to keep knocking.'

'Oh I'm sorry, the battery's flat. What are you doing in London?'

'Taking you out to lunch. Get your coat.'

Diana suddenly remembered she was in her working clothes.

'I can't go out like this. Give me a minute. Just sit there, I'll be back in a sec.' She raced to her bedroom to find something half decent to wear. Anything clean ... not much evidence of that, she thought, looking round the trail of her clothes that littered the floor, chair and bed. One thing she hadn't had to think of lately was clothes. Any old thing did for potting and gardening, and let's face it, she hadn't been doing much of anything else in the two weeks since they'd come back from Australia. Work, feeding the kids and getting them to holiday care, followed by more work—that had been about the sum of it. She spied her jeans at the bottom of the pile and grabbed a black T-shirt and a rather snazzy wide belt. She found a loose muslin top to go over it all and some red beads. This was so amazing, to be seeing Johann again, she could hardly believe it.

'You were quick,' said Johann. 'A definite improvement, I must say.'

He was seriously looking her up and down. Diana had to smile.

'You've lost weight, the beads are a good colour.'

She and Megs had learnt to value Johann's compliments. He always knew what looked good.

He proffered his arm. 'Where's the nearest pub?'

They walked out the door and Johann opened the gate for Diana. At her nod they turned right. 'I spoke to Megs last week. She said you and the kids had been to see her and that you were back here.'

'Megan is a good friend. I need to keep up with her, with you both. Let's not let go again.'

'That's exactly what we were saying.'

They were outside the pub. Johann smiled and held the door open for her. 'Sit, and I'll get you a beer.'

Diana found a table, and smiled at the burly owner, with the long white curls, following Johann with menus in his hand.

'I recommend the Ploughman's lunch, best in London,' said Diana. 'Bart, this is a friend of mine from Australia, Johann.'

'What's this, eh, best in London? You'd have to go a fair way before you get a Ploughman's to top it anywhere.'

'You're right. What am I thinking? How are you going, Bart?'

'All the better for seeing you, me darlin'. I haven't seen you for a while. Heard you'd gone back to Australia.'

'We got back last month.'

Diana watched his retreating back and turned to Johann. 'I feel so awful I never tried to contact you. I mean, I didn't hear about Paul for some time after he died. I wrote, but I couldn't find out where to send it. I'm so sorry. We all loved him so much.'

'Don't worry about it. I pretty much went into my shell. I travelled a lot before I looked up Megs again. When I heard about Charlie I wanted to see you. I emailed you and found out you were back in Australia. Sorry's a terrible word. Let's wipe it out. Why did you come back, Diana?'

She looked down at her pint of bitter, put her finger in the slight head on the top, swirled it around and tasted it. 'You've been talking to Megan.'

Johann waited patiently, looking at her through those long sooty lashes.

Diana gave a shaky sigh. 'Work. Sebastian was going crazy, I've got an exhibition in September. The kids wanted to come back. I'm not all that clear on it now. It seemed to be the right thing to do at the time. To find myself or to lose myself, it's all a bit the same.'

'That's a negative approach. Back to the bottom line, Diana, why did you come back?'

She took a drink, fiddled with the coaster. 'I don't know. I was confused. Things at home were messy. Going back home is never what you think it's going to be, is it? I met this guy, Patrick, who was pushing me a little too hard. I don't know.' She rubbed her temples with both hands.

Johann reached over and pulled her hands away. 'It's never easy thinking you can start again, but you should. At least give it a go.'

'You don't know the half of it, Johann. You were with Paul all the time, all those years. You got to say goodbye, and I love you.'

'Yeah, we got to say it a lot. But at the end it was the same—you were never going to get to say it again.'

They were both quiet for a minute and Johann reached out and took Diana's hand in both of his. 'The worst part was feeling so guilty just for being alive.'

Diana remembered that night.

Charlie hadn't come back for dinner so she was putting it in the oven when she heard voices outside at the door—loud voices, singing and laughter. They weren't only going to wake the kids, they'd be rousing the whole neighbourhood.

She walked quickly to the door and threw it open.

'Ah, Diana, my beautiful wife.' Charlie stood there, his arm draped around a young girl, waving his key at her. Six other people lounged against the wall or sat on the steps with wide smiles on their faces, clutching bottles and packets of chips.

'Come in. Come in.' He ushered them in waving expansively. 'Tell Diana your names. I've just met these wonderful fellas down at the pub. And this gorgeous girl is Poppy. Meet my wife Diana.'

She stood in the hall as the others trooped past. Poppy—who couldn't be twenty—disengaged herself from Charlie and stood looking embarrassed, like she didn't know what to do now. She was obviously very surprised to find a wife at home.

Charlie had brought strange people home before, many, many times, but not a young girl who looked positively horrified to meet her. What had she been expecting?

'Sorry,' the girl said.

'Sorry for what?' Diana was trying not to feel sick.

'I didn't know, that is, Charlie didn't tell me.'

'What, that he's married? Has three kids?'

'No.'

'Well, the others are in there.' Diana pointed to the sitting room.

'I think I have to go, could you tell Charlie.' She turned for the door and quickly disappeared.

'Where's Poppy?' Charlie ambled back into the hallway.

'She's gone. What was that all about?'

'Damn you, Diana, I promised to show her my paintings.' He grinned and tapped his nose. 'You know.' He wriggled his eyebrows and laughed. He was drunk.

'I don't understand.'

'No, you don't. Party pooper, that's what you are.'

'I think you'd better tell your friends to go home.'

'No, you go and get Poppy to come back.'

Suddenly Diana had had enough. She walked to the doorway and flung it open. 'Sorry everyone. There's no party here tonight.'

Six pairs of eyes stared at her with alarm. They trooped past her, mumbling apologies.

Charlie was furious. 'How dare you, those people were my friends.'

'I've had enough, Charlie, don't you dare do this again. I don't know what you were going to do with Poppy but you're not going to do it in our house.'

'You wouldn't care, you wouldn't give a damn who or what I brung,' he coughed, 'brought home.'

'I am so sick of this, Charlie. Sick of your Peter Pan ways. Grow up. And I think you'd better get out. Go and find Poppy for all I care. Just get out. Get out.'

The car keys were sitting on the hall table. Charlie swept them up and walked out the door.

*   *   *

The guilt swept over her now. Made her feel sick.

'He grabbed those keys and walked out the door and killed himself.' She took a breath. 'No, it was wet and he was drunk and he just skidded off the road into a tree. Oh Christ, I can't bear it.' The sob stuck in her throat. Through her tears Diana registered a plate full of salad and cheese slices and pickled onions sliding on to the table in front of her. 'I can't eat this, Bart, I'm sorry.'

She picked up her bag and raced outside before the huge racking sob erupted. Johann caught up to her on the street and wrapped her in another of his bear hugs.

Diana howled into his chest. 'It's entirely my fault. Can't you see? I killed him.'

'This is a mighty public confession you're making. Do you want to get us arrested?'

'Jesus, Johann, I deserve to go jail. I should be garrotted, tortured, hanged.'

'You exaggerate, surely. Anyway, they don't hang people any more. I'm not so sure about the garrotting.'

'Then I remember the kids. They need me. I can't say anything. I don't get to be punished.'

'No worse than you hating and punishing yourself, I'd be thinking.'

They came to a little park at the end of the street and Johann led her to a wooden bench where they sat down.

'Charlie was an idiot, he shouldn't have got into that car. It was an accident. Right, now listen to me. How do you think Paul caught AIDS?'

Diana looked at him in amazement. 'Not through you?'

'No, Diana,' Johann said. 'Do you think I'd still be here? I took him to a party one night, they were my friends. He felt I was neglecting him, we had a fight and he went off with one of them. And for the next three long years, I had to watch the love of my life die before my eyes. Every day thinking if only we hadn't gone, we hadn't fought, he hadn't ...' He shook his head. 'Well, you see, it's not much different, is it?'

'You seriously can't blame yourself for him getting AIDS.'

'Well, it's not much different to what you're suggesting, is it?'

'How do you cope?'

Johann shrugged. 'The first year after Paul died, not very well. Then you realise you're alive and Paul's dead. Then you ask yourself, would he want you to be miserable all the time? And you realise, no, he would not. He'd want you to be happy again, be all the things he loved about you, and he'd want you to love someone else.'

'I just wish I hadn't said those things,' Diana said miserably.

'And don't you think Charlie is wishing he hadn't drunk that bottle of red and walked out the door that night? He has to take responsibility for the things he did.'

'I just never got to say I didn't mean it.'

'Go on, then, say it now. Yell it out so he can hear you.'

Diana looked around her. The park looked nearly empty. There was a young woman with a huge pram over in the distance ... but so what if she did hear?

Diana stood facing the fast, rolling clouds as they gal-
loped past. He had to be up there. She shouted into the
summer sky, 'I'm sorry, Charlie, I didn't mean it. I didn't
mean any of it.' She took the handkerchief Johann offered
and blew her nose. 'I'm truly sorry,' she said, louder this
time.

Charlie didn't say anything. No thunder or lightening,
not even a gust of wind.

No voices in her head. She looked around, not even a
feather floating.

Johann smiled at her and she looked doubtfully at him.

'That's it?'

'Nope.' He slung an arm around her neck. 'It's just the
beginning. Better?'

She nodded.

'Good! Feel like eating the best Ploughman's in the
universe?'

She nodded again, managing a wobbly smile this time.
Strangely she did feel a tiny bit better. They got up and
walked back into the pub.

CHAPTER FORTY-EIGHT

Stella closed up her iPad with a sigh.

'Finished?' Tom didn't look up from his newspaper, spread out on the kitchen table.

'Yes. You didn't want to use it, did you?'

'No, I'll get on to that English chap tomorrow. Did the pictures go through?'

'Yes, Diana texted me back—perfect, she said. This is all so strange. "Australian sunsets, glorious colours" is what she wanted for her catalogues. So I take them with the iPad and send them straight across the world. It's completely bizarre. It's taken me an hour.'

Car lights striped across the windows.

'Who's this?' Stella went to the back door. 'It's Rosie.' She took a second look 'And Mal. They didn't say they were coming over, did they? I'll put the kettle on, or Mal would like a beer, probably.'

Tom grunted. Stella gave him a quick look. It had been ages since her daughter and her husband had just dropped in. They hadn't had much to say to each other. What could you say?

Rosie put her head round the door. 'Can we come in?' Without waiting for an answer she came bouncing in the door. 'It's still cold, isn't it? Mum, we just had to show you. Look what we've got.' And she waved something at them. 'Tickets to London. We're going too, to Diana's exhibition, and then we're doing the continent.'

'Whoa. You're coming over for the exhibition? In September?' Stella was astounded. She and Tom had bought their plane tickets weeks ago.

'Yes, but I don't want you to tell Diana, right? Keep it a secret.'

Stella felt like bursting into tears. 'Rosie, this is fantastic, I'm so thrilled. What's happened to change your minds? The last time I was talking to you there was no way you were coming.'

'A change of direction.' Rosie smiled at Mal and Mal's smile back spoke volumes. 'Go on, you tell them.'

'We've just signed the lease on a restaurant in town.'

'What?'

'It's Mal,' said Rosie. 'He's always wanted to run a restaurant. So we're researching, and we have to go overseas to do it properly. How fantastic is that? My job will be all the front of house stuff, and his will be in the kitchen. Isn't this just the best thing you've ever heard?'

'Who's going to do the cooking?'

'We'll put a chef on to begin with,' said Mal. 'And I'm putting my name down to take some courses next year.'

Stella sat down. 'Where did all this come from?'

'I'll put the kettle on,' said Rosie.

'We've been talking about it for months and we finally decided a couple of weeks ago,' Mal explained, 'but we wanted to wait for the lease to be signed.'

'And then our plane tickets arrived,' Rosie blurted, 'and we had to tell you or I was going to explode.'

'Rosie, Mal,' Stella said, 'I'm thrilled for you.'

Tom went to the fridge and got out two beers. 'Congratulations. Would you like a beer?'

Mal nodded, and the two men stepped out onto the verandah.

'I can't wait to tell Diana,' said Rosie, 'but I've got to tell her in person. I was such an idiot before she left. Everything was closing in on us, Mal and me. We were very unhappy. But this is what Mal has wanted to do for ages. We just couldn't work out how.'

The kettle boiled, its shrill whistle cutting across the kitchen. Rosie got up to make the tea.

'So what changed everything?' Stella asked.

'Well, you did.'

'When?' She was mystified, still trying to take it all in.

'Mum, Mal was so unhappy. He was doing it for me. Staying here, I didn't realise what was happening, only that he wasn't happy. I thought it was me he was unhappy with. But after the funeral we started to talk and ... you've got to keep talking to each other, don't you?'

'Yes,' Stella said faintly.

'Mum, he's changed. Look at him. This is our thing, not mine, not his—ours. Don't you see?'

Stella and Rosie looked out at their husbands, standing on the verandah. Mal was talking and Tom was listening intently.

Rosie, Rosie, Rosie. When had she ever stopped saying to her girls you've got to keep talking? A relationship, any relationship, needs work and keeping the lines of communication open.

'I'm so happy for you, darling. This is such good news. What are you going to call the restaurant?'

'The Bowerbird Cafe, and there's going to be lots of blue decor. What do you think?'

CHAPTER FORTY-NINE

September had arrived in a flurry of autumn leaves, bringing with it both excitement and dread. Diana's parents were arriving Thursday morning and the exhibition opening was on Friday evening. Patrick, good friend that he was, had arrived yesterday and Diana had conned him into helping deliver the pictures and pots she'd prepared round to the gallery tonight.

'So, it's all in.' He closed the door of the van she had hired.

'It's so good of you to do this. When you said you were arriving a couple of days early and then you offered to help.' Diana grinned at him.

'Why am I not so sure about this?' Patrick quizzed her.

'It won't take too long. The gallery's about fifteen minutes away. I'll just get the kids.'

*   *   *

The gallery was eerie with no one around. Open packing boxes littered the floor, pictures were stacked against the wall. It seemed to object heavily to the kids and Patrick and Diana interrupting its holy quiet time. Milo ran across the open floor, jumping two boxes and skidding to a stop in front of her.

Diana looked up from the crate she was jimmying open. 'Milo, if you do that again I'll, I'll fry you in oil. Please be careful.'

'Look, I found the catalogues,' said Milo.

'Thank goodness, put them on the desk near where you come in.' She turned to Patrick. 'That's the second batch. They had to be done again, the colour was simply dreadful and they'd left some of the prices out.'

'Where do you want me to put these?' he asked. 'They're marked Fragile.'

'Everything is fragile, including me.' Diana took a quick look. 'Ah, over in that corner, thanks.'

The girls came in carrying a box awkwardly between them.

'No, what are you doing?' She flew over towards them, scattering packing case straw as she went. Patrick was there before her and lifted it away from them.

'It's the last one, Mummy, and we thought we could do it.' Sienna looked so pleased with herself.

'Thank you, girls.' She let out a breath of relief. 'Now you can relax. That wasn't so bad, was it?' She looked at Patrick.

'I don't classify anything we do together as bad.' Patrick chuckled and sat on the floor. 'That's everything in from the truck. How much more do you want to do tonight?'

'Now it's all in, I can just fiddle. I can't thank you enough. Bill Sutton offered to help but he's really not strong enough.'

Patrick reached up and pulled her down beside him. 'Why don't you sit for a minute and tell me your plan.'

She was so aware of Patrick's arm. A restless energy made her want to spring back up but she made herself sit still for a minute.

'Charlie's pictures are going on that wall and over there. They'll look beautiful—you'll walk in and they'll hit you and draw you round the corner. See, where the window will throw light onto that little table, I'm draping a fabulous piece of material down the wall and over the table. It'll be a backdrop, a bit like a silken waterfall.'

'Two days will be enough?'

'Plenty. They'll have to be. Ask me again on Friday afternoon at four. Actually, I wouldn't advise that. No one talks to me the afternoon before.'

Patrick looked at her curiously. 'That isn't like you.'

'You forget, I'm an artist. Before an exhibition I can be moody, eccentric and insane. It's allowed.' She blinked and jumped to her feet.

'I'm so nervous. Mum and Dad are coming in two days. Somehow that scares me more than anything. Thank you for coming, Patrick. I wasn't sure, when I sent you the invitation, whether you'd be able to come.'

'It's my pleasure, that's what friends are for.'

Diana gave him a quick look.

'I can't face cooking or food, really. How about we all go out for dinner? It's on me.' She paused, looking around, just before she turned off the light. So much work. Now the empty spaces were filled with pots, jugs and crates. Two more days, she thought.

Moments later, they were all seated on gold-woven cushions at the Indian around the corner. Patrick was good at organising, she'd give him that.

'Thursday, after the opening, the Sutton's have asked us all round to dinner. Then they'll look after the children if we want to go out.' Diana stopped for a moment. Was that crossing the friendly line they'd established? Patrick may not want to go out with her.

'I think I like that idea.' He signalled the waiter.

Diana's pappadum broke in her hand. She swept up the bits and sprinkled them on her meal. 'Right. It will be good to see Mum. I know how much they're looking forward to this trip.'

Patrick smiled.

'And I can't wait to see them. Sienna, please don't eat all the chutney, pass it around. Sienna does love the hot mango chutney.'

'By the way,' said Patrick. 'I've a friend who has a mini-bus. I was wondering if I could take you all out to pick up your parents when they arrive on Thursday.'

'That would be wonderful. Perhaps we could come back via Buckingham Palace? I don't know how Mum and Dad will be, comatose probably, but I'm dying to show them around. We've got a trip planned for Dad to Grantham, where the Aveling-Barfords were made—you know Dad's got an old Aveling-Barford grader. That's after we get the exhibition over and done with.' She sounded like a babbling brook.

Patrick laughed. 'How did you unearth all that?'

'Not me. The internet! My parents have discovered the internet. We Skype, we email—we don't exactly do Facebook or Twitter yet, but it's a start.' Diana laughed.

'And Stella, I hope you have something organised for her?'

'Oh yes, Madame Tussauds, and the Victoria and Albert Museum. First on the list, isn't it, girls?'

'I can't wait, Mummy,' said Saskia. 'Stella is going to see my school too.'

'Absolutely. Two sleeps to go.'

They delivered the taxi truck back to its special car park. Walking home with Patrick and the kids, Diana felt tired. Not the desperate, numbing tiredness she suffered before—this was plain exhaustion, mixed with excitement that her parents would be there on Thursday. To see her work. She was absolutely terrified.

'Beer?' Diana asked. The kids were in bed and Patrick was standing in the hallway, his coat in his arms, obviously wondering whether to leave or not. She didn't want him to go.

'Thanks. Yes I will.'

Dinner had been so much fun. Milo teasing Patrick about the terrible scores the Aussie cricketers were getting. The girls telling Patrick about the concert they were in. He'd seemed very relaxed then; now she wasn't so sure. Maybe it was her making him nervous.

'Thank you for all your help.' She handed him a beer.

'Really, stop doing that.'

'What?'

'Thanking me.'

'You've come a long way, and you've been a great help.'

'I had fun,' he said. 'Are the kids settling back in okay?'

'I don't know. Everything's supposed to be getting closer with the internet but Mog's Hill still seems worlds away. It's just so different.' She studied her beer bottle. 'It's funny, sometimes Milo will ask about the farm and Tom. So we ring, and the girls love talking to Stella. Connections have been made. Our trip was not in vain.'

'I'm glad you all came out.' Patrick was looking at her intently. She felt a little flustered.

'I don't know, maybe I've made it worse. Milo gets this broken look on his face sometimes ...'

'He's lost his dad.'

'I know. I worry if we go back he won't have an identity—will he be Australian or English? Say Ireland's playing Australia, who do you really want to barrack for?'

Patrick laughed. 'Aussie, Aussie, Aussie, Oi, Oi, Oi. I appreciate my Irish heritage but it's Australia all the way for me.'

'What will Milo do?'

'Make up his own mind,' Patrick said. 'I'd better be going or I'll fall asleep on the carpet and I'll wake up with all these jungle animals roaring around me. It wouldn't be good. I won't see you tomorrow, but I'll be ready with the bus on Thursday morning. How about six?'

'If you're sure, that would be wonderful.'

A kiss on the cheek and he was gone. He was a great friend, that was for sure.

*   *   *

Diana was surprised the next morning to hear the front doorbell chime. She had the vacuum cleaner out and was trying to give the house a final spit and polish before her parents got in the next morning. The kids were at school and she had little time to spare. There was still so much to do at the gallery.

She flew to door and wrenched it open. Her sister stood there, wrapped in a woolly jacket with a red scarf wound around her throat.

It was, Rosie, slightly apprehensive, eyes filled with tears, standing there on the step.

'Rosie!'

They hadn't spoken for months, not since Peg's funeral, but Diana didn't hesitate. She opened her arms wide. 'Rosie, I don't believe it! What are you doing here?'

It was a long hug. Rosie still hadn't said anything, just rained tears down her face and onto Diana's T-shirt. Diana pulled her gently inside the door.

'Di, I'm so sorry,' Rosie hiccupped. 'I'm really sorry.'

'You dope. I'm so glad you're here. Why didn't you tell me? Damn, did everyone know except me? Where's Mal? Did he come too? I can't believe this.'

'Mal's here. He'll be back in an hour. I just wanted to clear up, you know, everything first.'

'And we both know he hates the waterworks. What a coward.'

'Di, I honestly don't know what got into me. I was so awful.'

'It's fine, don't worry, it's all forgotten. Now what are you doing here?'

Rosie sat on the sofa. 'We've got so much to tell you.'

Diana just looked at her expectantly.

'Mal and I are leasing a restaurant in Holbrook. Organic food, the whole shebang, meat, vegetables, bread, wine … everything.'

'What? Who's cooking?'

'That's the best part. Mal. We've got our feelers out for a chef, just to begin with and then Mal's going to do some courses, and I'm going to grow the vegetables. I must say I think I'd be good at the front of house stuff, don't you think?' Rosie laughed at the expression on Diana's face.

'And honestly, I haven't seen Mal so excited. It's like someone has released him from jail.'

Diana was speechless.

'It really is the best thing we've decided to do and we're so happy, and really it was all because of you, and I want to be talking to you again but I am so ashamed and I wasn't sure if you could forgive me.'

'Rosie, don't be an idiot,' said Diana. 'Mum didn't breathe a word of any of this.'

'Well, we didn't tell them till just a couple of weeks ago and it's nearly killed her to keep it a secret, I know.' Rosie dimpled. 'But I had to tell you in person.'

Her parents would be here tomorrow, and now this. It couldn't get much better, could it?

*　　*　　*

Muted conversations, every single person a critic. Diana knew exactly what the little experts were saying—how they'd have done it differently. How she hated them all. Before six o'clock she'd been chewing her fingernails, totally convinced no one would turn up. She'd be sitting there with all that champagne and food and not a soul to eat and drink it.

It was always like this.

Diana nursed her champagne and looked glumly round the small gallery. It was quite a coup to have got this gallery, Sebastian was right. The gallery owner had been very helpful. Grudgingly she admitted there was a satisfying amount of people here. A lot were relatives. Her children were behaving beautifully and were spending all of the time with their grandparents—all four grandparents—and it wasn't hard to see they were all jockeying for position. Who *was* the favourite granny?

It would be interesting to quiz her mother later, on what she thought of Charlie's pictures. They were looking good, she thought. Patrick was talking to Sebastian; it looked like they were discussing the pictures.

'I am so proud of you, Diana.' Her dad came up behind her. 'Everyone is rapt. I've been going round listening in on conversations.'

'Thanks, but I don't believe you. You look so much better, Dad, I can hardly believe you're the same person.'

'Diet and exercise. Worked a treat, I can tell you. I can't believe I could so easily have missed this—and I wouldn't have, not for the world. Congratulations.'

'I just get so nervous, and hate it all so much. It's like standing naked in front of everyone.'

'You must feel better when those little red dots start appearing ... and there goes one now.' Tom nodded to the table behind her.

Diana frowned. 'I hope Patrick isn't doing it.'

'Why not?'

'I don't need a sympathy vote.'

'I think it would be more like a case of getting in first.' He grinned. 'Or missing out.'

*   *   *

Stella pinched herself. She was at Diana's exhibition in London. Actually. Here. Seeing her daughter, *her daughter*, in this setting. The buzz, the excitement, all these arty people. Arty people were always the same, no matter whether you were in London or the local art gallery in her home town. She couldn't resist a little smile.

'Watch it, Stella, you're looking like the Cheshire cat.'

'What does the Cheshire cat look like, Tom?' she whispered back.

'Wasn't it the one that swallowed all that cream?'

'No actually, but it doesn't matter, I get the idea. You're not half wrong. Where are the girls?'

'Over with Patrick. Let's join them.'

Stella put an arm around the girls and gave them a smile. 'My goodness there's a lot of people. Tom, you should take the girls and get them a drink.'

'It certainly looks like a good crowd,' said Patrick. 'I'm interested in how these occasions work. Is it the quality of the purses or quantity of people in the door that works better?' he mused, as they watched Tom shepherd the girls over to the bar.

'Neither,' said Sebastian. 'It's who's here that's most important. See the tall thin man over there—he's one of the most voracious collectors in Europe. For him to have come is very good.' Sebastian was almost trembling with satisfaction.

'So Diana should be pleased. How are Charlie's pictures going?'

'Well, it wasn't my top priority,' Sebastian said confidentially. 'Diana insisted, and it took a lot of time yesterday to get them hung. The headaches—I tell you. But it's all looking good now.' He reached for another glass of champagne as a tray passed by.

'So what do you think of Charlie's pictures?' Patrick asked Sebastian.

'Well, just between you and me, Charlie was running a bit behind Diana, always had. And people were starting to notice, if you know what I mean. Diana was always sticking up for him, but Charlie was getting very jealous of her success.'

'A pity.'

'I asked her a couple of times but Diana wouldn't ever say there was a problem. Strong lady, she is. Always covered up for him and pushed him as much as she could.'

'Did you like Charlie?'

'Ah, everyone liked Charlie. Patrick, I want you to meet a friend of mine. Excuse us, Stella.'

Stella stood for a moment, thinking. It hadn't been easy for Diana. But, she looked around, it hadn't been all bad—their decision to get Diana to England. Look what she'd accomplished. But she had to wonder—how much had she wanted this for herself? Had she pushed Diana into coming because it was what she had wanted, so many years ago?

'You're looking pensive, Mum,' Diana came up beside her. 'I'm the only one who has an excuse to be worried tonight.'

'I'm so thrilled for you, but I am worrying if you still blame us for not talking it out with the two of you. Just assuming you would come here and Rosie would stay at Mog's Hill. Did we make the right decision?'

'Looking at it from twenty years on is very difficult. Circumstances have changed, we can't assume things are the same as they were then.'

'I just hope it wasn't some crazy wish to see you succeed, take up the chances I missed out on when I decided to marry your father.'

'In the end, Mum, I have to take ownership of the decision to accept that ticket and get on that plane.' Diana chinked her glass against her mother's. 'And here I am, for whatever the reason, so thank you.'

Stella watched her eldest daughter wander through the crowd. Yes, they'd given her a hefty push. And paid the price. No. She wouldn't change anything about her life. And then she wondered, given it to do all over again, would Diana have done the same thing too? Her children for a start, how could she even think of life without them?

'Brought you a champagne.' Tom arrived beside her.

She looked at his bright blue eyes behind the glasses. At the kindness and the honesty in that so familiar face. She rubbed her cheek against the roughness of his jacket. Breathed him in.

'Thank you, Tom Crawford.'

CHAPTER FIFTY

Gospel Oak, London, February.

The pot Diana was throwing began to get the death wobble. Her concentration was poor today. Frustrated, she clumped it down, scraped it back into the pugmill and waited for the clay to emerge as a fresh cylinder, ready to start again. Potting appealed to her frugal nature—mostly everything could be used again, all the rejects and end bits. Listening to the drone of the screw as it worked the clay back into a malleable form, Diana looked around her studio. It was all so comfortingly familiar—the recently fired set of bowls with the Chinese lettering, twenty large and twenty small, were ready to pack and be sent to China to the family that had commissioned them; some porcelain dishes she'd been experimenting in with an iron glaze; the kiln, cold and empty, waiting for her to finish the range of pots decorated with dancing figures that Sebastian said he could never get enough of. Well, he'd just have to wait a little longer.

Would spring never come? The winter she had dreaded had been dragging on and on and London was freezing, hopefully in the last cold snap before spring. They'd all had colds and coughs, and she was sure she'd bought the last bottle of cough syrup available in the UK. Pulling her cardigan round her and opening the window of her attic studio wider, she ignored the rush of cold air and looked out over the slate-grey roofs across to Hampstead Heath, the tracery of the leafless trees breaking up the monotony of the woolly sky. She could see the gorse bushes halfway up the hill and a few brave figures striding upwards.

Slowly she had come to accept Charlie's death as an accident. She'd been able to stop blaming him for being so careless, throwing away his life and leaving them. He'd been a great dad. And she'd begun to forgive herself, on a good day. There were still plenty of bad ones. Johann rang her often to remind her. Telling Milo on the beach that day had been the beginning for her. Accepting that it was an accident, that it could have happened to anyone. She'd had a bad time with Milo for a while but they'd come through it, with lots of hugs. It hadn't been her fault. It hadn't been his fault. That's what an accident was—nobody's fault.

A big change for her had happened just before Christmas, when Janet, Charlie's mother, had rung to ask what she wanted to do with Charlie's ashes.

Charlie's ashes hadn't been on her list. She'd left them with the Suttons. Or had she asked them to pick them up from the crematorium? It was all a bit of a blur and she couldn't remember exactly. Diana had sat looking at the phone for quite a while. The only sound she could hear was the relentless tick of the clock. It was one-thirty. She had an hour before the kids would be dropped off after various play dates. She didn't know what you did with ashes.

She didn't want to think about it.

Outside, it was iron grey skies and very cold. There'd been no snow yet. She started walking, head down, hands in her pockets to keep warm. Counting the odd dead leaf that hadn't blown away or been sucked up by the street sweepers. She set off on her favourite, well-trodden path, up the hill, past the brown gorse bushes, not wanting to think about what she should do.

All right, Charlie, what do you want me to do?

Silence. Unfortunately he wasn't answering her any more.

Cremating Charlie had been quite traumatic. And all those questions from the kids. Will it hurt? Does Daddy know? That had been hard to answer. She'd done it for him, so she'd hoped like hell he knew and appreciated the fact he'd been cremated. He would have hated being buried in the ground. Well, only half the job was done, she realised, suddenly stopping, watching as two matching poodles in tartan coats trotted past her, noses in the air.

It was time to let him go.

*   *   *

She'd turned the telly off, a very sure sign that something serious was afoot. Three faces warily looked up.

'Do you remember that Daddy was cremated? We said goodbye to Daddy in the church and then his body was taken away and he was cremated.'

Silence. Not a sound. Worse, they looked terrified.

Try again. 'When people die, you can do two things, bury them in the ground or have them cremated, burned. Then the people give you back the ashes in a container and you do something with them.'

'What do you do with them?' Milo found his voice.

'Well that's what I'm asking you. We have to decide what to do with Daddy's ashes.'

'Where are they?' Milo again.

'Pa and Grandma have them. They've been keeping them for us, but now I feel, they feel, it's time we said goodbye properly.'

'What do they look like?' Saskia asked wide-eyed, obviously imagining a life-size pile of ashes in Pa's backyard.

Diana didn't know either. She hadn't seen them. She'd quickly read the book upstairs about grief counselling when she'd got home, and although it hadn't been particularly forthcoming about this situation it had said, above all, be honest. 'I can't really remember, but its only small, a box about this size.' She shaped it with her hands. 'I've asked Grandma and Pa over to talk about this. They'll be here soon and then we all have to make a decision.'

Charlie's ashes were in an urn which Pa placed on the mantelpiece. The children couldn't take their eyes off it. Neither could Diana.

'I was thinking in the wall at the crematorium.' Janet Sutton sat managing her cup of tea with the two little girls cuddled up to her. 'So I know where he is. And if you go off to Australia to live, you'll know where to find him when you come back.'

Diana stared at her mother-in-law.

'Don't look so surprised, Diana. We know you'll probably go back there one day. And take that disapproving look off your face, Bill. I know I wasn't to say anything first but no one else had any suggestions. It's a starting point, that's all.'

'What about the Heath? We had some lovely picnics there—there's space and trees and grass,' Diana offered slowly.

Bill looked over his glasses at her. 'Diana, think about it, you were the one who needed space and trees. Our Charlie was a Londoner, through and through. I'm thinking the old Highbury Stadium.'

'It's not their ground anymore,' said Milo. 'They've built houses all over it.'

'I don't want him closed in.' Diana was adamant.

'But, Diana,' Bill said gently, 'don't you see he's not closed in, he's with us all the time. This is just a resting place, where he loved to be.'

Milo sat there with a set expression on his face and said simply, 'The ocean. Then we can share him. He'll be over in Australia or here, whenever he wants to be.'

The Atlantic Ocean it was then, or rather the English Channel. Hopefully Charlie would be able to find his way, Diana thought, as they piled into two cars and headed for the coast. Navigation had not been one of his strong points.

The day was beautiful, the sea a special vibrant blue, quite flat, looking as if it might go on forever, all the way to Australia. They'd hired a boat at a marina and all clambered in. Pa was quite at home with the controls. Sienna had written a poem and Saskia brought a jar of Charlie's favourite olives and his beloved old sable paintbrush. He'd always called it the magic one. Grandma and Pa brought a jumper he'd worn at school. But it wasn't till just after they'd scattered Charlie's ashes in the ocean that Milo pulled out Charlie's football scarf and dropped it in the water.

No sighs, no goodbyes, tossed around in the fresh breeze.

After that it all started to get better. They'd settled back into Saturdays being grandparents' day—the girls usually went off with Grandma and Pa took Milo. Sometimes they went to the football. It used to bring such a lump to her throat watching the two of them, Milo and his grandfather, setting off wreathed in Arsenal red.

Now her days were filled with kids' stuff, an eternal round of dropping off and picking up, washing clothes, cooking meals and working. Lots of work, trying not to think too much of home, Australia and Patrick. But that was a bit of a lost cause.

And then he'd ring or text. She loved those phone calls. Patrick would ring when it was late at night for her and he'd be at work somewhere, telling her about the pub and his day, or Lost Valley. That was fun, but the best ones reached her in the middle of her day when he was going to bed. She'd be full of chat and tell him about the kids and make him laugh.

She'd rung him just the other night before she got into bed.

'I hope this is a good time for you.'

'Sure, it's quiet today, I'm filling in for one of our bartenders and I've got three old pensioners sitting here, looking at the cricket, telling me all about the good old days when West Indies were king.'

'Jeez, that was a long time ago.'

'How're the kids?'

'Good. I have to tell you, though, what Milo said to me this morning. Out of the blue, it was, "Mum, you know how I'm going to play for Arsenal when I get big?" And I said "Of course," because we all know that's his main aim in life.'

She could hear Patrick laugh down the other end of the phone. 'I thought it depended on whether it was the cricket or football season?'

'And it's obviously football now. But then, he said "It's okay, Mum, because in my contract they can put, if Australia gets into the World Cup, they can release me, so's I can still play for Australia. Isn't that good?" You could have knocked me over.'

'Nothing wrong with dreaming.'

'Of course not. But it was an interesting thing to say, wasn't it?'

'Very interesting.'

'How would he know that?'

'Boys his age are obsessively manic about sport, they pick up a lot more than you think.'

'How do you know?'

'Well, I'm a boy, of course, and I have two nephews much the same age who can intelligently discuss what the Australian cricket team has for breakfast.'

'Weet-Bix. Everyone knows that.'

That phone call had only been a couple of weeks ago, and Diana couldn't stop thinking about it. Was Milo thinking they might go to Australia? Live in Australia? He'd have to if he was thinking of playing for Australia.

She closed the window. She yearned for the hills of home—Mog's Hill, with the paddocks silvery gold as they were at the end of summer. There'd been some rain, not enough, her mother had said yesterday, but at least there'd been something. Not that it would do them much good at the moment. They really needed it next month. And they had so much faith in the long-range weather forecaster. Why, she had no idea, he never seemed to be right. But the guru had forecast rain for March so they were happy. Diana had had to do some research for Patrick and had gone to Kent to check out some hop vines.

'It's fascinating, Patrick,' she'd told him on the phone one day. 'The kids thought we'd walked straight into the fairytale, *Jack and the Beanstalk*. There are these huge vines climbing up poles, and they lower the poles down to pick the flowers, which look like green artichokes, and then they chuck them straight into the beer. It gives the beer its flavour.'

'You're not doing me any good finding out all this information way over there,' he said. 'I need you here, tasting them, helping me choose which variety. I've decided on three. See if you can find them over there in a beer.'

'Okay.' She laughed. 'I'll try. I'm not sure it's so good for the kids to be racing around looking for different beer flavours.'

'I'm particularly interested in the "piney" and "citrus" flavours.'

'Right. I won't be able to get down to Kent again for a couple of weeks.'

'Whenever. Thanks, Diana, I'd really appreciate it.'

She must take the kids and follow it up soon. Milo was good at asking questions, too. Maybe Bart would have some ideas on how to taste-test the hops.

'How are you getting on with my beer mugs?' Patrick asked.

'Not bad. I'm basing the size on the glass jars they serve drinks in in cafes these days, but I haven't got it right yet. I think it's more a middy size.'

'I want my brand on the mug.'

'Sure. I'll send a photo when I've got something to show you.'

* * *

Diana missed her mother. Saskia did too; just the other day she'd asked when they were going back to see Stella and Tommo.

She sighed and, wrapping the clay in plastic sheeting, she decided to leave it for the night.

The door banged downstairs. The kids would be back from school. Food was all she had time to think of now. Heaven help her—she'd forgotten to do the shopping! She tore down the stairs, arriving at the bottom just as the first yells rent the air.

'Mum, there aren't any biscuits.'

'Hello, everyone, how was school? I've had a great idea, let's go out and get some donuts.' Grabbing the keys, she shepherded them outside again before they had time to take their coats off.

There was an off-license around the corner and the bell jangled as they trooped in and stood at the counter. Siena and Saskia pressed their noses as usual against the glass display counter, behind which lay pink, chocolate and banana iced donuts on china plates.

'Hello, Mrs Akhtar, I think the usual. No one's changing their minds today.'

Three donuts were put in three paper bags and they all walked slowly back to the house.

'How was your day, Saskia?'

'Bella wouldn't play with me so Anna and I went to the library.'

'That sounds a good idea,' Diana replied absently. The answer hadn't been all that different from the day before. Rounding the corner, they saw a brand-new black Saab parked in front of their house.

There was a figure wrapped in a coat, leaning against the car, and he raised his arm in greeting when he saw them. It took all of ten seconds before the kids recognised Patrick standing there.

'Patrick!' And they were running to greet him like he was some long-lost friend or relative they hadn't seen for ages. Well, they hadn't seen him since September.

Neither had she.

'What a surprise.' Diana slowed her steps to retain her composure. He was diving back into the car for a bag of presents. The kids were all over him. She was so jealous. 'What are you doing here?'

'Just passing and thought I'd drop in.'

'Very funny.'

'Sorry, it was a sudden decision. Is it a good time? Here are a couple of things I saw at the airport I thought the kids might like, some nougat and chocolates.'

Patrick leant down to hug the children, shaking hands with Milo, and Saskia, as usual, ending up in his arms. A kiss for Sienna. He looked so good standing there, his blue eyes smiling hello.

And all she wanted to do was jump his bones.

'It's so good to see you,' composure, slowing her pulse rate. She raised her cheek for his kiss. It was a perfunctory kiss, very friendly.

'Well, come on in.' She turned and walked inside.

CHAPTER FIFTY-ONE

Patrick was here and Diana didn't know why. He hadn't let her know he was coming. He hung his cashmere coat on the stand in the hallway. It looked incongruous beside their parkas. She stood there for a minute, just looking at him. The children had taken over and were showing him homework, bears and bicycles.

Things had changed between them again. The sparks were back, but she may be the only one to be experiencing it. Surely he could feel it—the damn air around them was electric.

'Would you like a coffee?' she asked.

'Thank you.' Patrick smiled at her and she nearly tripped over a backpack as she turned to go out.

'How long are you over for?' Diana picked up the jar of instant coffee she had on offer. 'I'm sorry, there's no milk.'

'I'm not sure, maybe a week or two. There's a couple of things I have to sort out. I've brought some things from your mother. They're in the car.' He looked distracted.

'How is she?' They knew he was coming and they hadn't mentioned it. But she hadn't talked to them for a few days.

'Very well, very happy, she sends her love. And Tom, too.' He was definitely on edge. What was the matter?

'I heard that his hops are in,' she said. 'And you talked Dad into using your new man, one day a week. Thank you, Rosie and I appreciate it. We're in awe actually—getting my stiff-necked father to accept help.'

'There's no help involved, he's paying for Mark's day.' Patrick frowned. 'Diana.'

'Yes.' She swallowed. He just looked so good. She wanted to walk straight into those strong arms and stay there. Heaven help her.

'Mum, I need food to take to cricket tomorrow and I can't find anything.' Milo walked into the room.

Diana suddenly remembered her empty cupboards. 'We'll go to the supermarket later.'

'Why don't we all go now?' Patrick said.

'Right. You've just survived a twenty-four hour flight and now you want to brave five o'clock rush hour in the super-market?' She looked at him curiously.

'You shop, the kids and I are going to have a milkshake.'

'Yeah,' was the general reaction. Three children ran for their coats.

'Can we go in Patrick's car?' said Milo.

'No problem. Are you right to go, Diana?'

She looked at him, slightly bemused.

'Okay.'

The supermarket was frantic, just as she'd thought. It was time to tell Patrick how she felt. This friendly thing wasn't working. At least not for her. *Eggs.* So, how did she feel? *Bread times two.* She was so glad to see him, and she couldn't take her eyes off him when he was there with her. *Oranges.* She had to give herself a chance, and that wasn't going to happen until she told him how she felt.

She'd been standing with a packet of blue cheese in her hand for a whole minute. What was he doing here? Was he going to say he'd found someone else? That he was getting married next week and just thought he'd let her know? No, he wouldn't do that ... She hated blue cheese. She put it back. *Cheddar cheese, little cheeses that Milo liked for tomorrow, margarine, butter.* So what did she want—a long-distance relationship? No. *Salami.* But that meant moving back to Australia and problems times three. *Bacon.* And potting— make that problems times four, having to start building a reputation all over again.

Now she was sinking into indecision. *Ice cream.* What was she—a woman or a mouse? Hell, everyone had problems. They'd sort it. *Muesli bars.* She wanted to love him. *Sausages.* And live with him, and care for him, for the rest of their lives. *Mince and chicken legs.* They could make it work, but all she felt now was that they were wasting time.

There she went again, jumping the gun. *Slow down and see how this visit goes.* Let things work themselves out. *Be patient.* She reached for a tray of some tantalising and very expensive rump steak.

Patrick just might stay for dinner.

*   *   *

Diana pushed her trolley over to the booth in the coffee shop to join Patrick and the children.

'Mummy,' Saskia's face was alight, 'Patrick said he would take me to the zoo to see Forrest.'

'Oh no, Saskia, Patrick will not do anything of the kind.'

'But he doesn't know what a kinkajou is.'

'No one knows what a kinkajou is. They've been learning all about kinkajous at school,' she apologised to Patrick. 'Move over, Sienna.'

'I ordered you a Coke too.'

'Are you all drinking Coke? At this time of night?'

'Sorry.' Patrick looked worried.

'Mmm. It's not your fault.' She looked round at three innocent faces in front of her. 'They should know better.'

'We're all right, Mum, it's only Sassy who goes hypo,' Milo said.

'I hope so. You've got homework to do, as well, remember.' She smiled at Patrick. 'Thank you.'

He passed over her Coke. 'Well, what is a kinkajou?'

Diana nudged Saskia, who was concentrating on finishing her glass as fast as she could, just in case someone might whisk it away.

'It's this cute little furry bear that comes from Brazil, and it loves eating honey, and it loves eating figs and peaches, and it can hang from the tree by its tail,' Saskia announced to them all. 'And Forrest is a kinkajou in the zoo here and Patrick said he wanted to see one.'

Diana looked at Patrick sceptically. 'I don't think you do, really.'

He cleared his throat. 'Actually, I do. Tomorrow's Saturday, let's go to the zoo.'

Sienna and Saskia glanced at each other. 'Saturday's our day with Grandma.'

'She could come too,' Saskia said firmly.

Patrick hesitated. 'Mmm, I was thinking just the five of us.'

Diana was interested in Patrick's hesitation, brief though it was. If she didn't know him better, she would say he looked nervous.

'My cricket's on tomorrow,' Milo said.

'All right.' Patrick definitely looked odd. 'I've been planning this all the way over in the plane, and I had thought tomorrow, somewhere special. But what the heck, now's as good a time as any.' He took a deep breath. 'I think I'd better get this over and done with, before I lose my nerve and you all disappear on your Saturday jaunts. So while we're all together, the thing is ...' He cleared his throat. 'I want to marry your mother.'

Everyone except Saskia had ceased drinking.

Diana's eyes flew to his. What she saw there took her breath away.

'I love your mother very much, but it is complicated. I haven't asked her yet. Generally, a man asks the woman's father first but Tom's not here and I felt you guys were more important. So before I ask your mother, I want to ask you, Milo, Sienna and Saskia, to give me permission to ask your mother to marry me, and say that I can come and be part of this family too. Which I want, very much.' Patrick took a large breath.

Diana felt frozen to the spot. The children looked at her and she felt her face turn beetroot. Noises of the cafe around her melted away. *What would they say?*

'Where are we going to live?' Sienna was the first to break the silence.

'Australia. But I'm thinking, how about one holiday a year in London, to catch up with your other grandparents and friends.'

'Where will we go to school?' Milo asked slowly.

'Sydney is where my business is, but I spend a lot of time at Lost Valley, so I think that's something we'll all have to decide. I know it's going to be difficult for you all ...' He paused uncertainly. 'I do know I'll be the happiest man in the world if you say yes. At least I will be if your mother says yes, too."

Patrick was looking at the children.

Her children were looking at each other.

Then Sienna smiled and got on her knees to whisper in Patrick's ear.

He smiled. 'I certainly do.' And he pulled a little black box out of his pocket and put it on the table.

They all looked at the little black box.

Then they all looked at Diana.

ACKNOWLEDGEMENTS

I salute those wonderful women of my mother's genera-tion. Born in the First World War, schooled through the depression and fighting in the Second World War, they pro-duced the baby boomers. They sailed from lamplight and wood stoves through to our world of computers and mobile phones—although maybe they didn't adapt quite so easily to the phones. They are the backbone of our country.

I thank the wonderful Harlequins Sue Brockhoff, Rachael Donovan and Annabel Blay. You have been so supportive and enthusiastic and made this journey such a delight. And a special thanks to Dianne Blacklock, my caring editor. I have been so lucky.

Then I wish to thank the people I have befriended in the wonderful farming community over these many years. Their humbleness and strength and generosity and wonder-ful sense of humour make them stand-out figures. To Skye, for being my 'agent' and steering me through the profes-sional swamp of publishing, I give a grateful thank you. To Richard, a very special thank you. I wouldn't be here if it wasn't for my beautiful husband who understands how important this is to me. And finally, a big hug to Mia San-dilands for sharing her story of the kinkajou.

BOOK CLUB DISCUSSION POINTS

1. What were the main themes throughout this book?

2. 'Miss him. It was hard to know what that meant. It was so difficult to comprehend or understand the concept of death. Charlie was gone and she'd never see him again.' What are your first impressions of Diana's relationship with Charlie? How does this change once she travels to Australia, and by the end of the book?

3. Diana keeps hearing Charlie's voice in her head, but gradually it fades until, by the end of the book, it has gone. Why do you think she is having these imagined conversations?

4. Diana's relationship with her mother is vastly different to that with her father. While personality plays a certain part, why do you think Diana seems to blame her mother for things that happened more than her father?

5. Rosie and Diana have a difficult relationship. Why do you think Rosie is so jealous of Diana, and why does Diana make excuses for Rosie's outbursts?

6. Families have various dynamics. Discuss the dynamics in the Crawford family as a whole, then discuss the dynamics of Diana's own young family.

7. How had Cody's death affected the Crawford family? Did they all deal with the death the same or differently?

8. It's obvious Mal was in love with Diana when they were younger. Do you think he still has any of those feelings for her?

9. We learn a lot about Patrick before we meet him. What was your first impression of him through third-party information? How did this change after Diana met him for the first time?

10. Why do you think Diana confided in Johann about the terrible night of Charlie's death, and not in her mother, father or sister?

11. Diana made it a condition that she would only display her works at the gallery if some of Charlie's paintings could be shown as well. Discuss what you think her reasons were.

12. Alzheimer's is a terrible disease for both the sufferer and their family. Diana was horrified by the deterioration and change in Peg, but there were times Peg was still present and behaving like her beloved grandmother. Diana herself remembers her past in Australia so clearly, but finds the happenings in the present confusing, not to mention her own mental dilemmas over Charlie's death. Do you think Peg's Alzheimer's disease was a metaphor for Diana's perspective when she arrives back in Australia?

13. The ending was quite sudden. Do you think it made sense or do you think the author could have resolved the story more completely?